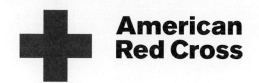

American Red Cross

American Red Cross
Lifeguarding

MANUAL

The following organizations provided review of the materials and/or support American Red Cross Lifeguarding:

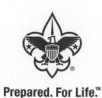

Prepared. For Life.™

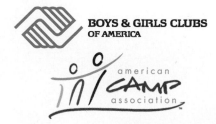

BOYS & GIRLS CLUBS OF AMERICA

american CAMP association™

USA SWIMMING

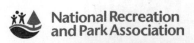

National Recreation and Park Association

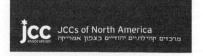

JCC JCCs of North America

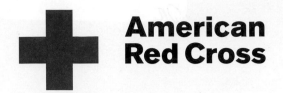
American Red Cross

This manual is part of the American Red Cross Lifeguarding program. By itself, it does not constitute complete and comprehensive training. Visit redcross.org to learn more about this program.

The emergency care procedures outlined in this book reflect the standard of knowledge and accepted emergency practices in the United States at the time this book was published. It is the reader's responsibility to stay informed of changes in emergency care procedures.

Published by Krames StayWell Strategic Partnerships Division

Printed in the United States of America

ISBN: 978-1-58480-487-1

Scan this code with your smartphone to access free skill refreshers, or visit **redcross.org/LGrefresher.**

Acknowledgments

This manual is dedicated to the thousands of employees and volunteers of the American Red Cross who contribute their time and talent to supporting and teaching lifesaving skills worldwide and to the thousands of course participants and other readers who have decided to be prepared to take action when an emergency strikes.

This manual reflects the 2010 Consensus on Science for CPR and Emergency Cardiovascular Care and the Guidelines 2010 for First Aid. These treatment recommendations and related training guidelines have been reviewed by the American Red Cross Scientific Advisory Council, a panel of nationally recognized experts in fields that include emergency medicine, occupational health, sports medicine, school and public health, emergency medical services (EMS), aquatics, emergency preparedness and disaster mobilization. This manual also reflects the United States Lifeguarding Standards: A Review and Report of the United States Lifeguard Standards Coalition, a collaborative effort of the American Red Cross, the United States Lifesaving Association and the YMCA of the USA.

Many individuals shared in the development and revision process in various supportive, technical and creative ways. The *American Red Cross Lifeguarding Manual* was developed through the dedication of both employees and volunteers. Their commitment to excellence made this manual possible.

The following members of the American Red Cross Scientific Advisory Council also provided guidance and review:

David Markenson, MD, FAAP, EMT-P
Chair, American Red Cross Scientific Advisory Council
Chief, Pediatric Emergency Medicine
Maria Fareri Children's Hospital
Westchester Medical Center
Valhalla, New York

Peter Wernicki, MD
Aquatics Chair, American Red Cross Scientific
  Advisory Council
Sports Medicine Orthopedic Surgeon
International Lifesaving Federation Medical Committee
  Past Chair
U.S. Lifesaving Association
Medical Advisor
Vero Beach, Florida

Roy R. Fielding
Member, American Red Cross Scientific Advisory Council
University of North Carolina–Charlotte, Department
  of Kinesiology
Coordinator, Exercise Science/Director of Aquatics
Charlotte, North Carolina

Terri Lees
Member, American Red Cross Scientific Advisory Council
Aquatic Supervisor
North Kansas City Community Center
North Kansas City, Missouri

Francesco A. Pia, PhD
Member, American Red Cross Scientific Advisory Council
Water Safety Films, Inc.
President, Pia Consulting Services
Larchmont, New York

S. Robert Seitz, M.Ed., RN, NREMT-P
Member, American Red Cross Scientific Advisory Council
University of Pittsburgh
Center for Emergency Medicine
Pittsburgh, Pennsylvania

The Sounding Board for this edition included:

Joyce A. Bathke
Chief Administrative Officer
American Red Cross St. Louis Area Chapter
St. Louis, Missouri

David W. Bell, PhD
National Aquatic Committee
National Health and Safety Committee
Boy Scouts of America
Ponca City, Oklahoma

Pete DeQuincy
Aquatic Supervisor
East Bay Regional Park District
Oakland, California

Shawn DeRosa, JD, EMT-B
Manger of Aquatic Facilities and Safety Officer for
 Intercollegiate Athletics
The Pennsylvania State University
University Park, Pennsylvania

Scott E. Gerding
Sales Manager
Mid-East Division
American Red Cross
Columbus, Ohio

Juliene R. Hefter
Deputy Director
Wisconsin Park & Recreation Association
Owner, Safety First Aquatics, LLC
Greendale, Wisconsin

Carolyn Hollingsworth–Pofok
Director of Recreation and Events
Millcreek MetroParks
Canfield, Ohio

William A.J. Kirkner, JD
Aquatics Director
JCC of Greater Baltimore
Reisterstown, Maryland

Joetta R. Jensen
Assistant Professor and Director of Aquatics
Hampton University
Hampton, Virginia

Rhonda Mickelson
Director of Standards
American Camp Association
Estes Park, Colorado

Edwin Pounds
Aquatics Manager
City of Pearland
Pearland, Texas

Clayton D. Shuck
Deputy Manager of Recreation
South Suburban Parks and Recreation
Centennial, Colorado

Thomas C. Werts
President
Aquatics Safety Consulting
Kissimmee, Florida

**The following individuals participated as Waterfront
and Waterpark Working Group members:**

Adam Abajian
Recreation Program Manager/Lakefront Operations
City of Evanston
Evanston, Illinois

Darwin DeLappa
Director of Water Safety
New York State Parks and Recreation
Queensbury, New York

Luiz A. Morizot-Leite
Captain, Ocean Rescue Lifeguard, Miami-Dade
Fire Rescue Department
Miami-Dade County, Florida

Robert E. Ogoreuc
Assistant Professor
Slippery Rock University
Slippery Rock, Pennsylvania

William J. Frazier
Aquatic Operations Manager
Massanutten Resort
McGaheysville, Virginia

Lee Hovis
Director of Recreation Operations
Nocatee Waterpark Recreation
Ponte Vedra Beach, Florida

Danial Llanas
Director of Support Services
Busch Entertainment Corporation
San Antonio, Texas

Scott Mersinger
Aquatics Director
Lost Rios Waterpark
Wisconsin Dells, Wisconsin

The following individuals provided external review:

Alex Antoniou
Director of Educational Programs
National Swimming Pool Foundation
Colorado Springs, Colorado

Jerome H. Modell, MD., D Sc (Hon.)
Emeritus Professor of Anesthesiology
Courtesy Professor of Psychiatry
Courtesy Professor of Large Animal Clinical Sciences
Colleges of Medicine & Veterinary Medicine, University
 of Florida
Gainesville, Florida

The American Red Cross thanks Jorge L. Olaves H., Ed S,
Florida A&M University, for his contributions to this manual.

Preface

This manual is for lifeguards, whom the American Red Cross profoundly thanks for their commitment to safeguarding the lives of children and adults who enjoy aquatic facilities. As the number of community pools and waterparks grows nationwide, participation in aquatic activities is also growing. With this growth comes the need for even more lifeguards.

To protect this growing number of participants, lifeguards must receive proper and effective training. Lifeguards also need to maintain their skills to ensure their ability to work effectively with others as a part of a lifeguard team. Participation in frequent and ongoing training is essential.

Lifeguards must be able to recognize hazardous situations to prevent injury. They must be able to supervise swimmers, minimize dangers, educate facility users about safety, enforce rules and regulations, provide assistance and perform rescues.

Being a lifeguard carries a significant professional responsibility, but lifeguarding also offers opportunities for personal growth. Experience as a lifeguard can help one develop professional and leadership skills that will last a lifetime—through college, career and family.

There are a half million American Red Cross-trained lifeguards working at swimming pools, waterparks and waterfronts across our country. Every day on the job, these lifeguards are part of a critical force for good—ensuring the safety of patrons and protecting lives.

CONTENTS

CHAPTER 9

Cardiac Emergencies

CHAPTER 10

First Aid

CHAPTER 11

Caring for Head, Neck and Spinal Injuries

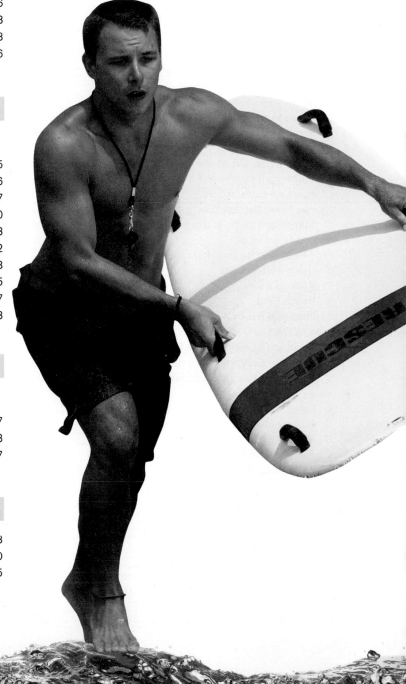

SKILL SHEETS

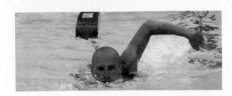
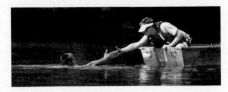
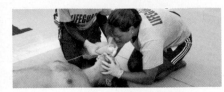

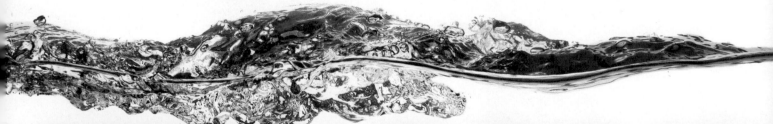

The Professional Lifeguard

CHAPTER 1

Lifeguarding can be a rewarding job. Being a lifeguard is:

- **Dynamic.** Each day on the job presents you with new situations.

- **Challenging.** You need to make quick judgments to do the job well.

- **Important.** You may need to respond to an emergency at any moment.

- **Inspiring.** With the knowledge, skills and attitude you acquire through your lifeguard training, you can save a life.

This chapter describes the characteristics, responsibilities and rewards of being a professional lifeguard. It also discusses the importance of maintaining lifeguarding knowledge and skills. ■

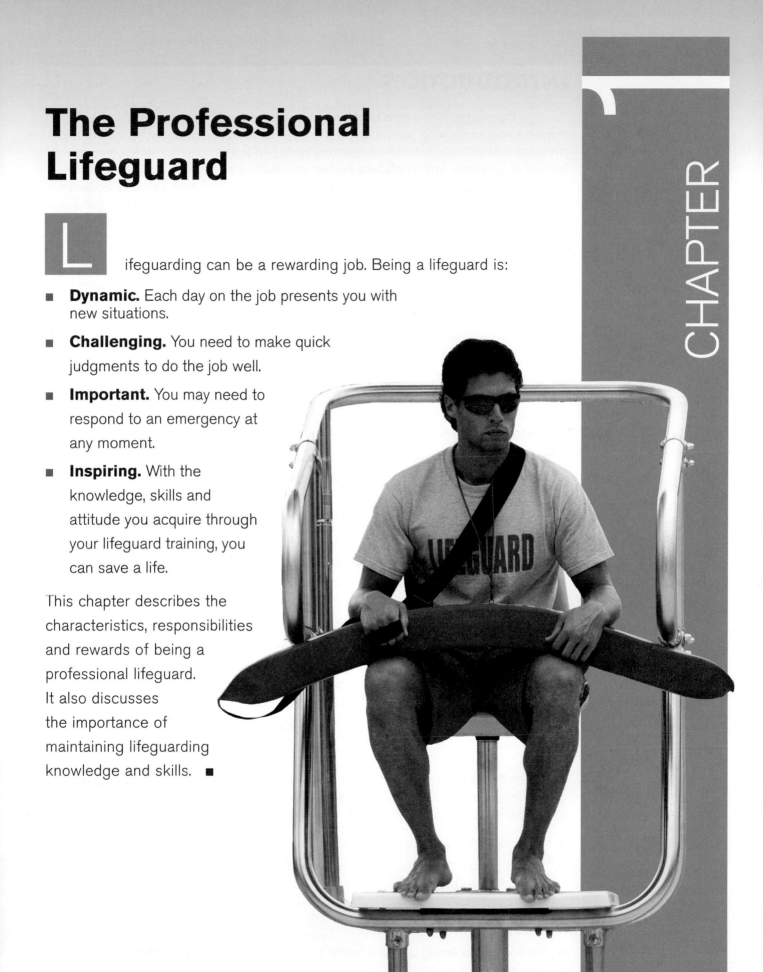

INTRODUCTION

You are training to become a professional lifeguard, taking responsibility for the lives of people who are participating in a variety of aquatic activities. As a professional rescuer with a legal responsibility to act in an emergency, you must be self-disciplined and confident in your knowledge and skills. You need to have solid public-relations, customer-service and conflict-resolution skills. In addition, you must be willing to be a leader as well as a good team member. Being a lifeguard requires maturity, professionalism and competence in specialized rescue techniques.

The purpose of the American Red Cross Lifeguarding course is to teach you the skills needed to help prevent and respond to aquatic emergencies. This includes land and water rescue skills plus first aid and CPR.

RESPONSIBILITIES OF A PROFESSIONAL LIFEGUARD

As a lifeguard, your *primary responsibility* is to prevent drowning and other injuries from occurring at your aquatic facility (Figure 1-1). Lifeguards do this in many ways, such as:

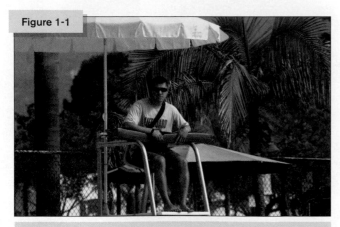

Figure 1-1

Patron surveillance is an important part of a lifeguard's primary responsibility.

- Monitoring activities in and near the water through patron surveillance.
- Preventing injuries by minimizing or eliminating hazardous situations or behaviors.
- Enforcing facility rules and regulations and educating patrons about them.
- Recognizing and responding quickly and effectively to all emergencies.
- Administering first aid and CPR, including using an automated external defibrillator (AED) and, if trained, administering emergency oxygen when needed.
- Working as a team with other lifeguards, facility staff and management.

A lifeguard also is responsible for other tasks, which are *secondary responsibilities*. Secondary responsibilities must never interfere with patron surveillance. Secondary responsibilities can include:

- Testing the pool water chemistry.
- Assisting patrons (conducting safety orientations, administering swim tests and fitting life jackets).
- Cleaning or performing maintenance.
- Completing records and reports.
- Performing opening duties, closing duties or facility safety checks and inspections.

CHARACTERISTICS OF A PROFESSIONAL LIFEGUARD

To fulfill the responsibilities of a professional lifeguard, you must be mentally, physically and emotionally prepared at all times to do your job (Figure 1-2). As a professional lifeguard you must be:

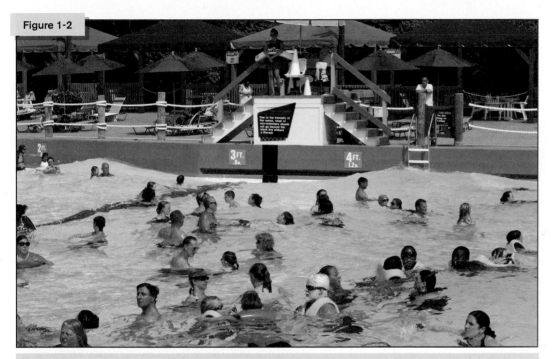

Figure 1-2

Lifeguards must be mentally, physically and emotionally prepared to carry out their duties.

- **Knowledgeable and skilled.** Have the appropriate knowledge and skills to help prevent and respond to emergencies. Successful completion of this Lifeguarding course is your initial training. You must maintain your knowledge and skills through annual or preseason orientation and training, and through regular, frequent in-service training.
- **Reliable.** Arrive at work on time, accept assignments willingly, be committed to your work and respond to all incidents quickly and effectively.
- **Mature.** Be a leader but also be a good team member, act responsibly, take initiative and obey all facility rules, leading others by example.
- **Courteous and consistent.** Be polite and enforce the rules firmly and equally for everyone (Figure 1-3).
- **Positive.** Show a positive attitude in all job activities.
- **Professional.** Look professional and be prepared to respond appropriately to any situation by:
  - o Wearing the lifeguard uniform only when on duty.

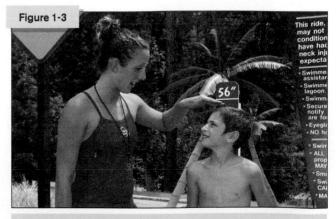

Figure 1-3

Lifeguards should be courteous and consistent with patrons when enforcing rules.

o Sitting or standing upright at the lifeguarding station.

o Being well groomed.

o Keeping rescue equipment positioned for immediate use when on duty.

o Keeping your eyes focused on your assigned zone of responsibility at all times.

o Keeping interactions with others brief and not letting them interrupt patron surveillance.

o Transferring and handling equipment carefully.

o Observing all facility rules, regulations and policies.

o Eating only when on break or off surveillance duty.

■ **Healthy and fit.** To stay in good physical condition, a professional lifeguard must:

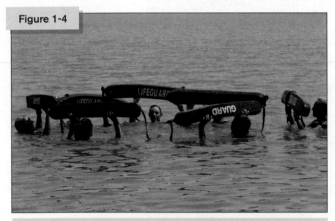

Figure 1-4

Regular exercise helps lifeguards stay physcially fit.

o **Exercise.** An exercise program should include swimming and water exercises that focus on building endurance and developing strength (Figure 1-4). Regular exercise helps you to stay alert, cope with stress and fatigue and perform strenuous rescues.

o **Eat and hydrate properly.** Good nutrition and a balanced diet help to provide the energy needed to stay alert and active. Drink plenty of water to prevent dehydration.

o **Rest adequately.** Proper rest and sleep during off-duty hours are essential for staying alert while on duty.

o **Protect yourself from sun exposure.** Overexposure to the sun's ultraviolet (UV) rays can cause many problems, such as fatigue, sunburn, skin cancer, dehydration, heat exhaustion and heat stroke. To prevent these problems:

● Use a sunscreen with a sun protection factor (SPF) of at least 15, re-applying at regular intervals.

● Use an umbrella or shade structure for sun protection and to help keep cool.

● Wear a shirt and hat with a brim that shades your face, ears and the back of your neck and use polarized sunglasses with UVA/UVB protection.

● Drink plenty of water.

● Take breaks in cool or shaded areas.

As a professional lifeguard, there are also some things you must *not* do. Keep the following in mind:

■ Do not leave your lifeguard station while on surveillance duty.

■ Do not use mobile phones or other devices for personal calls, texting or other types of communication when on duty.

■ Do not slouch in a lifeguard stand. Always be attentive and sit or stand upright when on surveillance duty.

■ Do not participate in conversations at the lifeguard station.

■ Do not eat at the lifeguard station.

- Do not leave the facility while on duty.
- Do not use alcohol or drugs. Alcohol or drugs can negatively affect job performance and can jeopardize the safety of patrons, co-workers and yourself.

SWIMMING FOR FITNESS

Getting to a victim, executing water-based rescues and moving the victim to safety, and performing life-sustaining resuscitation require you to have adequate strength and endurance at a moment's notice. This means that you need to constantly maintain or improve your personal level of fitness. Luckily, most lifeguards have access to one of the most versatile pieces of fitness equipment available, the water.

There are two main approaches to improving your level of fitness: improving endurance and increasing intensity. You can improve your endurance by practicing more, whether by swimming longer distances or for longer periods of time.

When exercising to increase endurance, you must commit to a regular, consistent workout schedule. Count the number of pool lengths that you can swim without having to stop to take a break. Your goal should be to increase this amount slightly each time you practice. At the beginning, you should be able to swim at least 300 yards without stopping. Try to build up to a competitive mile, which is about 1650 yards, or 66 lengths of a 25-yard pool. Once you build your endurance to this level, you will find it easy to practice even longer distances.

If your practice time is limited, you may choose to focus on the intensity of your swim. Typically, when a person is doing an activity for a long period of time, he or she begins to slow down as muscles become fatigued. Strength is built by forcing muscles to work at or beyond their current peak level, which requires maintaining— or increasing—your level of effort over your period of exercise.

In swimming, this can be done through interval training. *Intervals* are a series of repeat swims of the same distance and time interval, each done at the same high level of effort. There is a rest period between the time spent swimming that depends on the speed of the swim. The entire swim series is a set. As an example, an interval set is "5 x 100 on 1:30." This means that the 500-yard swim is broken up into five 100-yard swims, with 1:30 being the total amount of time for the swim and rest. In this example, a swimmer who swims the 100 in 1:15, has 15 seconds available for rest. This short rest period keeps the heart rate within the target range without dropping back to a resting heart rate. Interval training is the best all-around method to develop both speed and endurance.

As your level of fitness improves, you should combine the endurance and intensity approaches. Breaking down a larger endurance workout into smaller parts allows you to keep up your level of intensity, and it also helps to make the workout more interesting.

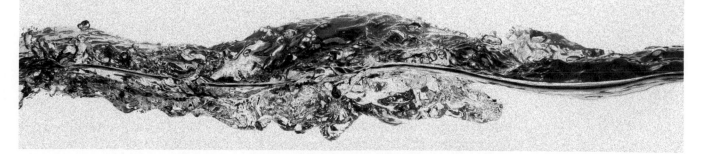

DECISION MAKING

Decision making is an important—and sometimes difficult—component of lifeguarding. In an emergency, such as a situation requiring a possible rescue or CPR, you must make critical decisions quickly and act quickly. Your facility should have established emergency action plans (EAPs), which are the written procedures that guide the actions of lifeguards and other staff members in emergencies.

In a non-emergency situation, such as how to work with your facility's management or how to interact with patrons, you can take more time for deliberation. In these kinds of situations, when time is not a critical factor, a decision-making model can help guide you through the process. The FIND decision-making model can be applied to lifeguarding situations to help you clearly understand what is involved in a decision. FIND means:

- F = Figure out the problem.
- I = Identify possible solutions.
- N = Name the pros and cons for each solution.
- D = Decide which solution is best, then act on it.

LEGAL CONSIDERATIONS

To avoid liability, it is important to understand the following legal principles that apply to your role as a professional lifeguard.

- **Duty to act.** While on the job, you have a legal responsibility to act in an emergency. Failure to adhere to this duty could result in legal action.
- **Standard of care.** You are expected to meet a minimum standard of care, which may be established in part by your training program and in part by state or local authorities. This standard requires you to:
  o Communicate proper information and warnings to help prevent injuries.
  o Recognize someone in need of care.
  o Attempt to rescue those needing assistance.
  o Provide emergency care according to your level of training.
- **Negligence.** When a person is injured or suffers additional harm because lifeguards failed to follow the standard of care or failed to act at all, the lifeguards may be considered negligent. Negligence includes:
  o Failing to control or stop any behaviors that could result in further harm or injury.
  o Failing to provide care.
  o Providing inappropriate care.
  o Providing care beyond the scope of practice or level of training.
- **Abandonment.** Once care is initiated, it must be continued until emergency medical services (EMS) personnel or someone with equal or greater training arrives and takes over. You can be held legally responsible for abandoning a person who requires ongoing care if you leave the scene or stop providing care.
- **Confidentiality.** While making a rescue or providing care, you may learn something about the injured or ill person, such as information about medical

conditions, physical problems and medications taken. This person's right to privacy is protected by laws that require you to keep information learned about the person confidential. Reporters, insurance investigators or attorneys may ask questions following an incident. This information should not be shared with anyone except EMS personnel directly associated with the person's care, facility management or the facility's legal counsel. Sharing personal information with individuals not directly associated with an injured person's medical care may constitute a breach of the victim's privacy.

- **Documentation.** Properly documenting injuries and incidents is very important. If legal action occurs later, your records and reports can provide legal documentation of what was seen, heard and done at the scene. Complete the required forms as soon as possible after the incident, preferably, immediately after the incident has wrapped up. As time passes, critical details may be forgotten. When completing a report, state the facts of the incident without including your opinion. Once the report is complete, sign and date it and have all responders read the report, then sign and date it as well. A copy of the report should be kept by the facility.

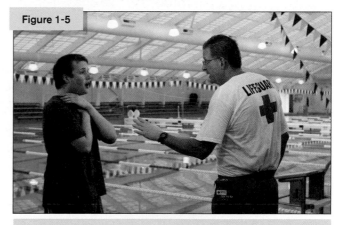

Figure 1-5

You must ask for a victim's consent before giving care.

- **Consent.** An injured or ill person must give permission before responders can provide first aid and emergency care (Figure 1-5). To obtain consent:

  - State your name.
  - State your level of training.
  - Ask if you may help.
  - Explain that you would like to assess him or her to find out what you think may be wrong or what you can do to help.
  - Explain what you plan to do.
  - With this information, an ill or injured person can grant his or her informed consent for care. Someone who is unconscious, confused or seriously injured or ill (such as in a nonfatal drowning) may not be able to grant consent. In these cases, the law assumes the victim would give consent if he or she were able to do so. This is called *implied consent*. Implied consent also applies to a minor who needs emergency medical assistance and whose parent or guardian is not present.

- **Refusal of care.** Some injured or ill people may refuse care, even if they desperately need it. Parents also may refuse care for children. Even though someone may be seriously injured, his or her wishes must be honored. In these situations, you should explain why he or she needs care. For significant injuries, you should call EMS personnel to evaluate the situation. For non-life-threatening emergencies, when care is refused and you

Good Samaritan Laws

Most states and the District of Columbia have Good Samaritan laws that protect people against claims of negligence after having provided emergency care in good faith without having accepted anything in return. These laws differ somewhat from state to state but generally help to protect people who act in good faith, within the scope of their training, and who are not negligent.

Some Good Samaritan laws, however, do not provide coverage for individuals who have a legal duty to act, which includes professional lifeguards. Therefore, it is important that lifeguards consult a lawyer or the facility's legal counsel to determine the degree of protection provided by their state's Good Samaritan laws.

are asked not to call EMS personnel, make it clear that you are neither denying nor withholding care and that you are not abandoning the victim. You must document any refusal of care. Someone else, such as another lifeguard, should witness the person's refusal of care and sign a report. Ask the person who refuses care to sign the report as well; if he or she refuses to sign, note that on the report.

Did You Know?

You may be evaluated periodically while on the job by your employer or through a contracted agency, such as the Red Cross or a combination of both. These evaluations may be announced or unannounced and may include how you perform patron surveillance and lifeguarding skills.

CONTINUING YOUR TRAINING

Earning a lifeguarding certification means you have successfully completed a training course and passed written and skill evaluations on a given date. It does not mean that you have learned everything there is to know about lifeguarding. Once hired as a lifeguard, you should expect that you will be required to continue your training.

It is the responsibility of facility management to provide direction and help lifeguards maintain and build on skills and to perform effectively as a team. Expect facility management to provide a pre-service evaluation, annual or preseason orientation and training, a policies and procedures manual and regular in-service training.

Pre-Service Evaluation

Facilities often require lifeguard applicants to hold a current training certificate from a nationally recognized agency, such as the American Red Cross. State codes, insurance company rules and standards of organizations to which your facility belongs may require your employer to evaluate your current skill level. Your employer may have you participate in rescue scenarios to ensure that you understand your responsibilities within your team and are familiar with your facility's layout and equipment.

Annual or Preseason Orientation and Training

Lifeguards should have annual training. This is especially important for seasonal lifeguards, who can forget knowledge and skills between seasons. Annual training can include review courses or a review of first aid, CPR/AED and lifeguarding knowledge and skills (Figure 1-6).

Figure 1-6

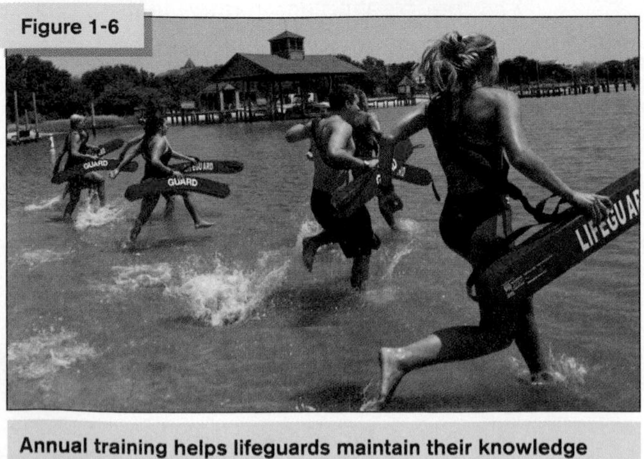

Annual training helps lifeguards maintain their knowledge and skills.

An orientation session about facility operations and lifeguards' responsibilities helps both new and returning lifeguards understand the facility, their responsibilities and management's expectations. The orientation is critical for learning what is unique about your workplace and how it differs from the environment in which you were trained. Ask your employer questions about your facility and become completely familiar with your facility's operations.

Policies and Procedures Manual

A policies and procedures manual should provide the information that you need to understand what is expected of you, to be able to work safely and to perform your duties effectively. This manual usually includes administrative policies and procedures, personnel policies and guidelines and standard operating procedures.

Regular In-Service Training

In-service training takes place while you are employed as a lifeguard and is designed to help you maintain your knowledge and skills at a professional level (Figure 1-7). It also gives you a chance to practice with other lifeguards at your facility. This will help you to efficiently respond as a team in an emergency.

BEING PART OF THE TEAM

There are two teams at most aquatic facilities: the *lifeguard team* and the *safety team*. The lifeguard team is formed whenever two or more lifeguards are on duty. The lifeguard team is part of a larger safety team, which is a network of people who prevent, prepare for, respond to and assist in an emergency at an aquatic facility. To be effective, members of both teams must know, understand and practice the roles that they are assigned in an emergency.

Lifeguard Team

If you work at a facility where two or more lifeguards are on duty at a time, you are part of a lifeguard team. To learn what you should expect from other team members, it is critical that you communicate and practice together. Your ability to respond to an emergency depends in large part on how much you have practiced the facility's EAPs together and how well you communicate.

By practicing with your team, you will learn how staff members work together in a variety of circumstances (Figure 1-8). Team practice also gives teammates the chance to work on different responder roles together. This is particularly important because team rescues are an integral part of lifeguarding. Several of the rescues presented in this course require more than one rescuer to provide care.

In-Service Training

It is a best practice of many well-managed facilities that lifeguards participate in a minimum of 4 hours of in-service training each month. The facility manager, lifeguard supervisor, a head lifeguard or an individual who is an expert in a particular subject matter, such as a public health official, risk manager or human resources representative, may conduct in-service trainings. Training sessions will address issues, such as surveillance and recognition, water and land rescue skills, emergency response drills, decision-making protocols, facility rules and regulations, customer service, records and reports and physical conditioning.

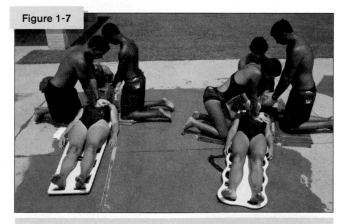

Figure 1-7

In-service training allows lifeguards to practice their skills.

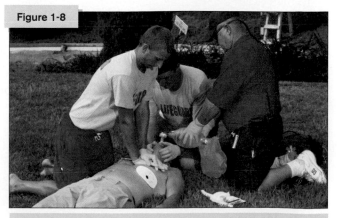

Figure 1-8

Practicing together helps lifeguard teams be better prepared for an emergency.

In addition to practicing rescues and response, it is important that the team works to maintain a climate of teamwork. Effective communication, trust, mutual respect, commitment and cooperation are crucial elements for working effectively as a team. Some ways that you can have a positive effect on your team include:

- Arriving to work on time.
- Rotating stations on time.
- Attending in-service trainings.
- Enforcing safety rules in a consistent manner.
- Communicating clearly while treating others with respect.
- Being prepared by maintaining your knowledge, skills and physical fitness.
- Completing secondary responsibilities in a timely and acceptable fashion.

The Emergency Action Plan

The lifeguard team and other staff members must practice the facility's EAPs together until everyone knows their responsibilities and can perform them effectively.

Because conditions can change throughout the day, you may need to adapt the EAP to a particular situation. Some facilities have created more than one EAP to cover specific situations or conditions. Factors that may affect the steps of an EAP include the number of lifeguards on duty. the number and availability of other safety team members on duty and the types of patron activities occurring.

Safety Team

After your lifeguard team activates the facility's EAP, the safety team needs to back you up and provide assistance. The main objective of the safety team is to assist you in maintaining a safe environment and providing emergency care.

In addition to the lifeguard team and other facility staff members, the safety team is composed of local emergency service personnel. Other members of the safety team may work off-site and often include upper-level management personnel. Chapter 5 discusses safety team members and their roles and responsibilities.

WRAP-UP

Being a professional lifeguard means being fully prepared for this challenging and important work. Looking and acting professional indicates readiness to do the job. Maintaining professional conduct requires practice and commitment. No one is a natural-born lifeguard; it takes hard work. A lifeguard can meet the challenges and gain the rewards of being a professional through practice, hard work and dedication.

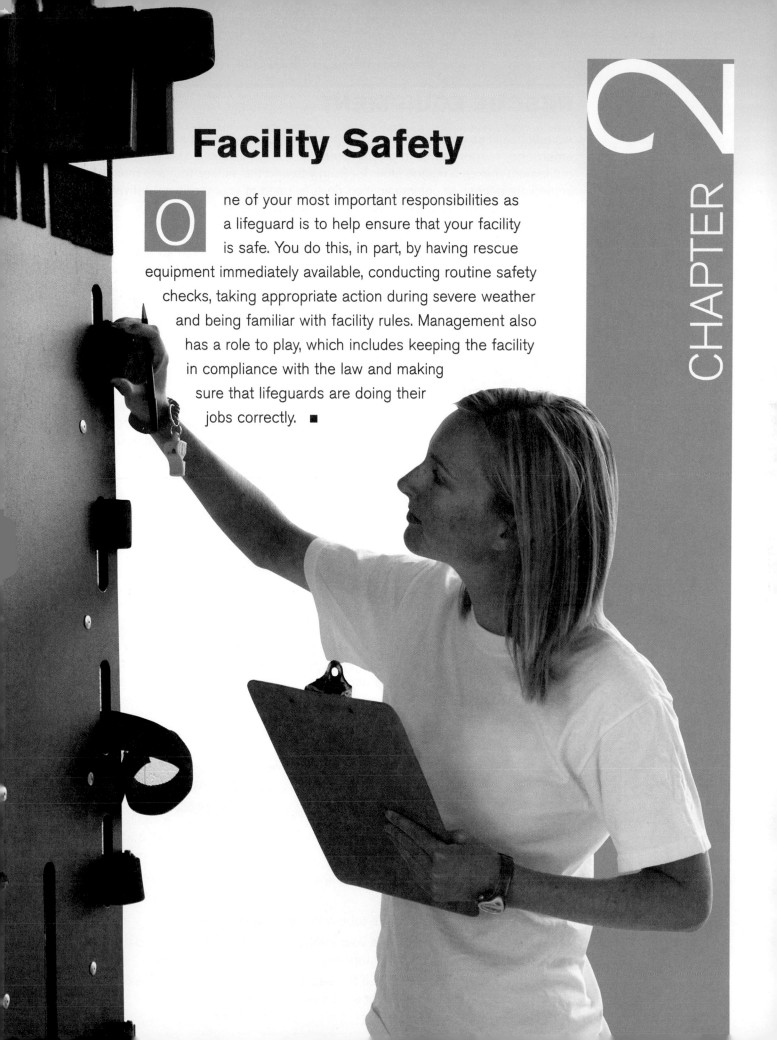

Facility Safety

One of your most important responsibilities as a lifeguard is to help ensure that your facility is safe. You do this, in part, by having rescue equipment immediately available, conducting routine safety checks, taking appropriate action during severe weather and being familiar with facility rules. Management also has a role to play, which includes keeping the facility in compliance with the law and making sure that lifeguards are doing their jobs correctly. ■

RESCUE EQUIPMENT

Aquatic facilities must have the appropriate rescue equipment available for emergency response and in proper working order at all times. Using rescue equipment makes a rescue safer for both you and the victim. You also must have immediate access to communication devices used at your facility to activate an emergency action plan (EAP), which may include a whistle, megaphone, radio, flag or other signaling equipment.

As a lifeguard, you must always wear or carry certain equipment so that it is instantly available in an emergency. The primary piece of rescue equipment used to perform a water rescue is the rescue tube. Another piece of equipment that must be immediately accessible is the backboard, which is used to remove victims from the water. Some facilities, like waterfronts, may use specific or specialty rescue equipment to meet the needs of their particular environments.

Equipment That You Wear or Carry

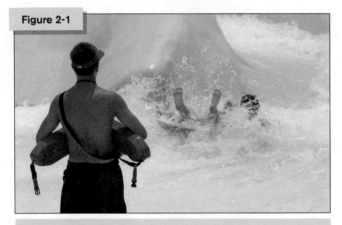

Figure 2-1

It is important to wear your lifeguard gear properly.

To respond quickly and appropriately to an emergency, a rescue tube, resuscitation mask and gloves must be instantly available. The best way to ensure this is to always keep the strap of the rescue tube over your shoulder and neck and wear a hip pack containing the gloves and resuscitation mask (Figure 2-1). You should wear the hip pack at all times, even when not on surveillance duty.

Rescue Tubes

The rescue tube is used at pools, waterparks and most non-surf waterfronts. It is a 45- to 54-inch vinyl, foam-filled tube with an attached tow line and shoulder strap. A rescue tube is capable of keeping multiple victims afloat.

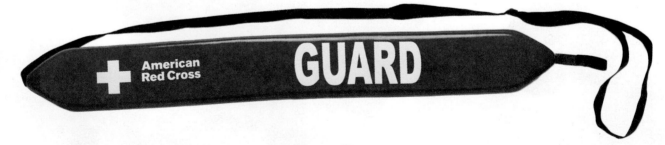

When performing patron surveillance, always keep the rescue tube ready to use immediately.

- Keep the strap of the rescue tube over the shoulder and neck.
- Hold the rescue tube across your thighs when sitting in a lifeguard chair or across your stomach when standing.
- Hold or gather the excess line to keep it from getting caught in the chair or other equipment when you move or start a rescue.

Resuscitation Masks

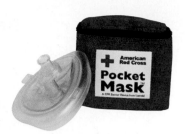

A resuscitation mask is a transparent, flexible device that creates a tight seal over the victim's mouth and nose to allow you to breathe air into a victim without making mouth-to-mouth contact. All masks should have a one-way valve for releasing exhaled air. Some masks also have an inlet for administering emergency oxygen. Masks come in different sizes to ensure a proper fit and tight seal on adults, children and infants.

Gloves

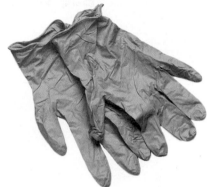

Disposable (single-use) gloves are used to protect employees that may be exposed to blood or other body fluids. Gloves should be made of non-latex materials, such as nitrile. Gloves also should be powder free.

Equipment You Can Easily Reach

Other first aid and rescue equipment should be easily accessible for emergency use. This additional equipment may include backboards, rescue buoys, other personal protective equipment (PPE), other resuscitation equipment, an automated external defibrillator (AED), first aid supplies and rescue boards.

Backboards

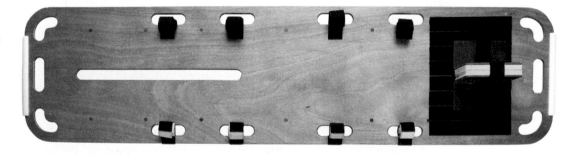

A backboard is the standard piece of equipment used at aquatic facilities to remove victims from the water when they are unable to exit the water on their own or when they have a possible injury to the head, neck or spine. Some backboards have runners on the bottom that allow the board to slide easily onto a deck or pier. A backboard must have a minimum of three body straps to secure a victim in cases of head, neck or spinal injury, in addition to a device for immobilizing the head. Additional straps may be necessary for special removal situations, such as steep inclines or vertical lifts.

Rescue Buoys

A rescue buoy (Figure 2-2), also known as a rescue can or torpedo buoy, often is the primary piece of rescue equipment used at waterfronts and surf beaches. Most rescue buoys are made of lightweight, hard, buoyant plastic and vary in length from 25 to 34 inches. Molded handgrips along the sides and rear of the buoy allow the victim to keep a firm hold on the buoy. Rescue buoys are buoyant enough to support multiple victims.

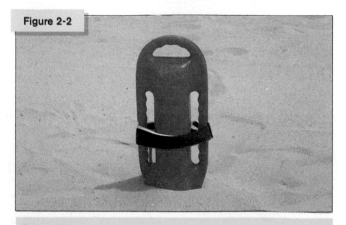

Figure 2-2

Rescue buoy

Personal Protective Equipment

Personal protective equipment (PPE) is the specialized clothing, equipment and supplies used to prevent you from coming into direct contact with a victim's body fluids. In addition to gloves and resuscitation masks, other PPE may be available at your facility, including gowns, masks, shields and protective eyewear. A blood spill kit should also be available to safely clean up blood.

Bag-Valve-Mask Resuscitator

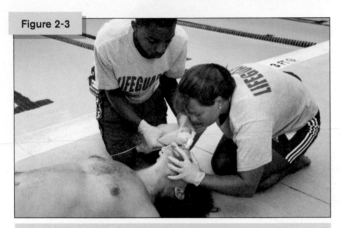

Figure 2-3

Giving ventilations using a bag-valve-mask resuscitator.

A bag-valve-mask resuscitator (BVM) is a hand-held device attached to a resuscitation mask that is used to ventilate a victim in respiratory arrest or when performing CPR. BVMs come in various sizes to fit adult, children and infants. The appropriately sized BVM should be used based on the size of the victim. Using a BVM requires two rescuers: one to maintain a tight seal for the mask, and one to squeeze the bag (Figure 2-3).

Other Resuscitation Equipment

In addition to resuscitation masks, other resuscitation equipment is effective in responding to breathing and cardiac emergencies. Use of all of the following supplemental resuscitation equipment is not covered in the Lifeguarding course and requires additional training. This equipment may or may not be used at your facility.

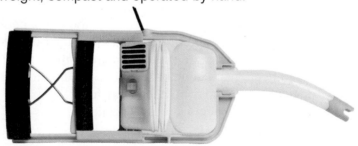

- **Oxygen cylinders and delivery devices.** In a breathing or cardiac emergency, oxygen cylinders and delivery devices are used to administer emergency oxygen to the victim.
- **Suctioning devices.** Manual suction devices are used to remove fluids and foreign matter from the victim's upper airway. They are lightweight, compact and operated by hand.

- **Airways.** Oropharyngeal and nasopharyngeal airways come in a variety of sizes and are used to help maintain an open airway in a nonbreathing victim. They do this by keeping the tongue away from the back of the throat during resuscitation.

Automated External Defibrillators

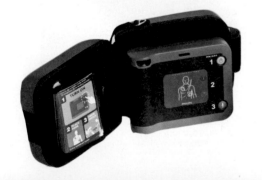

An AED is a portable electronic device that analyzes the heart's rhythm and can deliver an electrical shock, which helps the heart to re-establish an effective rhythm. This is known as defibrillation.

It is used in conjunction with CPR on unconscious victims with no obvious signs of life (movement and breathing). An AED should be available at your facility.

First Aid Kit and Supplies

An adequate inventory of first aid supplies must be available at all aquatic facilities. Common contents of a first aid kit include items used to treat bleeding and wounds and to help stabilize injuries to muscles, bones and joints. Ice packs and rescue blankets also may be included since they may help to treat heat- and cold-related emergencies. Your state or local health department may establish specific requirements for the contents of your first aid kit.

Rescue Board

Some waterfronts use rescue boards as standard equipment. Rescue boards are made of plastic or fiberglass and may include a soft rubber deck. They are shaped similarly to a surf board but usually are larger to accommodate a lifeguard plus one or more victims. Rescue boards are fast, stable and easy to use. They may be used during rescues to quickly paddle out long distances. They also may be used by lifeguards as a patrolling device, with the lifeguard paddling along the outer boundary of the swimming area.

Ring Buoys, Reaching Poles, and Shepherd's Crooks

A ring buoy, reaching pole and shepherd's crook often are required by the health department for swimming pools and waterparks. This equipment is not typically used by lifeguards to perform the professional rescues taught in this course. This equipment usually is used by untrained bystanders. If your facility has any of these items, you should learn how to use them.

FACILITY SAFETY CHECKS

Facility safety checks are the primary tool used by aquatic facility staff to ensure overall safety for their facilities. These checks may be performed by lifeguards or by staff that are trained to handle facility operations and maintenance, or by a combination of both (Figure 2-4). A lifeguard supervisor or facility manager will instruct you about the specific procedures for your facility. You should never perform safety checks while also performing patron surveillance. If you identify an equipment problem during your surveillance or if a problem is reported to you, notify a lifeguard supervisor or another lifeguard who is not performing surveillance. If the condition is hazardous, follow your facility protocols and stop patrons from using the equipment or prohibit them from entering a potentially hazardous area.

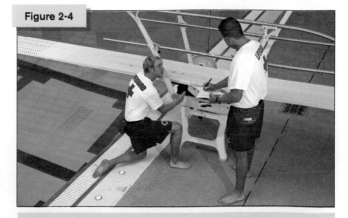

Figure 2-4

When performing facility safety checks, report any unsafe conditions found.

TYPICAL ITEMS FOUND ON A FACILITY CHECKLIST

The facility safety checklist should include the status of the following items (if they are okay or not okay) and any action required.

Equipment:

Verify that all equipment is in good working order, there is a sufficient number and equipment is in the proper location.

Rescue Equipment

- Rescue tubes and/or buoys
- Rescue board
- Non-motorized craft
- Motorized craft
- Masks and fins
- Reaching pole
- Ring buoy

First Aid Equipment

- Hip packs
  o Resuscitation masks
  o Disposable gloves
  o First aid supplies
- Backboard(s) with head immobilizer and straps
- First aid kit
- AED(s)
- Suctioning equipment
- Emergency oxygen delivery system

Safety Equipment

- Lifeguard stands/stations
- Communication devices – whistles, radios, E-stop(s)
- Telephone – directions for emergency calls posted
- PPE – extra gloves, gowns, face shield, blood spill kit
- Life jackets
- Umbrellas or shade structures
- Sunscreen

Operational Conditions:

As applicable for the environment and facility type.

- Bottom free of hazards
- Water clarity (pools and waterparks should see the bottom)
- Water level
- Water temperature – within specified range
- Air temperature – within specified range
- Weather conditions – safe
- Lighting – underwater and above ground working properly
- Water chemical ranges – within specified range
- Drain covers undamaged and secured
- Suction fittings undamaged and secured
- Circulation system – within range and proper operational condition
  o Flow rates
  o Filter differential
  o Hair/lint strainer
  o Gutter/skimmer baskets

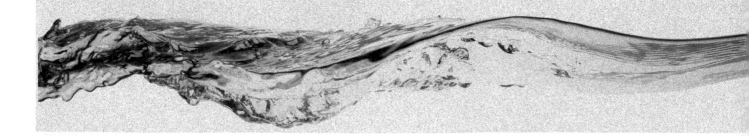

Risk Management:

In place, visible, secure, clean, ready for use.

- Depth markings clearly visible
- Swim area sections set up with ropes and/or buoys
- Signage in line of sight for patrons
- Fences and barriers, gates and doors secure
- Walkways/decks clear, accessible, non-slip and free of hazards
- Handrails or guardrails secure
- Ladder rungs or steps secure
- ADA accessibility equipment secure and ready for use
- Diving boards – secure and non-slip
- Starting blocks – secure and non-slip
- Floating features – tethered and secure, undamaged
- Fire extinguishers – charged and ready for use
- Emergency exits – clear, accessible with working lights and alarms

Facility Sanitation:

Clean, non-slip and ready to use

- Pool shell – free of algae, free of scum line
- Deck or shoreline – clean and free of environmental debris, such as animal droppings
- Restrooms/locker rooms
  - o Warm, running water
  - o Soap
  - o Paper products adequately stocked
- First aid station – adequately stocked
- Tables and seating
- Trash receptacles

Administration:

Posted or filed as applicable.

- Zones of surveillance diagrams posted
- Lifeguard rotation plans posted
- EAPs available
- MSDS sheets available
- Staff certifications – copies on file for all staff
- Training records – on file
- Water quality test results
  - o Daily results posted
  - o Records on file
- Rescue and/or incident reports on file
- AED inspection checklist – up-to-date
- Emergency oxygen system checklist – up-to-date

Aquatic Attractions:

- Rides and slides – inspected and test run complete
- Rafts, tubes and/or sleds – properly inflated and handles secure
- Landing areas free of rough surfaces and debris
- Water level and flow appropriate for attraction

Waterfronts:

- Shoreline is clean and free of sharp objects
- Bottom conditions are free from hazards
- Water conditions are safe for swimming
- Piers or docks are anchored, stable, and free from trip or injury hazards
- Lifeguard stands – surrounding area clear of objects

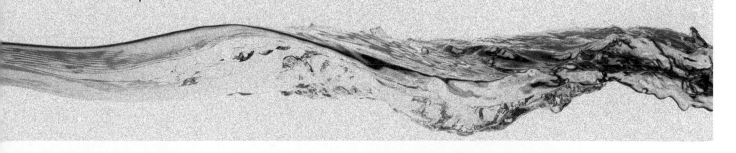

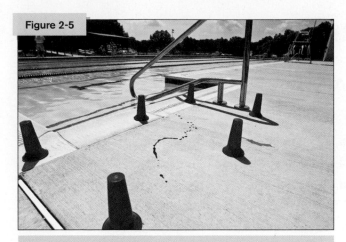

Figure 2-5

Use signs, ropes or cones to keep patrons away from unsafe conditions or areas not open to the public.

Safety checks are conducted before the facility is opened, during daily operations and at closing. Checks conducted before the facility is opened may include a physical inspection of all features, such as a test ride of all attractions. If you find an unsafe condition, you should correct the condition before the facility opens, if possible. If you cannot correct the problem, you should inform a supervisor immediately. If the condition is serious, the supervisor or facility manager may close or delay the opening of the facility, attraction or area until the condition is corrected. Signs, ropes or cones can keep patrons away from an area of the facility not open to the public (Figure 2-5). Inform other lifeguards about the hazard so that they can direct patrons away from the area. You also should record incidents in the daily log or on the appropriate form or report.

RIP CURRENTS

This course is not intended to prepare lifeguards to work at surf waterfront environments; however, it is important for all lifeguards to understand the dangers of rip currents and to help educate others about these dangers.

A rip current is a strong channel of water that flows offshore beginning near the shore and often extending well beyond the breaking waves. Rips currents are often associated with underwater features, such as sandbars, that may cause a channel in the bottom of a body of water, allowing water to escape from the near shore through a narrow channel. They also commonly occur near physical structures, such as piers, groins and natural outcroppings. Rip currents can create fast moving currents that may exceed 8 feet per second—this makes it

extremely difficult for even a strong swimmer to swim against.

According to the National Weather Service, common indicators of a rip current include:

- A channel of churning, choppy water.
- An area having a noticeable difference in water color.
- A line of foam, seaweed or debris moving steadily away from shore.
- A break in the incoming wave pattern.

Although these are good indicators, they are not always present. Consequently, it is not always possible even for an experienced lifeguard to spot a rip current. Rip currents can occur in any surf or weather condition.

The United States Lifesaving Association (USLA) estimates that each year more than 100 people

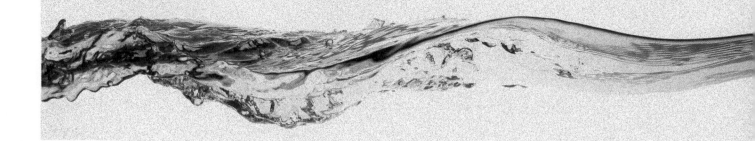

Specific Areas to Inspect for Safety

The facility's safety checklist is a guide for performing a safety check. The purpose is to verify that equipment has been tested, is working properly and is ready for use and that the facility is clean and safe for patrons. Your facility should have a checklist specific to your facility. General areas and equipment to inspect include:

- Rescue equipment (hip pack contents, rescue tubes, backboards and first aid supplies).

- Communication equipment.

- Pool decks or waterfront shorelines.

- Pools, waterfront swimming areas or waterpark attractions.

- Locker rooms (dressing areas, shower areas and restrooms).

- Equipment and structures (ladders, diving boards and starting blocks).

- Recreational equipment and play structures.

drown in rip currents. Rip currents are believed to account for more than 80 percent of rescues performed by surf lifeguards. This makes rip currents one of nature's most deadly natural forces. Many beaches and waterfront areas use color-coded flags to indicate the presence of hazardous water conditions and rip currents. Any time a red or double red flag is visible, stay out of the water; use extreme caution when there is a yellow flag.

If caught in a rip current, do not panic. Never attempt to swim against the current—fighting the current will cause you to become exhausted and possibly drown. Allow the current to take you away from shore. Once the current weakens, swim parallel to the beach then back to shore at an angle. Try to swim in the direction of least resistance to the current. If you are too exhausted to swim to shore, signal by calling and waving for help.

If you are lifeguarding at a waterfront area where there is the possibility of rip currents, it is critical to receive specialized training in the specific conditions and hazards that exist in your area and to learn how to identify rip currents and to help someone who is caught in them. For more information on rip currents, visit ripcurrents.noaa.gov and usla.org.

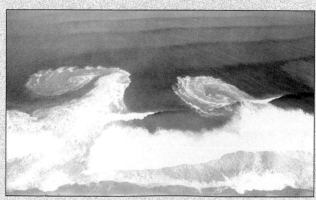

Photo courtesy John R. Fletemeyer

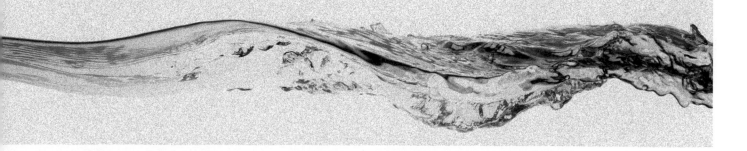

Inspecting Aquatic Attractions and Features

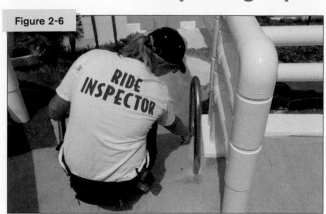

Figure 2-6

Safety checks are a primary method of facility surveillance and help prevent injuries to patrons.

Facilities should follow the manufacturer's guidelines for installation, safe inspection, maintenance and use of its various attractions and features (Figure 2-6). Your employer should provide you with a specific set of guidelines and training if you are responsible for these inspections. In some cases, maintenance personnel, rather than lifeguards, will be responsible for inspections. Even if the attraction or feature has been inspected already, stay alert for any problems that may develop, such as loose or rusted bolts; cracks; broken or missing pieces; frayed, loose or mildewed safety nets; unusual noises; and an area with increased frequency of injury to patrons.

Hazards at Waterfront Facilities

You should be aware of the specific potential hazards presented by some waterfront facilities. These include underwater hazards, physical structures and changing water conditions.

Dangerous conditions may develop with changing winds, tides and weather. On some days, the water may be totally calm and flat. On other days, there may be large waves. Checking for potentially hazardous conditions specific to your facility should be covered during your orientation. If they are not, ask your facility management to discuss procedures for any situation for which you do not feel adequately prepared.

Underwater Hazards

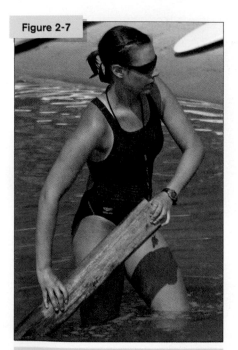

Figure 2-7

Remove any underwater hazards at waterfront facilities.

Common underwater hazards may change throughout the day and include:

- Holes in the swimming area and sudden drop-offs.
- Submerged objects, such as rocks, tree stumps and underwater plants (Figure 2-7).
- Bottom conditions (sand, rock, silt, weeds and mud).
- Slope of the bottom and water depth.
- Shells, barnacles and marine life.
- Broken glass or other sharp objects.

You should check for and, if possible, remove underwater hazards. If hazards cannot be removed, swimming areas should be re-positioned away from them. Alternatively, the shape and size of swimming areas may need to be changed to avoid underwater hazards. Floating buoys can be used to mark underwater hazards to warn patrons of their danger.

Physical Structures

Piers and docks in the water often are used for different activities (Figure 2-8, A–D). The following precautions should be taken with these structures:

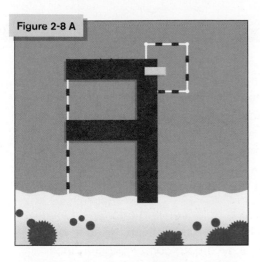
Figure 2-8 A

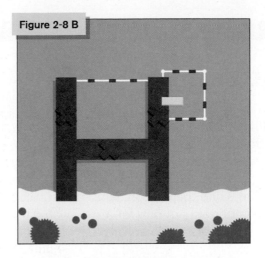
Figure 2-8 B

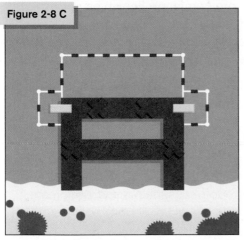
Figure 2-8 C

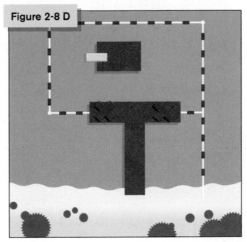
Figure 2-8 D

Dock formations: (A) "F" dock, (B) "H" dock, (C) "A" dock, (D) "T" dock.

- Ensure the floating piers, docks and rafts are anchored securely.
- Adjust attachment points between floating sections to minimize hazards.
- Be aware of and take steps to eliminate blind spots (obstructed views) caused by structures.
- Ensure that patrons dive only in designated areas. Check the water depth daily. Be aware of bottom and tidal changes before allowing head-first entries.
- Prohibit swimming in fishing areas around piers or docks or adjacent to boat activity.

Changing Water Conditions

Many factors can influence water conditions, which in turn can affect patron safety. These factors include:

- Water depth and currents. Changes in the water level may lead to increased currents that make standing difficult and could sweep swimmers beyond area boundaries. Examples include:
  - A dam that releases water, causing the water depth above the dam to drop and the river depth below the dam to rise.
  - Heavy rainfall that makes a lake or river rise, or a long, dry period that makes it too shallow for diving.
  - Tidal changes.

WATER QUALITY

The quality of water in spas and swimming pools constantly changes. It is affected by many factors, including the concentration of disinfectant in the water; the water's pH level, chemical balance and saturation; air temperature; sunlight; and contaminants from bathers and the environment. All of these factors are important not only for a safe swimming environment but also to ensure crystal-clear water clarity.

Additional training is needed, and a certification in pool operations often is required, to learn how and when to make chemical adjustments to the pool water. If you work at a swimming pool or waterpark, your responsibilities probably will include monitoring the water to make sure that it is safe, clean and clear. You may be asked to assist by periodically testing the water's chlorine or bromine and pH levels. You should receive training on how to properly test the pool water chemistry if this is included in your job responsibilities.

Disinfectant and pH Levels

Chlorine is one of the most common chemicals used to disinfect pools and spas. When dissolved in pool or hot tub water, chlorine produces a chemical called *hypochlorous acid*, also known as *free chlorine*. Free chlorine disinfects and sanitizes the water by killing germs and contaminants. To work most effectively, the free chlorine-to-water ratio should be 2 to 4 parts per million (ppm). This concentration of free chlorine, called a *residual*, should be maintained at all times throughout the water.

Free chlorine is colorless and odorless. However, it reacts with certain contaminants, such as human waste, to create *combined chlorines*, which are more commonly known as *chloramines*. Chloramines cause the chlorine-like smell found in indoor pools. Chloramines also can irritate the skin and mucous membranes.

The pH of the pool and hot tub water must be maintained at the appropriate level for free chlorine to be effective and for bathers to be comfortable. As the pH level goes down, free chlorine works better as a disinfectant. However, when the pH drops below 7.2, the water may irritate eyes and skin and corrode pool surfaces and equipment. Human tears have a pH of about 7.5; therefore, the ideal pH in pool and hot tub water is 7.4 to 7.6.

Bromine is another chemical commonly used to kill germs and contaminants in pool and hot tub water. It often is used in hot tubs instead of chlorine because it is more stable in hot

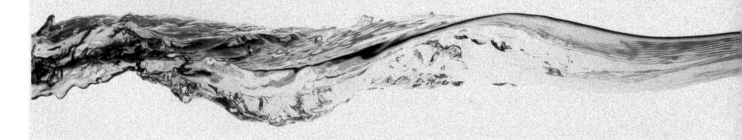

- Seiche, which is a standing wave of water that oscillates in large lakes usually created by strong winds and/or large barometric pressure gradients.
- Sandbars that can move and shift from season to season or from heavy rain that produces strong currents. These changes in the waterfront floor can create unexpected drops or new shallow-water features.
- Water quality. Insufficient flow may lead to stagnant water and compromise water quality.
- Debris or cloudiness in the water.

temperatures and does not burn away as quickly. It also does not leave a chemical odor in the water.

Testing and Adjusting

A supervisor, or another staff member trained and certified in pool operations, typically monitors and adjusts chemical levels throughout the day. However, you may be trained to test the chlorine or bromine and pH levels of the water. The water quality will need to be tested and the results recorded at periodic intervals throughout the day. Your facility should have a test kit available that measures free chlorine or bromine and pH levels. Some measure other water-balance levels as well. N,N-diethyl-p-phenylenediamine (DPD) is the most common test chemical used to test for free chlorine or bromine. DPD reacts with chlorine and turns the water test sample shades of light to dark pink. Phenol red is a dye used to test the water's pH. Its color changes from yellow to orange to red based on the pH level. The water test result color is compared with the colors on the test kit.

Your facility will have guidelines for the minimum, maximum and ideal ranges for chlorine or bromine and pH levels for safe swimming. Alert the appropriate staff member immediately if the water test results are not within the proper ranges for safe swimming at your facility. Adjustments may need to be made as soon as possible or the pool or hot tub may need to be temporarily closed until the chemical ranges are correct for safe swimming.

Waterfront Considerations

(Source: http://water.epa.gov/type/oceb/beaches Accessed September 6, 2011)

Water quality is also important at natural bodies of water. Swimming in unsafe water may result in minor illnesses, such as sore throats or diarrhea or more serious illnesses, such as meningitis, encephalitis or severe gastroenteritis. Children, the elderly and people with weakened immune systems have a greater chance of getting sick when they come in contact with contaminated water. The quality of natural bodies of water can be impacted by pollutants, such as runoff from animal waste, fertilizer, pesticides, trash and boating wastes and especially storm water runoff during and after heavy periods of rain. The Environmental Protection Agency recommends that state and local officials monitor water quality and issue an advisory or closure when beaches are unsafe for swimming.

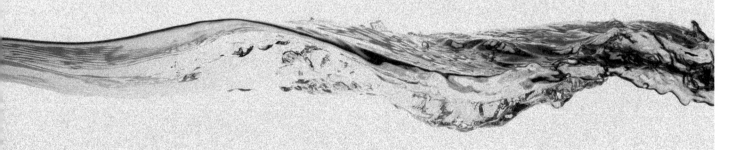

■ Water temperature, which usually is colder early in the summer and after rain. Although surface water may be warm and comfortable, water at a depth of several feet can be much colder. This condition, called a *thermocline*, can cause *hypothermia* (low body temperature).

When dealing with changing water conditions:

■ Warn patrons of hazards by using signs, buoys and safety announcements.

■ Check for objects that may have washed into the area.

■ Check for changes in bottom conditions, water depth and water quality.

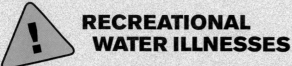

RECREATIONAL WATER ILLNESSES

Illnesses that are spread by swallowing, breathing or contacting contaminated water are called *recreational water illnesses* (RWIs). Typical RWIs include earaches, rashes and diarrhea. RWIs generally are not severe, but in rare cases they can result in serious outcomes, including pneumonia, neurological damage and even death.

Gastroenteritis, a stomach ailment that causes diarrhea, nausea, vomiting and abdominal pain, is one of most commonly documented RWIs. It occurs when feces are released into the water and swallowed by other swimmers before having been killed by chlorine or another disinfectant.

Cryptosporidium is the parasite that causes most gastroenteritis outbreaks. *Crypto* can remain infectious, even when exposed to disinfectant levels for several days; therefore, people suffering from diarrhea should not enter the water. Those diagnosed with cryptosporidiosis should not enter recreational water for 2 weeks after symptoms have ceased.

Fecal Incident Response Recommendations

During orientation or in-service training, your facility should provide training on how to respond to accidental fecal releases (AFRs). If an AFR occurs, you should direct all patrons to leave all of the pools that use the same filtration system. Remove as much of the fecal material as possible with a scoop or net, trying not to break formed stool apart. Dispose of the feces using the sanitary procedures. Do not vacuum the feces. Clean and disinfect the scoop and net and then place them in the pool during the following disinfection procedures.

Formed stool

- Continue to operate the filtration system.
- Adjust the pH to below 7.5.
- Raise the free chlorine level to at least 2 ppm.
- Maintain those levels for 25 minutes before reopening the pool.

Diarrheal discharge

- Continue to operate the circulation system.
- Adjust the pH to below 7.5.
- Raise the free chlorine level to at least 20 ppm.
- Maintain those levels for 13 hours.
- Backwash the filter.
- Return the chlorine level to normal levels before re-opening the pool.

Vomit in Pool Water

Patrons are unlikely to contract RWIs by swallowing, breathing or contacting pool water contaminated by vomit or blood. The vomit that a person produces after swallowing too much water probably is not infectious; however, if a person vomits and it contains any solid matter or food particles, you should respond the same way as you would to a formed stool incident.

To learn more about prevention practices, healthy swimming and recreational water topics, and to download free outbreak response toolkits and publications, visit CDCs website at cdc.gov/healthywater/swimming. You can learn even more by enrolling in a pool operator course.

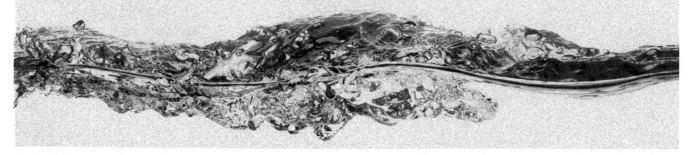

- Alert patrons to cold water and watch for signs of hypothermia in patrons.
- Check and document scheduled high and low tides in the daily log each morning before opening, and plan for changes in water depth.

WEATHER CONDITIONS

Weather affects the safety of swimmers both outdoors and indoors. You should be aware of the weather conditions in your area and know how to act when severe weather occurs.

The National Oceanic and Atmospheric Administration (NOAA) Weather Radio All Hazards is a good source of information about potentially hazardous weather. This nationwide radio network provides detailed weather information 24 hours a day to most areas. A special radio receiver is needed to receive the signal and can be set to sound an alarm when a warning is issued for a specific area. These radios have battery back-up in case of power failure. Local up-to-date forecasts and weather warnings also are available from Internet sites, such as the National Weather Service at www.nws.noaa.gov. Local radio stations, television channels and cable services also provide forecasts and emergency weather warnings.

Always follow your facility's EAP for severe weather conditions.

Lightning and Thunderstorms

In most parts of the United States, lightning and thunderstorms happen more often in the summer. Follow the facility's procedures for clearing patrons from the water before an impending storm. Patron or employee safety never should be put at risk. If a storm or other bad weather is predicted, stay alert for signs of the coming storm, such as thunder and lightning or high winds.

If thunder or lightning occur:

- Clear everyone from the water at the first sound of thunder or first sight of lightning. If you are in an elevated station, get down immediately. Move everyone to a safe area free from contact with water, plumbing or electrical circuits. For outdoor facilities, move everyone inside, if possible. Large buildings are safer than smaller or open structures, such as picnic shelters or gazebos.
- Keep patrons and staff out of showers and locker rooms during a thunderstorm as water and metal can conduct electricity.
- Do not use a telephone connected to a landline except in an emergency.
- Keep everyone away from windows and metal objects (e.g., doorframes, lockers).
- Watch for more storms and monitor weather reports on a radio or TV broadcast, weather radio or website.

Lightning

Lightning is the result of the build-up and discharge of electrical energy, and this rapid heating of the air produces the shock wave that results in thunder. 25 million cloud-to-ground lightning strikes occur in the United States each year. Lightning often strikes as far as 10 to 15 miles away from any rainfall with each spark of lightning reaching over 5 miles in length and temperatures of approximately 50,000° F. Even if the sky looks blue and clear, be cautious. One ground lightning strike can contain 100 million volts of electricity. The National Lightning Safety Institute recommends waiting 30 minutes after the last lightning sighting or sound of thunder before resuming activities.

Source: National Weather Service Web at www.lightningsafety.noaa.gov.

If caught outside in a thunderstorm and there is not enough time to reach a safe building:

- Keep away from tall trees standing alone and any tall structures.
- Keep away from water and metal objects, such as metal fences, tanks, rails and pipes.
- Keep as low to the ground as possible: squat or crouch with the knees drawn up, both feet together and hands off the ground.
- Avoid lying flat on the ground; minimize ground contact.

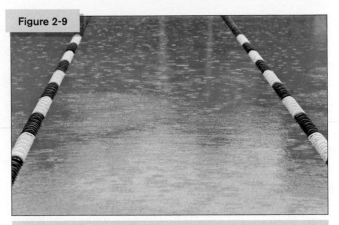

Figure 2-9

Rain can obscure the bottom of a pool.

Heavy Rain and Hail

Heavy rain and hail can be dangerous. Rain can make it difficult to see the bottom of the pool or beneath the surface. If you cannot see the bottom of the pool (Figure 2-9), clear the pool of all patrons. In addition, hail can cause serious physical injury. If it is hailing, clear patrons from the water and direct them to shelter.

Tornadoes

If the aquatic facility's locale is prone to tornadoes, facility staff should monitor weather forecasts. A *tornado watch* means that tornadoes are possible. Some facilities may decide to close once a watch is issued and before the arrival of wind, rain and lightning, which also may occur when tornado formation is likely. A *tornado warning* means that a tornado has been sighted or indicated on radar and is occurring or imminent in the warning area. Some communities activate sirens during a tornado warning. Everyone should take shelter immediately.

If a tornado warning is issued:

- Clear the water and surrounding area.
- Move everyone to the location specified in the facility's EAP, such as a basement or an inside area on the lowest level of a building.
- Keep everyone away from windows, doors and outside walls.
- Have everyone lie flat in a ditch or on a low section of ground if adequate shelter is unavailable at or near the facility.

If a tornado siren warning is heard, keep patrons in the safe location. Continue listening to local radio or television stations or a NOAA Weather Radio for updated instructions from the authorities.

High Wind

High wind may cause waves or turbulence that makes it hard to see patrons in the water. Wind also increases the risk of hypothermia, especially for small children and the elderly. Safety guidelines for high wind include:

- Clearing the pool or waterfront if visibility is impaired by waves or increased turbidity.

- Moving all patrons and staff indoors.
- Securing all facility equipment that could be blown around and become dangerous, but only if it is possible and safe to do so.

Fog

In some areas, fog can occur at any time of the day or night with changing weather conditions. If fog limits visibility, your facility may need to close.

Weather Conditions and Indoor Facilities

Indoor facilities are safe from most weather problems but still may be affected. Severe weather can cause a power failure; therefore, the facility should have some type of portable or emergency lighting. In the event of a power failure, you should clear the pool because circulation and filtration of pool water will not be possible. If weather conditions cause safety concerns, you also should clear the deck. Follow the facility's EAP for severe weather conditions.

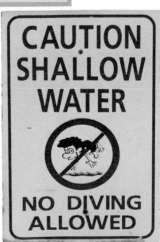

RULES AND REGULATIONS

Every aquatic facility establishes its own set of rules and regulations, some of which are required by the state or local health department, whereas others are determined by the facility management. This course concentrates on common rules aimed at keeping patrons safer and preventing injuries; however, you should be familiar with and enforce all rules at your facility.

Common Rules

Every facility should post its rules and regulations for patron behavior in plain view of all patrons and staff. Rules do not keep patrons from having fun. Rules exist for everyone's health and safety. Posted rules help patrons to enjoy their experience without endangering themselves or others. Facilities that attract numerous international guests or those that are located in multicultural communities also may post rules in other languages or use international signs or symbols.

Common rules posted at aquatic facilities may include:

- Swim only when a lifeguard is on duty.
- Swim diapers are required for small children or people with incontinence.
- No swimming with open or infected wounds.
- Obey lifeguard instructions at all times.
- No running, pushing or rough play.
- No hyperventilating before swimming underwater or breath-holding contests.
- No sitting or playing near or with drains or suction fittings.
- Dive only in designated areas (Figure 2-10).

Figure 2-10

To help prevent injuries, post signs, markings and warnings to inform patrons about dangers.

- No glass containers in the pool area and locker rooms.
- No alcoholic beverages or drug use allowed.

Waterfront Rules

Waterfront facilities often adopt additional rules that are specific to the waterfront environment. These may include:

- No playing or swimming under piers, rafts, platforms or play structures.
- No boats, sailboards, surfboards or personal water craft in swimming areas.
- No running or diving head-first into shallow water.
- No fishing near swimming areas.
- No umbrellas at the waterline (umbrellas present a surveillance obstruction).
- No swimming in unauthorized areas.

Waterpark Rules

At waterparks, rules and regulations should be posted, but they also may be recorded and played over a public address system. Rules may vary based on the type of attractions available. For example, U.S. Coast Guard-approved life jackets may be required on certain attractions but not allowed on others.

Waterparks should have signage at every attraction stating the depth of the water, height or age requirements and how to safely use the attraction. This is to prevent patrons from finding themselves in water that is deeper or shallower than they expected. For example, some pools at the end of a slide are shallow so that patrons can stand up, but others are very deep. Without signage to warn them, patrons may expect a shallow catch pool and be surprised to find themselves in deep water.

Additional rules for each attraction typically cover:

- The minimum or maximum number of people allowed on an attraction or a tube at a time.
- The maximum height or age requirements in areas designated for small children.
- The minimum height or weight requirements for patrons using an attraction (Figure 2-11).
- Common rules for winding rivers, such as:
  - Enter and exit the winding river only at designated places.
  - No jumping or diving into the water.
  - No people on shoulders.
  - Stay in tubes at all times if tubes are used.
  - No walking or swimming in the winding river if tubes are used.
  - Only one properly fitted life jacket per patron.
  - No stacking of tubes or life jackets.
  - No forming chains of tubes or life jackets.
  - Only one patron allowed per tube, except for an adult holding a small child. The child must be wearing a U.S. Coast Guard-approved life jacket in case the adult tips over.

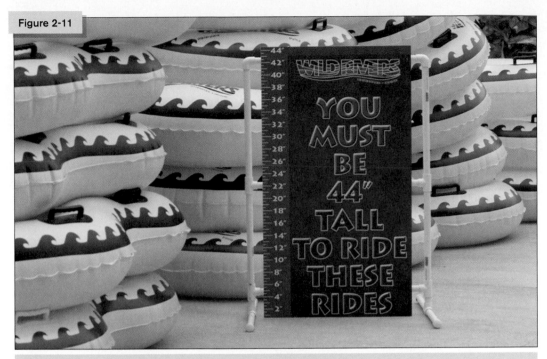

Figure 2-11

Use a measuring pole or line to ensure patrons are the proper height to use a ride.

- Common rules for waterslides, such as:
  - Enter, ride and exit the slide feet-first.
  - No stopping in the slide, and no running, standing, kneeling, rotating or spinning on the slides. Keep hands and feet inside the slide.
  - No metal objects, locker keys, jewelry, metal snaps/zippers, eyewear or watches, including metal rivets, buttons or fasteners on swimsuits or shorts.
  - No aqua socks or aqua shoes, eyeglasses, sunglasses or goggles.

Rules for Facility Equipment and Structures

Other rules for specific equipment and structures depend on the facility and may include:

- One person at a time on a ladder or attraction.
- Do not sit or hang on lifelines or lane lines.
- Do not climb on lifeguard stands or towers.
- Starting blocks may be used only by swim team members in scheduled practices, competitions and instruction when supervised by a certified coach or instructor.

Diving-Area Rules

Rules for diving boards and dive towers should be posted in the diving area. The rules may include:

- Patrons must demonstrate their swimming ability before entering deep water.
- Only one person on the diving board at a time and only one person on the ladder at a time.
- Look before diving or jumping to make sure the diving area is clear.

- Only one bounce allowed on the diving board.
- Dive or jump forward, straight out from the diving board.
- Swim immediately to the closest ladder or wall.

Rules for Spas, Hot Tubs and Therapy Pools

Spas, hot tubs and therapy pools are popular, but their hazards include drowning, hyperthermia (high body temperature) and disease transmission. Rules common to these areas include:

- Use only when a lifeguard is present.
- Shower with soap and water before entering the water.
- People with heart disease, diabetes, high or low blood pressure, seizures, epilepsy or other medical conditions are cautioned against using a spa or hot tub.
- Pregnant women and young children should seek their health care provider's approval before using a spa or hot tub.
- No unsupervised use by children.
- Do not use the spa or hot tub while under the influence of alcohol or other drugs.
- No diving, jumping or rough play in the spa or hot tub.
- Do not allow anyone to sit or play near or with the drain or suction fittings.
- Secure or remove any loose or dangling items, including hair, swimwear and jewelry.
- Limit time in the spa to 10 minutes. Patrons then may shower, cool down and return again briefly. Prolonged use may result in nausea, dizziness, fainting or hyperthermia.
- Remove swim caps before entering the spa or hot tub.

MANAGEMENT AND SAFETY

As a lifeguard, your job is to follow and enforce your facility's rules and regulations. The job of your facility's management is to ensure that the facility is in compliance with local, state and federal regulations and to make sure that you are enforcing the rules correctly. Management is responsible for:

- Creating, reviewing and revising a facility's policies and procedures, rules and regulations and EAPs as needed.
- Addressing unsafe conditions.
- Complying with federal, state and local laws and regulations for facility operations and employment.
- Maintaining records on the facility and its employees.
- Assisting after an emergency.

Policies, Regulations and Emergency Action Plans

Facility management is responsible for ensuring that policies, rules and procedures, and emergency action plans are in place. Management also is responsible for reviewing and revising these plans as necessary to address any changes that may have occurred, such as new programming, new features or attractions or emerging codes and industry standards.

Addressing Unsafe Conditions

Lifeguards work with management to address unsafe conditions at a facility. Management tells lifeguards what to check during safety checks and relies on them to find and report dangers. When an unsafe condition is found and reported, management is responsible for correcting the condition. You should always report unsafe conditions to your supervisor. In some instances you may be asked to take action to limit use of an unsafe area or to help correct the unsafe condition, such as by sweeping up broken glass or by removing a piece of equipment from use.

Complying with Regulations

Government regulations protect patrons and employees. The facility and staff must comply with all regulations. Federal, state and local regulations affect the operation of aquatic facilities in many ways, such as lifeguard certification requirements, facility design and safety features, pool capacities, staff training requirements and lifeguard competencies, ratio of lifeguards to patrons, water sanitation procedures, first aid equipment and supplies, lifeguarding equipment and diving depths.

Regulations are specific to individual areas. You should be familiar with those that affect your facility. Facility management should provide this information during orientation or in-service training.

The following sections describe some federal regulations that may affect you.

Age Limitations for Employment

Federal and state departments of labor set conditions on the number of hours and the types of tasks that employees younger than 18 years are allowed to perform. The requirements typically are more stringent for 15 year olds than for those 16 and 17 years of age. A facility's policy and procedures manual should cover how these regulations affect your duties.

Hazard Communication Standard

Federal regulations protect people from chemical hazards in and around a facility. For example, the Hazard Communication Standard is designed to prevent injury and illness caused by exposure to hazardous chemicals in the workplace.

Employees must be trained about the chemicals stored and used in the workplace for jobs that involve handling such items. Each chemical has an information sheet called a Material Safety Data Sheet (MSDS), and the information for each hazardous chemical must be easy to find and use. Each MSDS includes procedures for handling each substance and provides information about the dangers of exposure as well as first aid and medical follow-up if exposure occurs. Be sure to learn about all hazardous materials are at your workplace and know where to find and access your facility's MSDSs (Figure 2-12). Employees have a right to know:

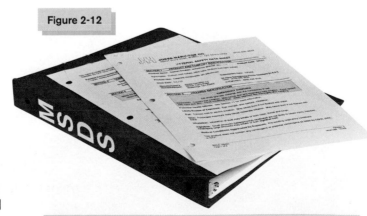

Figure 2-12

Every chemical stored at a facility should have a Material Safety Data Sheet.

- Which hazardous chemicals are in the facility.
- Where those chemicals are stored in the facility.
- The specific dangers of those chemicals.
- How to identify chemical hazards in the facility.
- How to protect themselves and others from being exposed to hazardous chemicals.
- What to do if they or others are exposed to such hazards.

Hazardous chemicals must be handled properly and with care, and stored properly, as specified in the Hazard Communication Standard. Unauthorized personnel should be kept away from chemical storage areas.

Bloodborne Pathogens Standard

The federal Occupational Safety and Health Administration developed the Bloodborne Pathogens Standard to reduce the risk of disease transmission while on the job. This standard helps to protect employees from contact with body fluids that may contain disease-causing bacteria and viruses, called *bloodborne pathogens*. Your employer must provide an exposure control plan to help protect employees from being exposed to bloodborne pathogens and let employees know what to do if an exposure occurs. Additional information is provided in Chapter 7, Before Providing Care and Victim Assessment.

WRAP-UP

Your top priority as a lifeguard is helping keep patrons safe and free from injury so that they can safely enjoy aquatic activities. Lifeguards prevent injuries by enforcing the safety rules. Lifeguards also prevent injuries by conducting safety inspections of the facility, water, equipment and attractions. Lifeguards also need to recognize and respond to the changing water conditions and weather conditions that can occur. Together with management and your fellow lifeguards, your job is to set the stage for this safe experience by helping to create and maintain a safe aquatic facility.

Surveillance and Recognition

Y our primary responsibility as a lifeguard is to help ensure patron safety and protect lives. The main tool used to accomplish this is *patron surveillance*—keeping a close watch over the people in the facility and intervening when necessary. You will spend most of your time on patron surveillance. To do this effectively, you must be alert and attentive—and ready to react—at all times as you continuously supervise patrons. ■

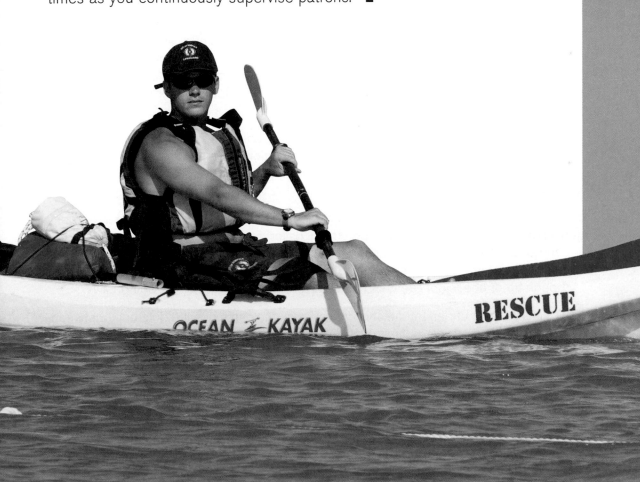

AN OVERVIEW OF THE PROCESS OF DROWNING

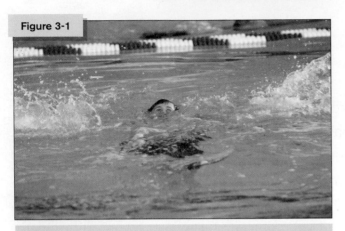

Figure 3-1

A conscious drowning victim struggles to breathe and cannot call out for help.

Drowning is a continuum of events that begins when a victim's airway becomes submerged under the surface of the water (Figure 3-1). The process can be stopped, but if it is not, it will end in death. The process of drowning begins when water enters the victim's airway. This causes involuntary breath holding and then *laryngospasm* (a sudden closure of the larynx or windpipe). When this occurs, air cannot reach the lungs. During this time, the victim is unable to breathe but may swallow large quantities of water into the stomach. As oxygen levels are reduced, the laryngospasm begins to subside and the victim may gasp for air but instead inhales water into the lungs.

Due to inadequate oxygen to body tissues, cardiac arrest may occur. This can happen in as little as 3 minutes after submerging. Brain damage or death can occur in as little as 4 to 6 minutes. The sooner the drowning process is stopped by getting the victim's airway out of the water, opening the airway and providing resuscitation (ventilations or CPR), the better the chances are for survival without permanent brain damage.

No two drownings are alike—there are many intervening variables that can affect the outcome, including any underlying medical conditions of the victim and the time until advanced medical care intervenes. However, in general, giving ventilations often will resuscitate the victim if they are given within 1½ to 2 minutes of submerging.

When you are providing care, an unconscious victim may have isolated or infrequent gasping in the absence of other breathing, called agonal gasps. Agonal gasps can occur even after the heart has stopped beating. Normal, effective breathing is regular, quiet and effortless. Agonal gasps are not breathing. Care for the victim as though he or she is not breathing at all by giving ventilations or providing CPR.

Lifeguards must understand that only a few minutes can make the difference between life and death. To give a victim the greatest the chance of survival and a normal outcome, you must recognize when a person needs help or is in danger of drowning and you must act immediately. If there is any question whether a person in the water is beginning to drown or merely playing games, it is essential that you intervene, and if necessary, remove the person from the water immediately and provide care.

EFFECTIVE SURVEILLANCE

With effective surveillance, you can recognize behaviors or situations that might lead to life-threatening emergencies, such as drownings or injuries to the head, neck or spine, and then act quickly to modify the behavior or control the situation. Effective surveillance has several elements:

- Recognition of dangerous behaviors
- Victim recognition

- Effective scanning
- Zone of surveillance responsibility
- Lifeguard stations

Recognition of Dangerous Behaviors

A focus of preventive lifeguarding is to intervene quickly to stop potentially dangerous behaviors that could result in an emergency. This may include redirecting a child to shallower water, stopping a group of teens from having breath-holding contests or stopping swimmers from *hyperventilating* (breathing rapidly and deeply) and swimming underwater for extended periods. Swimmers and nonswimmers, regardless of age, can become victims quickly because of dangerous behaviors or other situations (Figure 3-2, A–E). Examples include:

- A weak swimmer or nonswimmer who is:
  - Bobbing in or near water over his or her head.
  - Crawling hand-over-hand along a pool wall.
  - Beyond arm's reach of a supervising adult, even if wearing a floatation aid.

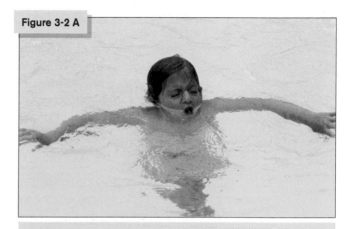

Figure 3-2 A

A child bobbing in water over her head.

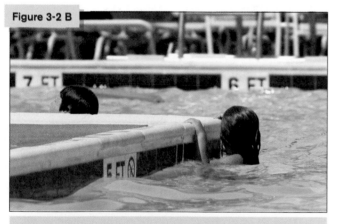

Figure 3-2 B

A small child crawling hand-over-hand toward deep water.

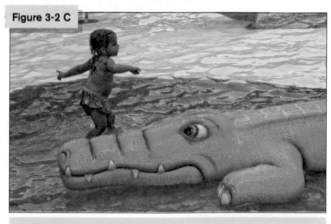

Figure 3-2 C

A toddler left unattended.

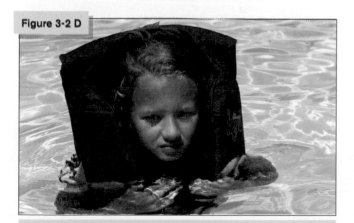

Figure 3-2 D

A child wearing an improperly fitting life jacket.

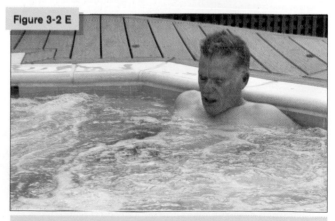

Figure 3-2 E

A victim experiencing a medical emergency.

- ○ Clinging to something or struggling to grab something to stay afloat.
- ○ Wearing a life jacket improperly.
  - ■ A person who is:
- ○ Breath-holding or swimming underwater for an extended period after hyperventilating.
- ○ Participating in a high-risk/high-impact activity, such as diving.
- ○ Experiencing a medical emergency, such as a sudden illness.

Victim Recognition

Another element of effective surveillance is being able to recognize when someone is in trouble in the water. It is important to understand the behaviors that a victim shows when in distress or drowning. Someone in trouble may struggle at the surface for just a short time or may quickly disappear beneath the surface without any signs of distress. Others may be submerged already when the process of drowning begins, such as the person who has jumped or slipped into water over his or her head and is struggling to reach the surface.

A swimmer may be in distress or actively struggling to survive. Others may be passive and therefore unable to help themselves, showing little or no movement. Understanding these behaviors enables lifeguards to recognize quickly when someone needs help. Lifeguards should be able to recognize and respond to a drowning victim within 30 seconds.

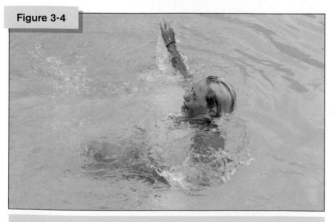

Figure 3-3

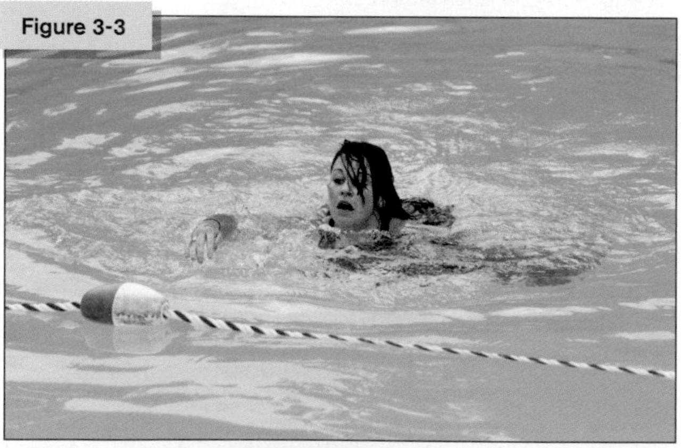

A distressed swimmer may reach for a rescue device, such as a rescue tube or a rope line.

Figure 3-4

A distressed swimmer may wave for help, float on the back, scull or tread water.

Swimmers in Distress

A swimmer can become distressed for several reasons, such as exhaustion, cramp or sudden illness. Quick recognition is key to preventing the distressed swimmer from becoming a drowning victim. A distressed swimmer makes little or no forward progress and may be unable to reach safety without assistance. Distressed swimmers may be:

- ■ Able to keep their face out of the water.
- ■ Able to call for help.
- ■ Able to wave for help.
- ■ Horizontal, vertical or diagonal, depending on what they use to support themselves.
- ■ Floating, sculling or treading water.

The distressed swimmer generally is able to reach for a rescue device, such as a rescue tube (Figure 3-3). If a safety line or other floating object is nearby, a distressed swimmer may grab and cling to it for support. As conditions continue to affect the distressed swimmer, such as fatigue, cold or sudden illness, he or she becomes less able to support him or herself in the water (Figure 3-4). As this occurs, his or her mouth moves closer to the surface of the water, and anxiety increases. If a distressed swimmer is not rescued, he or she may become a drowning victim; therefore, you need to immediately initiate a rescue.

Drowning Victim–Active

A drowning victim who is struggling to remain at the surface of the water has distinctive arm and body positions. These are efforts to try to keep the mouth above the water's surface in order to breathe (Figure 3-5). This universal behavior is called the *instinctive drowning response*. Once it is recognized that a victim is drowning, the lifeguard must perform a swift or immediate rescue.

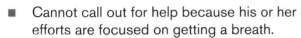

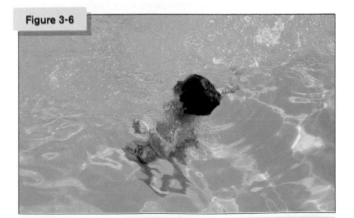

A drowning victim may become unable to support themselves and struggle at the surface of the water.

Some victims cycle through these behaviors quickly and might submerge within seconds, whereas others are able to remain near the surface of the water for a short time. A drowning victim who is struggling:

- Cannot call out for help because his or her efforts are focused on getting a breath.
- Works to keep the face above water in an effort to breathe. A young child may be in a horizontal face-down position during the struggle because he or she is unable to lift the face out of the water.
- Has extended the arms to the side or front, pressing down for support.
- Is positioned vertically in the water with no supporting kick. A young child may tip into a horizontal face-down position.
- Might continue to struggle underwater once submerged.
- Eventually will lose consciousness and stop moving.

Drowning victims who are struggling to breathe may not always look the same. For some, the mouth sinks below the surface and reappears, sometimes repeatedly. While the mouth is below the surface, the drowning victim attempts to keep the mouth closed to avoid swallowing water. When above the surface, the drowning victim quickly exhales and then tries to inhale before the mouth goes below the surface again. While the victim is gasping for air, he or she also might take water into the mouth (Figure 3-6). For a young child who is in a horizontal face-down position, he or she is not able to keep the mouth above the surface of the water at all.

Figure 3-6

A drowning victim may struggle to breathe and cannot call out for help.

Often, a drowning victim at or near the surface is unable to call out for help. He or she can take in only enough air to breathe, so no air is left to call out. A drowning in progress often is silent.

A drowning victim does not make any forward progress in the water. A young child may appear to be doing a "doggy paddle" but has no forward progress; all efforts are devoted to getting air. The victim might be able to stay at the surface for only 20 to 60 seconds, if at all. He or she may continue to struggle underwater but eventually will lose consciousness and stop moving.

A victim may slip into water over his or her head, incur an injury, or experience a sudden illness and struggle underwater to reach the surface. If unable to swim or make progress, he or she will be unable to reach the surface. This drowning victim may appear to be a person who is playing or floating underwater. It may be easier to recognize a swimmer in distress or a victim struggling on the surface than to recognize a victim who has submerged already or is submerging.

Never assume that anyone exhibiting these behaviors is playing or faking; it is essential that you intervene, and if necessary, remove the person from the water immediately and provide care.

Drowning Victim–Passive

Some drowning victims do not struggle. They suddenly slip under water due to a medical condition or another cause, such as:

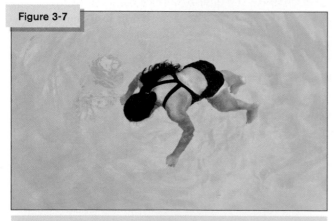

Figure 3-7

A drowning victim may float face-down at or near the surface of the water.

- A heart attack or stroke.
- A seizure.
- A head injury.
- A heat-related illness.
- Hypothermia (below-normal body temperature).
- Hyperventilation and prolonged underwater breath-holding activities.
- Use of alcohol and other drugs.

These drowning victims:

- Might float face-down at or near the surface or might sink to the bottom (Figure 3-7).
- May be limp or have slight convulsive-type movements.
- Have no defined arm or leg action, no locomotion and no breathing.
- May appear to be floating, if at the surface of the water.
- May be face-down, on one side or face-up, if at the bottom (Figure 3-8).

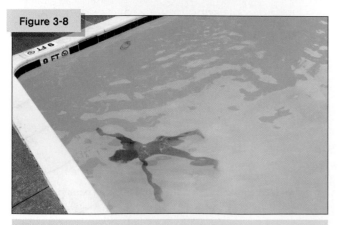

Figure 3-8

A drowning victim may be face-down at the bottom of a pool.

Anyone who is exhibiting one or more of these signals for 30 seconds should be considered a drowning victim and responded to immediately. It can be difficult to clearly see a victim who is underwater or at the bottom of a pool because of glare, reflections, or water movement from the wind or other swimmers. The victim may appear to look like a smudge, an object like a towel, or a shadow. Do not expect to see a clear outline of a person on the bottom. At waterfronts, submerged victims may not be visible, depending on the water depth

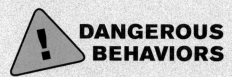

⚠ DANGEROUS BEHAVIORS

Hyperventilation and Extended Breath-Holding

Voluntary hyperventilation (rapid, deep breathing) is a dangerous technique used by some swimmers to try to swim long distances underwater or to hold their breath for an extended period while submerged in one place. They mistakenly think that by taking a series of deep breaths in rapid succession and forcefully exhaling that they can increase the amount of oxygen they breathe, allowing them to hold their breath longer underwater. This is not true. Hyperventilation does not increase the amount of oxygen or allow a swimmer to hold his or her breath longer; instead, it lowers the carbon dioxide level in the body. The practice is risky because the level of carbon dioxide in the blood is what signals a person to breathe. As the level of carbon dioxide increases, a person normally takes a breath. When a person hyperventilates and then swims underwater, the oxygen level in the blood can drop to a point where the swimmer passes out before the body knows it is time to breathe. Then, when the person finally does take a breath instinctively, water rushes in and the drowning process begins.

Do not allow swimmers to participate in contests, games or repetitive activities to see who can swim underwater the farthest or hold their breath underwater the longest. Hyperventilation, prolonged underwater swimming for distance and breath-holding for time are extremely dangerous. If you see these dangerous activities, you must intervene. Explain to patrons that they should only take a single inhalation before submerging when swimming and playing underwater. In addition, instructors must prevent these activities during instructional periods, such as swim lessons, lifeguard classes, SCUBA classes and competitive swimming.

Alcohol

The following are some ways that alcohol can affect a person in the water and lead to drowning or head, neck or spine injuries:

- Alcohol affects balance. Some people with alcohol in their body have drowned in shallow water when they lost their balance and were unable to stand up. "Ordinary" actions on steps, ladders, diving boards or play structures become hazardous for an intoxicated person.

- Alcohol affects judgment. A person might take unusual, uncharacteristic risks, such as diving into shallow water.

- Alcohol slows body movements. It can greatly reduce swimming skills, even those of an excellent swimmer.

- Alcohol impairs ones ability to stay awake and respond appropriately to emergencies.

One of the biggest myths about alcohol is that an intoxicated person can sober up by going swimming. Splashing water on a person's face or immersing a person in water will not reduce the amount of alcohol in the bloodstream or reduce the effects of alcohol.

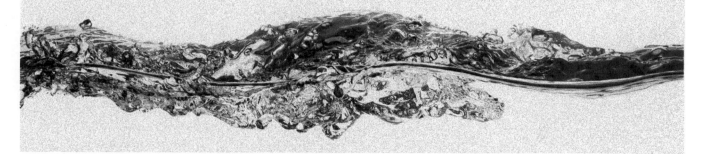

or because of poor water clarity. If you see something on the bottom that should not be there, do not delay, go right away.

Specific Behaviors

When conducting surveillance, look for behavior that indicates a patron in need of immediate assistance. It is important to recognize the behaviors of

Table 3-1: **Behaviors of Distressed Swimmers and Drowning Victims**			
	Distressed Swimmer	**Drowning Victim– Active**	**Drowning Victim– Passive**
Head Position	Above water	Tilted back with face looking up	■ Face-up or face-down in the water ■ Submerged
Appearance and, if visible, Facial Expressions	■ Trying to support self by holding or clinging to a lane line or safety line ■ Expression of concern for personal safety	■ Struggling to keep or get the head above the surface of the water ■ Struggling to reach the surface, if underwater ■ Expression of panic/ wide eyed	■ Limp or convulsive-like movements ■ Floating or submerged ■ Eyes may be closed ■ If submerged, may look like a shadow
Breathing	Is breathing	Struggles to breathe	Not breathing
Arm and Leg Action	■ Floating, sculling or treading water ■ Might wave for help	Arms to sides or in front, alternately moving up and pressing down	None
Body Position	Horizontal, vertical or diagonal, depending on means of support	Vertical, leaning slightly back	Horizontal or vertical
Locomotion	■ Little or no forward progress ■ Less and less able to support self	None	None
Sounds	Able to call for help but may not do so	Cannot call out for help	None
Location	At the surface	At the surface, underwater or sinking	Floating at the surface, sinking or submerged on the bottom

a drowning victim (Table 3-1). Notice:

■ Breathing.

■ Appearance or facial expression (if the face is visible to you).

■ Arm and leg action.

■ Head and body position.

■ Body propulsion or locomotion (movement) through the water.

Understanding these behaviors helps you to quickly recognize when someone needs help. When you see some or all of these behaviors, react. Do not spend time second-guessing yourself, immediately initiate a rescue. Quick action can mean the difference between life and death for a distressed or drowning victim.

Effective Scanning

Knowing *what* to look for to determine if a victim is in trouble in the water is a first step, but you also need to know *how* to look. *Scanning* is a visual technique for watching patrons in the water (Figure 3-9). When scanning, you should not just passively watch patrons in the water. Effective scanning requires you to deliberately and actively observe swimmers' behaviors and look for signals that someone in the water needs help. You must actively scan all patrons in the water, regardless of the type of activities taking place.

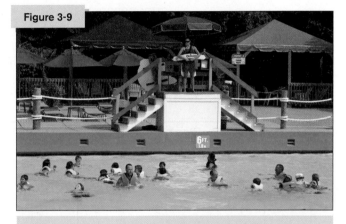

Figure 3-9

Scanning is a surveillance technique for watching patrons.

Guidelines for Effective Scanning

Drowning and injuries can happen in an instant, often silently. Scanning your entire area of responsibility quickly and thoroughly is important. You cannot prevent or save what you cannot see. When scanning:

■ Scan all patrons in your assigned area of responsibility.

■ Stay focused—do not let your attention drift.

■ Scan the entire volume of water—the bottom, middle and surface.

■ Move your head and eyes while scanning and look directly at each area rather than staring in a fixed direction. You may notice movement with your peripheral (side) vision, but to recognize that a person is in trouble, you must look directly at him or her.

■ Scan from point to point thoroughly and repeatedly. Do not neglect any part of the assigned area, including any deck or beach areas and those areas under, around and directly in front of the lifeguard station.

■ Focus on effective patron surveillance instead of the scanning pattern itself.

■ Scan for signs of potential problems: arm and leg action, body position and movement through the water may indicate that a patron is a weak swimmer and is in trouble in the water.

■ Scan crowded and high-risk areas carefully. Partially hidden arm movements might indicate that a victim is actively drowning.

■ Pay close attention to nonswimmers or weak swimmers. Excitement or lack of knowledge may lead nonswimmers or weak swimmers to become unknowingly careless. They might try things they would not otherwise do, or they might accidentally enter deep water.

- Maintain an active posture. Slouching, leaning back, sitting back with legs crossed, or resting your head in your hand may cause you to become too relaxed and lose focus.

- Adjust your body position or stand up to eliminate blind spots. Be aware of areas that are difficult to see. Areas might be blocked when patrons cluster together; or water movement, such as from fountains or bubbles, may distort the view underwater.

- Change your body position regularly to help stay alert. For example, switch between seated and standing positions while in an elevated station.

- While scanning, do not be distracted by people or activities outside of your area of responsibility. Keep focused on the assigned zone.

- Do not interrupt scanning an area if a patron asks a question or has a suggestion or concern. Acknowledge the patron and quickly explain that you cannot look at him or her while talking, but you are listening to the patron. Politely but briefly answer the patron's question, suggestion or concern, or refer him or her to the head lifeguard, facility manager or another staff member.

Scanning Challenges

There are many challenges to scanning (Figure 3-10, A–D). You must be aware of the challenges and actively employ tactics to combat them. The lives of patrons

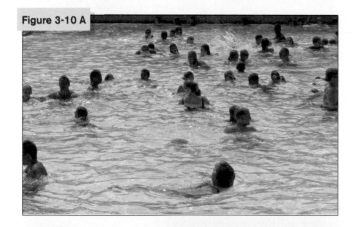

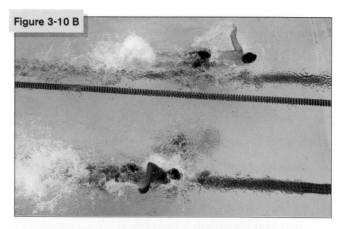

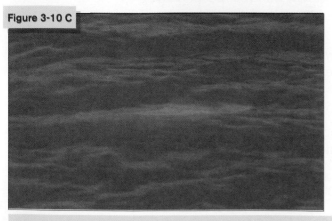

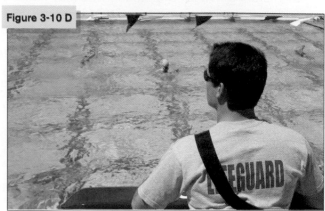

Scanning challenges include: (A) glare on the water, (B) water movement obscuring the bottom of the pool, (C) cloudy water and (D) fatigue

Table 3-2: **Scanning Challenges**

Challenge	Tactics
Monotony	■ Stay fully engaged in what you are seeing—do not let your attention drift. ■ Change body position and posture periodically. ■ Sit upright and slightly forward. ■ Rotate stations.
Fatigue	■ Request additional lifeguard coverage. ■ Keep hydrated, cool off and get out of the sun when on break. ■ Exercise during one of your breaks.
Distractions	■ Stay focused on patron surveillance. ■ Do not daydream, have conversations with co-workers or patrons or watch events outside of your area. ■ Keep patron activities safe and orderly. Signal for an additional lifeguard or supervisor if assistance is needed.
Blind spots	■ Adjust your location or body position or stand up. ■ Check all potential blind spots: under the stand, at play features or any part of the zone.
Glare (from the sun or overhead lights)	■ Use polarized sunglasses. ■ Change body position—stand up and look around and through glare spots. ■ Reposition your lifeguard station with permission of your supervisor.
Water movement and surface distortion of the water	■ Adjust your body position. ■ Be aware of the normal appearance of the bottom of the pool; know the appearance of drains, colored tiles or painted depth markings. ■ Scan the bottom carefully.
Murky water	■ Adjust your location or body position. ■ Stay alert for high-risk activities. ■ Signal for additional assistance to get extra coverage for the area.
Heavy patron loads	■ Stand up frequently. ■ Signal for additional assistance to get extra coverage for your area.
Low patron loads	■ Change body position and posture frequently. ■ Change to a ground-level station, if appropriate.
High air temperature	■ Use fans to cool the surrounding air in an indoor setting. ■ Stay in the shade; use umbrellas. ■ Cool off by getting wet during your break. ■ Rotate more frequently. ■ Stay in cooler areas during breaks. ■ Stay hydrated by drinking plenty of water.

depend on it. Table 3-2 presents some scanning challenges that you may encounter and tactics to overcome them.

Zones of Surveillance Responsibility

Your lifeguard supervisor or facility manager will establish each lifeguard's *zone of surveillance responsibility*—referred to as *zones*. These are the specific areas

THE RID FACTOR

If an active victim drowns while lifeguards are on duty, it is probably due to one or more of the following causes:

- Lifeguards fail to recognize the victim's instinctive drowning response.
- Secondary duties intrude on lifeguards' primary responsibility of patron surveillance.
- Lifeguards are distracted from surveillance.

This set of causes often is referred to as the "RID factor," where the acronym, RID, stands for recognition, intrusion and distraction.

Recognition

Knowing how to recognize that a swimmer is in distress or a person is drowning is one of the most important lifeguarding skills. You must be able to distinguish such behavior from that of others who are swimming or playing safely in the water. You must recognize when someone needs to be rescued. You cannot expect the victim or others to call for help in an emergency.

With good surveillance and scanning techniques, you can recognize even a passive victim who has slipped underwater without a struggle, if the victim is in clear water.

Intrusion

Intrusion occurs when secondary duties, such as maintenance tasks, intrude on your primary responsibility of patron surveillance. Lifeguards often have to sweep the deck, empty trash cans, pick up towels, check locker rooms and perform other maintenance duties. While these duties might be part of the job, you should not perform them while conducting patron surveillance. Before you begin these duties, you must be sure that another lifeguard has taken over surveillance for your assigned area of responsibility.

Similarly, you cannot perform adequate surveillance duties while also coaching a swim team or teaching a swimming lesson. These additional responsibilities should be performed by a different lifeguard, coach or instructor, even if there are no other patrons in the water.

Distraction

Distractions also affect patron surveillance: for example, a lifeguard talking with other lifeguards or friends. A brief conversation might seem innocent, but during that time, you could miss the 20- to 60-second struggle of a young child at the water's surface. The child could die because you were distracted. You should not engage in social conversation while are on duty.

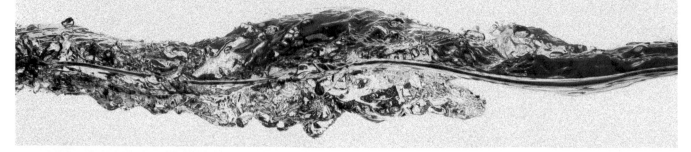

of the water, deck, pier or shoreline that are your responsibility to scan from your lifeguard station (Figure 3-11).

When establishing coverage, supervisors or managers must ensure that:

■ All areas of the water—from the bottom through to the surface—are covered and can be seen by a lifeguard.

■ There is overlapping coverage when more than one lifeguard is performing surveillance.

■ Lifeguards have unobstructed views of their zones from each station.

■ The size and shape of each zone allow lifeguards to respond quickly, within 30 seconds, to victims in the water.

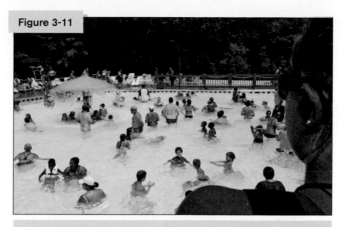

Figure 3-11

The zone of surveillance responsibility refers to the specific area a lifeguard is responsible for scanning.

Supervisors or managers should post diagrams or charts showing the size, shape and boundaries of each zone. These can change throughout the day, depending on the following:

■ Number of patrons

■ Types of activities

■ Variety of activities

■ Time of day

■ Environmental conditions, such as glare from the sun

To ensure that all areas of the pool are covered adequately, you might be assigned *zone coverage,* *total coverage* or *emergency back-up coverage.*

Zone Coverage

In zone coverage, the swimming area is divided into separate zones, with one zone for each lifeguard station (Figure 3-12, A–B). Zones can be designated by markers, such as ladders, lane lines, lifelines, buoys, or the shape of the pool. Zone coverage is effective for high-risk areas or activities, avoiding blind spots and reducing the number of patrons watched by each lifeguard. When zone coverage is being provided, each lifeguard needs to know the zone for each guarding position.

At a minimum, zones should overlap by several feet so that the boundaries between them have double coverage. This prevents any area from not being scanned. When zones overlap, it is important that each lifeguard react to an emergency; that is, you should not assume that the other lifeguard will notice a problem and react. However, if the

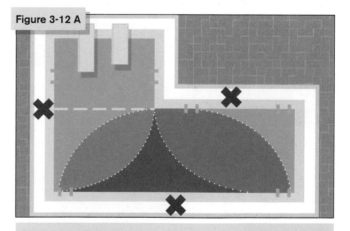

Figure 3-12 A

Zone coverage at a pool

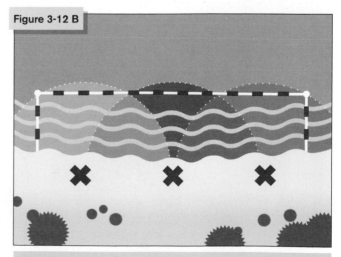

Figure 3-12 B

Zone coverage at a waterfront

position of the other lifeguard allows a significantly quicker rescue, your emergency action plan (EAP) should establish how lifeguards communicate as to who enters the water and who provides back-up coverage.

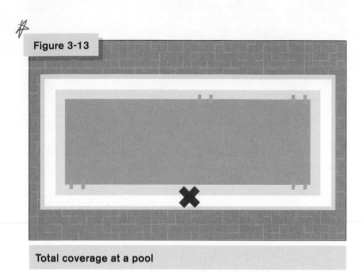

Figure 3-13

Total coverage at a pool

Figure 3-14 A

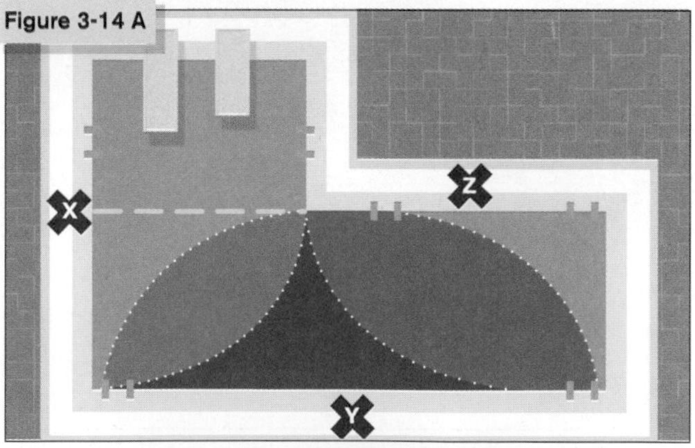

Zone coverage with three lifeguards

Figure 3-14 B

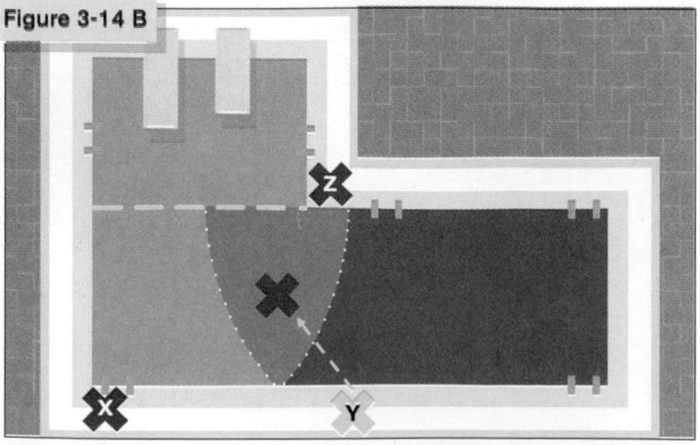

Back-up coverage during a rescue at a three-zone facility

Total Coverage

Read before test

When you are assigned total coverage, you will be the only lifeguard conducting patron surveillance while you are on duty. Some facilities, such as a small pool, always assign their lifeguards total coverage. Other facilities use total coverage for specific situations, such as when there are a limited number of patrons present. When only one lifeguard is conducting patron surveillance, that lifeguard has to scan the entire area, control the activities of patrons in and out of the water and recognize and respond to emergencies (Figure 3-13). If adequate coverage cannot be provided for all patrons, inform a supervisor that help is needed.

Emergency Back-Up Coverage

In emergency situations when two or more lifeguards are on duty and one lifeguard must enter the water for a rescue, lifeguards who remain out of the water must now supervise a larger area. They might need to move to better vantage points or close part of the swimming area, depending on the facility's design.

Figure 3-14, A illustrates zone coverage when three lifeguards are on surveillance duty. **Figure 3-14, B** shows an example of emergency back-up coverage for the same three-zone facility. **Figure 3-14, B** depicts lifeguard Y as the primary rescuer. He or she signals and enters the water (indicated by a dotted line). The other two lifeguards (lifeguards X and Z) stand in each of the lifeguard chairs and divide the responsibility for scanning the pool. Meanwhile, additional lifeguards or safety team members monitor the rescue and prepare to assist with additional equipment and call emergency medical services (EMS) personnel, if appropriate.

Lifeguard Stations

Lifeguards perform patron surveillance from a variety of positions including elevated, ground-level, roving and floating stations. Additional coverage at waterfront areas some-times is provided by foot patrols, boat patrols and four-wheel-drive vehicles. The goal is to provide optimum coverage for the whole facility by placing lifeguards in positions to quickly recognize and respond to emergencies. To ensure that lifeguards stay alert, periodic rotations and breaks from surveillance are built into their surveillance schedules.

The location of any lifeguard station must allow you to see your entire zone. The lifeguard stand may need to be moved or the position adjusted during the day to adapt to the changing sun, glare, wind or water conditions. It is critical for you to have a clear view of your entire zone.

Elevated Stations

Elevated lifeguard stations generally provide the most effective position for a broad view of the zone and patron activities (Figure 3-15). This is especially important at a facility where a single lifeguard at a time performs patron surveillance. When you are scanning from an elevated station, be sure to include the area under, around and directly in front of the stand. Movable stands should be positioned close to the edge of the water with enough room to climb up and down from the stand.

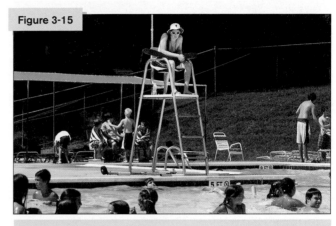

Figure 3-15

An elevated lifeguard station

The area surrounding an elevated stand must be kept clear of patrons or objects that might interfere with your ability to respond. You must know how to safely exit the stand, both in the course of a normal rotation as well as in an emergency. Be sure to practice with the rescue tube so that you are able to do so quickly and without getting injured. A safety zone should be established that allows access to the water in case of an emergency. At a waterfront, the safety zone should be thoroughly inspected with rakes and shovels before opening each day. This helps to prevent injuries to lifeguards during emergency exits from the lifeguard stand.

Ground-Level Stations

Lifeguards sometimes are assigned to a fixed location on a deck or in shallow water (Figure 3-16). These stations allow for quick response and are common around winding rivers, in shallow-water areas with play structures, and at the end of slides. The primary purpose of ground-level stations is to be close to patrons so you can easily make assists and enforce safety rules for patrons in the water and on the deck. While maintaining surveillance, you also can educate patrons about the reasons behind the rules; however, you should never become distracted from surveillance duties by talking socially with patrons or other staff.

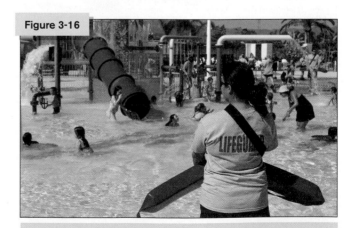

Figure 3-16

A ground-level lifeguard station

Roving Stations

When a facility becomes unusually crowded, such as during a special event or activity, supervisors or managers might assign a lifeguard to a *roving station*. The roving lifeguard is assigned a specific zone, which also is covered by another lifeguard in an elevated station. These roving, or walking, lifeguards are mobile and able to position themselves where needed within the zone. Combining the views from elevated stations with the mobility of the roving lifeguard provides extra coverage to help ensure effective patron surveillance.

Floating Stations (Rescue Watercraft)

In many waterfront facilities, lifeguards are stationed to watch swimmers from a water craft, usually as extra coverage. Rescue watercraft typically are used to patrol the outer edge of a swimming area. Often, someone in trouble in the water can be reached more quickly from watercraft than from a lifeguard station on the shore.

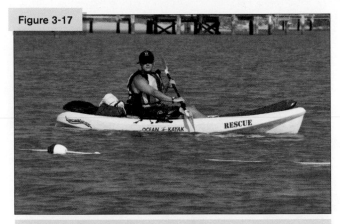

Rescue water craft, such as kayaks, may be used at waterfront areas.

In a small, calm area, a rescue board, kayak or flat-bottom rowboat might be used (Figure 3-17). When patrolling on a rescue board, sit or kneel on the board for better visibility (Figure 3-18). Some protocols may require you to keep the rescue tube or buoy strapped across your chest or attached to the board. In rough water, rowboats might be used. Powerboats, inflatable boats and personal watercraft also can be used as rescue watercraft. Facility management normally provides on-the-job training in the use of watercraft at a facility.

If stationed on watercraft in water with a current, you might have to row or paddle to stay in position. Some watercraft have a special anchor line with a quick release for lifeguards to make a rescue. In some larger watercraft, one lifeguard maintains the craft's position while a second watches the swimming area.

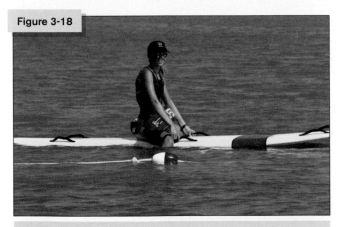

A rescue board may be used to help with patron surveillance at waterfront areas.

Make sure that you are well trained in operating the facility's watercraft before using it for surveillance or to make a rescue. Use caution with motorized watercraft to avoid injuring swimmers or damaging lifelines when crossing into the swimming area to make a rescue.

Lifeguard Rotations

All facilities should have a defined rotation procedure. Rotations include moving from one station to another as well as breaks from surveillance duty. Lifeguards should get regular breaks from surveillance duty to help stay alert and decrease fatigue. Typically, you might perform patron surveillance for 20 or 30 minutes at one station, rotate to another station for 20 or 30 minutes, and then rotate off of patron surveillance duty to perform other duties or take a break for 20 or 30 minutes, thereby getting a break from constant surveillance. Rest and meal breaks should be factored into the rotation.

An emergency back-up coverage "station" often is included as a part of the rotation. The location may be a staff room or on the pool deck, pier or shoreline within sight of the swimming area(s). The lifeguard at this station is not responsible for patron surveillance but is expected to be able to immediately respond to the EAP signal in an emergency. (Chapter 5 covers information about emergency action plans.)

Your supervisor will establish a plan for lifeguard rotations, usually based on:

- Locations of stations.
- Type of station (elevated, ground-level, roving or floating).
- The need to be in the water at some stations.
- The number of patrons using an attraction.
- The activity at the station, such as wave durations at a wave pool.
- EAPs.

The rotation begins with the incoming lifeguard. While rotating, each lifeguard should carry his or her own rescue tube, and both lifeguards must ensure there is no lapse in patron surveillance, even for a brief moment. Each lifeguard must know who is responsible for scanning the zone—"owning the zone"—and at what time during the rotation. You will be transferring scanning responsibilities back and forth as the incoming lifeguard gets into position and the outgoing guard prepares to leave the station. Keep any necessary conversations brief and make sure that eye contact remains on the water.

As the incoming lifeguard, you should be aware of the patrons and activity level of the zone you will be watching. Begin scanning your zone as you are walking toward your station, checking all areas of the water from the bottom to the surface.

The outgoing lifeguard should inform you of any situations that need special attention. The exchange of information should be brief, and patron surveillance must be maintained throughout the entire rotation. Once in position, with the rescue tube strapped in place, make any adjustments needed, such as removing shoes or adjusting an umbrella before confirming to the outgoing lifeguard that you own the zone. The outgoing lifeguard should continue scanning as he or she is walking toward the next station. The skill sheet at the end of this chapter outlines the steps for rotations for ground-level and elevated stations.

WRAP-UP

A lapse in coverage—even for just a few seconds—could result in injury or death. A lifeguard must be alert for dangerous behaviors and able to recognize a distressed swimmer and a drowning victim who is active or passive. Effective scanning techniques and lifeguard stations are needed both to prevent incidents and locate people in trouble.

ROTATIONS—**Ground-Level Station**

At a ground-level station, you (the incoming lifeguard) should:

1 Begin scanning your zone as you are walking toward your station. Note the swimmers, activities and the people on the deck. In a pool or waterpark setting where the water is clear, check the entire volume of water from the bottom of the pool to the surface of the water.

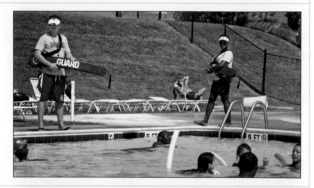

2 Walk to the side of the lifeguard being relieved and begin scanning the zone.

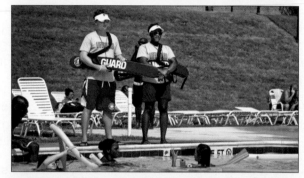

3 Exchange information. Ask the lifeguard being relieved whether any patrons in the zone need closer than normal supervision.

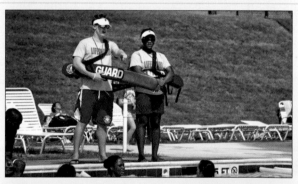

4 Once scanning has started, signal or tell the outgoing lifeguard that you have the zone covered and he or she can rotate.

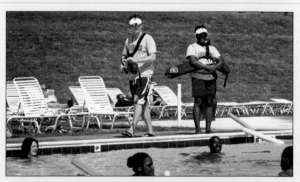

5 The outgoing lifeguard continues scanning as he or she is walking toward the next station.

ROTATIONS—**Elevated Station**

At an elevated station, you (the incoming lifeguard) should:

1 Begin scanning your zone as you are walking toward your station. Note the swimmers, activities and the people on the deck. In a pool or waterpark setting where the water is clear, check the entire volume of water from the bottom of the pool to the surface of the water.

2 Take a position next to the stand and begin scanning the zone. After a few moments of scanning, signal the lifeguard in the stand to climb down.

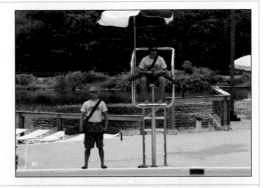

3 Once on the deck, the outgoing lifeguard takes a position next to the stand and is responsible for surveillance of the zone. Climb up in the stand, make any adjustments to equipment or personal items and begin scanning.

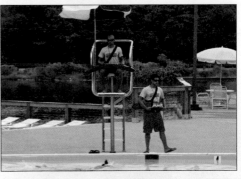

4 Exchange information. Ask the lifeguard being relieved whether any patrons in the zone need closer than normal supervision.

5 Signal or tell the outgoing lifeguard that you have the zone covered and he or she can rotate.

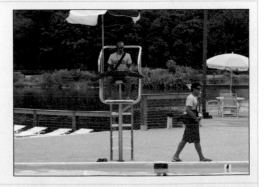

6 The outgoing lifeguard continues scanning as he or she is walking toward the next station.

Injury Prevention

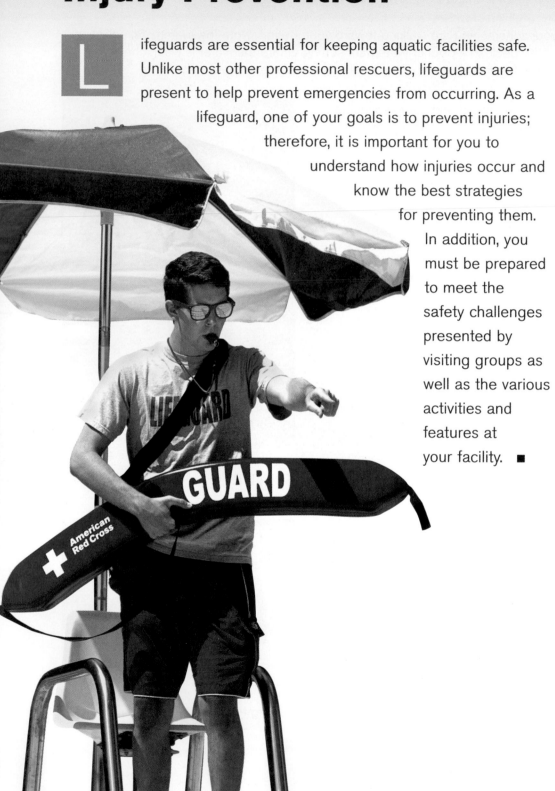

L ifeguards are essential for keeping aquatic facilities safe. Unlike most other professional rescuers, lifeguards are present to help prevent emergencies from occurring. As a lifeguard, one of your goals is to prevent injuries; therefore, it is important for you to understand how injuries occur and know the best strategies for preventing them. In addition, you must be prepared to meet the safety challenges presented by visiting groups as well as the various activities and features at your facility. ■

CHAPTER 4

HOW INJURIES HAPPEN

Aquatic injury prevention is part of your facility's risk management program. *Risk management* involves identifying dangerous conditions or behaviors that can cause injuries and then taking steps to minimize or eliminate those conditions or behaviors. Even though lifeguarding requires performing emergency rescues, far more time is spent on *preventive lifeguarding*—trying to make sure emergencies do not happen in the first place.

Although not all emergencies can be prevented, knowing what causes life-threatening injuries can help you to prevent many of them. Injuries either are life threatening or non-life-threatening. Examples of life-threatening injuries include drowning and injuries to the head, neck or spine. Life-threatening conditions that can result from an injury include unconsciousness, breathing and cardiac emergencies, severe bleeding and drowning.

Drowning begins when a person's mouth and nose are submerged and water enters the airway, regardless of the water depth. Drowning can occur in shallow or deep water. In shallow water a toddler may fall over and be unable to stand or unable to raise the head up. Drowning also may result when a nonswimmer enters or falls into water over his or her head, when a poor swimmer becomes exhausted and cannot stay afloat or when a patron is incapacitated in the water due to a medical emergency, such as a seizure or cardiac emergency.

Most head, neck or spinal injuries at aquatic facilities result from a high-risk/high-impact activity, such as head-first entries into shallow water. If a victim's head strikes the bottom or the side of the pool, the spinal cord can be damaged, causing paralysis or death.

Non-life-threatening injuries also occur in aquatic facilities. Examples of non-life-threatening injuries include fractures or dislocations, abrasions (scrapes), superficial burns (sunburns), muscle cramps (caused by overexertion), heat exhaustion, dehydration and sprains and strains.

Non-life-threatening injuries can occur by slipping, tripping, falling when running or getting cut on sharp objects. They also can occur when patrons do not follow rules when using play equipment or slides. If you understand how most injuries occur, you can help prevent them by increasing your awareness of risks and hazards, helping patrons to avoid risky behavior and developing a safety-conscious attitude at your facility.

INJURY-PREVENTION STRATEGIES

As you learned earlier in this course, your injury-prevention responsibilities include taking steps to ensure that the facility is safe and providing effective patron surveillance. Another important injury-prevention responsibility is communicating with patrons, which involves educating and informing patrons as well as enforcing your facility's rules.

Communicating with Patrons

Communicating with patrons is an important injury-prevention strategy. It requires you to inform and educate patrons about inappropriate behaviors and the potential for injury. Communication also includes consistently enforcing rules and regulations in a positive, customer-friendly manner.

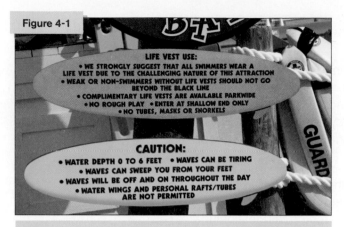

Figure 4-1

LIFE VEST USE:
- **WE STRONGLY SUGGEST THAT ALL SWIMMERS WEAR A LIFE VEST DUE TO THE CHALLENGING NATURE OF THIS ATTRACTION**
- **WEAK OR NON-SWIMMERS WITHOUT LIFE VESTS SHOULD NOT GO BEYOND THE BLACK LINE**
- **COMPLIMENTARY LIFE VESTS ARE AVAILABLE PARKWIDE**
- **NO ROUGH PLAY** • **ENTER AT SHALLOW END ONLY**
- **NO TUBES, MASKS OR SNORKELS**

CAUTION:
- **WATER DEPTH 0 TO 6 FEET** • **WAVES CAN BE TIRING**
- **WAVES CAN SWEEP YOU FROM YOUR FEET**
- **WAVES WILL BE OFF AND ON THROUGHOUT THE DAY**
- **WATER WINGS AND PERSONAL RAFTS/TUBES ARE NOT PERMITTED**

Signs provide instructions to patrons on how to use equipment and list rules and regulations of the facility.

Did You Know?

The precise way that you will use your whistle in an emergency should be spelled out in your facility's plan. Typically, an emergency action plan (EAP) will specify that a certain number and type of whistle blasts should correspond to a certain emergency situation. You should practice your whistle-blowing technique during orientations and in-service trainings to cover all of the variations and numbers of whistle blasts.

Informing and Educating Patrons

Patrons need to know about risks that could cause injury. Signs communicate warning, provide instructions on how to use equipment and list rules and regulations to prevent behaviors that can lead to injury (Figure 4-1). Part of your role, too, is to inform patrons about the potential for injury; therefore, you need to understand the rules and regulations of your facility and the rationale behind them.

Patrons may be unfamiliar with a facility's features or get so excited that they do not read signs or pay attention to the rules. If patrons are not following the rules, it is your job to inform them of the possible consequences. Explaining rules in a positive way encourages patrons to behave safely. The following steps can prevent a patron from engaging in risky behavior:

- Get the patron's attention, for example by blowing a whistle, and saying, "Excuse me." (Figure 4-2)
- Explain the hazard or danger, for example, "If you dive into shallow water, you might hit your head on the bottom and get injured." Or say, "You may slip and hurt yourself if you run." Simply telling someone not to do something often does not work. People usually understand and cooperate when they know why something is dangerous.
- Explain a safe option. For example, say, "If you want to dive, please go to the deep end of the pool where it is safe." Or say, "Excuse me, diving into shallow water is dangerous and can cause a head injury. Please use the deep end." Or say, "Walk, please." This type of explanation gets the patron's attention, clarifies the danger, emphasizes the consequences of the risky behavior and offers safe options, if available and appropriate.

Enforcing Rules

By enforcing the rules, you help to prevent injuries and encourage safe patron behavior. When conducting patron surveillance, keep rule enforcement brief by using only a few words or short phrases, such as, "Slow down," or by giving a hand signal. When enforcing rules, be consistent, fair and respectful. In some cases the patron may not know the facility's rules or may not understand them. Always use age-appropriate enforcement methods that are approved by the facility's policies.

If certain patrons repeatedly break the rules even after you have attempted to correct their behavior, you could direct them to leave the water for a set time. Signal for someone who is not engaged in patron surveillance, such as another lifeguard or

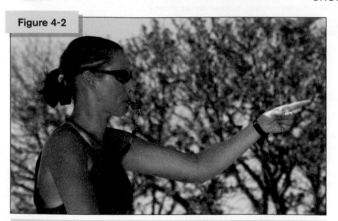

Figure 4-2

When enforcing rules, use your whistle to get patron's attention.

INTERACTING PROFESSIONALLY WITH THE PUBLIC

When you are on duty, your actions should promote an atmosphere of professionalism, safety, trust and goodwill. The following general guidelines will help you display a professional image and maintain a positive relationship with patrons:

- When conducting patron surveillance, any verbal interaction should be brief and your eyes should remain on the water. Politely refer the patron to a staff member who is not conducting surveillance if necessary.

- When not conducting patron surveillance:
  - Treat people as you would like to be treated. Make every patron feel welcome, important and respected.
  - Be professional at all times. Be courteous, mature and responsible. Never insult or argue with a patron.
  - Speak clearly and calmly, at a reasonable pace and volume.
  - Use appropriate language, but do not patronize or speak down to anyone, including children.

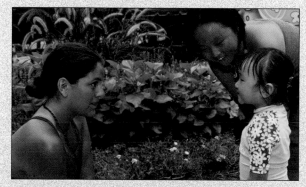

Lifeguards should interact with the public in a professional manner.

- When interacting with patrons, make frequent and direct eye contact. Remove your sunglasses, if necessary. When speaking to small children, kneel down to be at eye level with them.
- Take all suggestions and complaints seriously, and follow up as necessary. Avoid blaming anyone. If you cannot resolve a complaint, take it to your facility's management. Always follow the facility's procedures.
- Repeat the concern expressed by the patron back to him or her to ensure that you understand the concern correctly.
- Do not make promises that cannot be kept.
- Enforce rules fairly and consistently. Be positive and nonjudgemental. Reinforce correct behavior.
- Take a sincere interest in all patrons.

Nonverbal Communication

Spoken words make up a surprisingly small part of overall communication. A listener automatically tends to make judgments about a speaker's attitude based on the volume, pace, tone and pitch of the speaker's voice. A listener also reacts positively or negatively to visual cues or body language. You can gauge a person's attitude as cooperative or confrontational by evaluating these cues; know that the listener will be doing the same.

Nonverbal communication also is expressed while you are on duty, whether you are conducting patron surveillance or performing secondary responsibilities. Patrons may make judgments about your professionalism by observing your appearance, demeanor, posture and behavior. Lifeguards are "on stage" and set the tone while on duty.

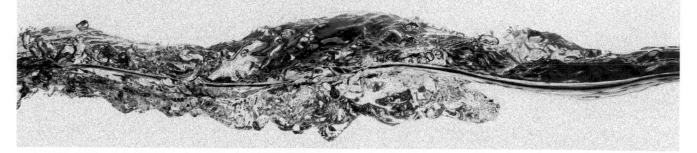

DEALING WITH UNCOOPERATIVE PATRONS AND VIOLENCE

No matter how fairly you enforce the rules, you may encounter an uncooperative patron. Before assuming that a patron is being uncooperative, you should make sure that he or she hears and understands you.

If a patron breaks the rules and is uncooperative, you should take action right away because breaking the rules can be a danger to the uncooperative patron and to others. Most facilities have procedures for handling uncooperative patrons; however, if your facility does not have a procedure, you should call the lifeguard supervisor or facility manager for help as soon as possible.

A patron may threaten to or commit a violent act. You must be realistic about what can be done in a violent situation. If violence is likely to erupt, call the supervisor or facility manager immediately. If violence does erupt, do not try to stop it. Never confront a violent patron physically or verbally and do not approach a patron who has a weapon. In such a situation, the best approach is to retreat and follow the facility's EAP for violence. Safety for patrons and facility staff should be your main goal.

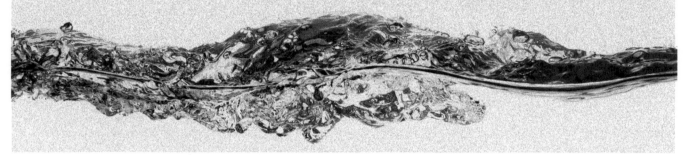

a supervisor, to explain the rules and their rationale. If the patron is a child and a parent or guardian is available, the rules should be clearly explained to the adult as well. Since most people want to be treated with respect, simply explaining and enforcing the rules usually is sufficient. If a parent or guardian is uncooperative, do not argue, but instead ask a supervisor or facility manager to assist you.

A patron may become uncooperative and defiant, compromising his or her safety and the safety of others. If this happens, you should summon a supervisor or facility manager, who may ask the patron to leave the facility. Use this approach only when other methods have failed.

If a patron refuses to leave after being told to leave for repeatedly breaking the rules, the supervisor or manager may choose to call the police or security personnel. Every facility needs a procedure for removing someone from the facility. This procedure should have specific steps and guidelines to follow. Any such action should be recorded in the facility's daily log and on the appropriate form or report.

EFFECTIVE GUARDING—INJURY PREVENTION CHALLENGES

Lifeguards should be conducting patron surveillance anytime the facility is being used by patrons or staff. A major goal of patron surveillance is looking for behaviors that indicate someone may need assistance. As part of your patron surveillance, you also may have specific responsibilities based on the facility's activities or features, such as enforcing age or height requirements, helping patrons with equipment or ensuring that riders are in the proper position. These responsibilities will vary and may include guarding:

- A variety of activities occurring simultaneously.
- "Kiddie" areas, play structures, special attractions, water slides, winding rivers and wave pools.
- Organized recreational swim groups and youth camps.

Guarding Activities

Facilities often have a variety of activities taking place simultaneously, all of which require your surveillance. Examples include:

- Open or recreational swim.
- Water exercises, such as water walking and lap swimming.
- Instructional classes, such as swim lessons, water therapy, water exercise and SCUBA lessons.
- Swimming, water polo, synchronized swimming and other team practice.
- Competitive events, such as swim meets and triathlons.
- Special events, such as movie nights and pool parties and after-hour rentals.

To help you identify patrons who may need assistance, be aware of the age and ability levels of those participating in the activity. For example, you may notice a young child in beginner-level swim lessons moving toward water over his or her head or an elderly man stopping frequently as he swims laps.

Each activity has its own unique characteristics and risks. Some activities, such as SCUBA classes, may require that you receive special training on what to look for specifically or be aware of while you are on surveillance duty. Considerations and questions that need to be answered for effective guarding include:

- What things could go wrong that are unique about this activity?
- What is the swimming ability or comfort level in the water of patrons involved in this activity?
- Are there any unique challenges or obstacles to recognizing an emergency, approaching a victim or performing a rescue?
- Do participants have any medical conditions that increase the chances for sudden illness or injury due to the nature of the activity?

Instructional Classes

Instructional classes are a type of general activity but have the benefit of supervision by trained personnel. Although the instructor is responsible for the safety of the class, that does not relieve you of your responsibilities. You must still scan every person in the water and enforce rules, perform rescues and provide first aid as appropriate. However, with proper preparation, instructors may become valuable members of your safety team. Facility management should share and practice emergency action plans (EAPs) with instructors, clarify their roles during an emergency and share those roles with you. Some instructors will have lifeguard training and specialized rescue skills; others will not.

Having an instructor present may help you to ensure patron safety because he or she may be:

- Familiar with special equipment. Therapy classes may use wheelchairs, lifts and special flotation devices. Instructors for those classes should be able to recognize and deal with potential problems with such devices.

- Familiar with the behavior of specific types of patrons. Instructors may be able to recognize subtle signs of potential problems that may not be obvious to you. For example, a water exercise instructor may detect the early signs of overexertion of a patron in that class.

- Able to help in an emergency related to the specialized class. For example, a SCUBA instructor should know how to deal with and respond to a victim wearing a SCUBA tank and buoyancy control device.

Guarding Areas for Young Children

Many facilities have shallow pools for young children. It is common for these areas to have play equipment, including slides, fountains, inflatable play equipment and climbing structures (Figure 4-3). Effective patron surveillance at these areas is essential, even though the water may be shallow. Enforce rules, such as height and age requirements, fairly and consistently. Note that:

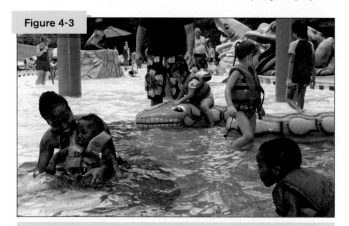
Figure 4-3

Many facilities have play equipment for young children.

- Older children might be too large for some structures, or their play might be too rough for young children.

- Toddlers who are still learning to walk may fall easily. If they fall down in water, they usually cannot lift themselves to an upright position, even if the water is ankle or knee deep.

- Children often get lost. Remind adults to supervise their children at all times.

- You must watch out for young children using the pool as a toilet. The facility should have procedures for preventing and addressing the situation, including handling fecal incidents, which follow local health department guidelines.

- Children usually do not think about overexposure to the sun or hypothermia. If a child is becoming sunburned or overly cold, immediately inform the child's parent or guardian.

Guarding Zones with Play Structures

Facilities may have play structures that are either permanent or removable (Figure 4-4). Permanent structures include sprays and fountains, interactive water-play structures and dumping buckets. Removable structures include large floating toys, inflatable play structures and water basketball and volleyball nets. Some play

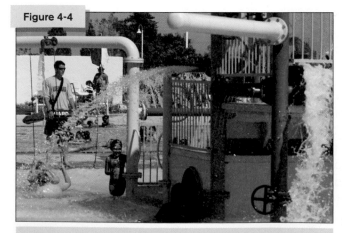
Figure 4-4

Sprays and fountains are a common feature at many facilities.

structures require their own lifeguards, whereas others are watched by lifeguards surveying a larger area.

While guarding at play structures:

- Do not let a play structure become overcrowded. Be prepared to restrict the number of patrons using it at one time.
- Do not allow patrons to swim underneath structures.
- Watch that patrons return to the surface after dropping into the water from a floating feature. Swimmers can be surprised by the fall or become disoriented, especially if they do not realize they will be dropping into deep water.
- Pay close attention to children playing in and around sprays, fountains and interactive water-play structures. These attractions usually are in shallow water. Excited children may run and fall. A very young child who falls might not be able to get back up or may strike his or her head.
- Pay close attention to patrons in moving water. Moving water can surprise people. They might lose their balance and be unable to stand up again.
- Watch for overcrowding and horseplay on floating structures. These structures are tethered to the bottom of the pool; some allow patrons to walk from one floating structure to another while holding onto an overhead rope (Figure 4-5).
- Keep play safe and orderly.
  - Patrons may climb onto floating toys and jump back into the water. They may not notice what is around them and jump onto other swimmers or into water that is over their heads.
  - Patrons may throw balls and other toys and hit unsuspecting swimmers, resulting in injury.

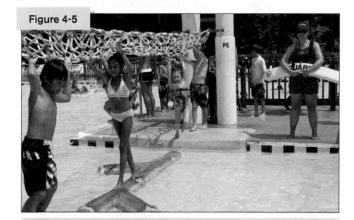

Figure 4-5

Floating structures are a special attraction at waterparks.

Guarding Special Rides and Attractions

Special attractions create a lot of excitement and can include rides, such as bowl slides, multi-person raft rides, uphill water coasters and high-speed water slides. Some attractions found at deep-water pools also include diving platforms, cable swings and hand-over-hand structures like ropes, nets and rings. In a waterpark setting, there are multiple attractions designed for a variety of age groups and abilities. Regardless of the patron's swimming ability, patrons may become fearful, disoriented or off-balance, thus requiring assistance.

Follow these general principles when guarding attractions:

- Watch patrons as they enter and exit an attraction. Dispatch patrons safely on a ride at set intervals. Dispatching is the method of informing patrons when it is safe for them to proceed on a ride.
- Carefully watch both the water below and the activities overhead.
- Keep patrons in view as long as possible. Keeping patrons in view can be

a problem on some attractions: structures, such as caves, enclosed tubes, bridges and buildings, might prevent you from seeing patrons at all times. When a patron goes out of sight, watch to make sure that he or she emerges safely on the other side.

■ Ensure that patrons who submerge return to the surface. The excitement may cause weak swimmers or nonswimmers to overestimate their abilities or underestimate the water's depth.

■ Be aware of special risks. Structures designed to have patrons sit or climb on them, or swim over or under them, pose hazards. Supervise patrons carefully. Someone who falls off of a mat, raft or tube might be injured or pose a hazard to another patron.

Guarding at Water Slides

On some water slides, patrons ride on an inner tube, raft, mat or sled. On others, riding equipment is not allowed. On some slides, only one person is allowed on an inner tube or a raft. On others, two or more people can go together on a special tube or raft. On an inner tube or raft, patrons ride in a sitting position. If no equipment is used, the proper riding position typically is face-up and feet-first. Lifeguard stations may be positioned at the top, middle and/or bottom of a slide.

Follow these guidelines when lifeguarding at a water slide:

■ When dispatching at the top of a slide:

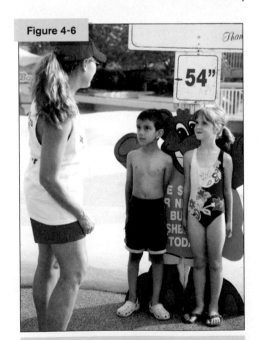

Figure 4-6

When guarding at a water slide, be sure patrons meet the minimum height requirements.

o Check that patrons are tall enough to use the slide by using a measuring pole or line on a wall (Figure 4-6).

o Instruct riders how to ride down the slide according to manufacturer's instructions and facility protocols and make sure they are in the correct riding position.

o Instruct riders not to stop on the slide.

o Help riders with the equipment.

o Confirm that the riders are ready to go and signal them to start.

o If assisting riders to take off, use tube handles when available. Avoid pushing or pulling riders by their shoulders, arms or legs.

o Dispatch the next rider(s) at the proper intervals. For drop-off slides, speed slides and free-fall slides, ensure that the previous rider has left the runout end of the slide or the catch pool and the lifeguard at the bottom has signaled for the next rider.

o If you can see the lifeguard at the bottom, he or she can use a hand signal or whistle.

o If you cannot see the lifeguard at the bottom, a mechanical system, such as light signals, can be used.

■ When stationed at the middle of a slide:

o Watch for riders who:

• Stop, slow down, stand up or form a chain.

• Lose their mat, tube or raft or have trouble getting down the slide.

- • Hit their heads on the side of the slide.
  - ○ Alert the dispatcher and lifeguard at the end of the slide of the situation and assist patrons as necessary.
- ■ When stationed at the bottom of a slide:
  - ○ Observe all riders exiting the slide into the catch pool (Figure 4-7). Patrons might not realize the depth of the catch pool and may need assistance.
  - ○ Assist riders who appear to be off balance or get caught underwater in the strong downward flow of water in the catch pool. This strong force can knock a person off balance or hold a small person or nonswimmer under water.
  - ○ Help riders, if needed, from the runout or catch pool. Some patrons might be disoriented or frightened from the ride (Figure 4-8).
  - ○ Ensure that riders do not cross in front of any slide when getting out of the runout or catch pool.
  - ○ Signal the lifeguard at the top when each rider has moved out of the catch pool or runout and it is clear to send the next rider.

Guarding Winding Rivers

In a winding river, water flows in a long circular or twisting path through a facility. Depending on the winding river, patrons may be floating on tubes, walking or swimming. Some wear life jackets, some do not. Water speeds may vary. Lifeguards may be positioned at the entrance and exit. They also may be positioned at several elevated or ground-level stations or at a combination of both with overlapping zones around the river (Figure 4-9).

When guarding a winding river:

- ■ Ensure that patrons enter and exit at designated locations.
- ■ Watch for inexperienced swimmers falling off their inner tubes or inflatable rafts. It will be difficult for you to see all patrons or the bottom of the winding river if there are a lot of tubes and rafts in the water. Similarly, it can be difficult for someone who falls off a raft or tube to come up for air if the surface is blocked. In addition, someone who is hit by an inflatable raft might be knocked down, hit the bottom and get into trouble.
- ■ Watch for patrons around features in winding rivers, such as fountains and waterfalls, which can catch patrons off-guard or cause patrons to gather.
- ■ Watch carefully for, and correct, risky behavior.

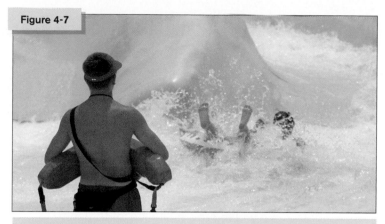

Figure 4-7

Watch for riders to exit the slide into the catch pool.

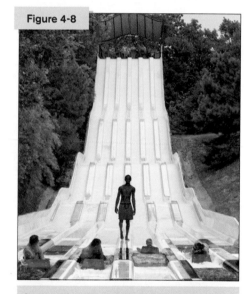

Figure 4-8

Assist riders to exit the speed slide, if needed.

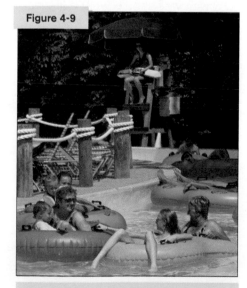

Figure 4-9

Lifeguards may be stationed in multiple zones around a winding river when performing patron surveillance.

LIFE JACKETS

The U.S. Coast Guard has categorized personal flotation devices (PFDs) into five categories. They are rated for their buoyancy and purpose. Types I, II, III and V are referred to as life jackets, whereas Type IV is a throwable device.

Swimming ability, activity and water conditions help determine which type of life jacket to use. For any type, it should be U.S. Coast Guard approved and in good condition. The U.S. Coast Guard label is stamped directly on any approved device (see image below).

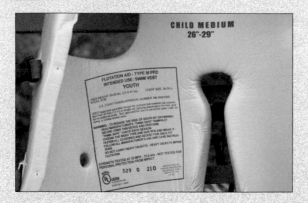

Facilities may have policies addressing the use of life jackets in a pool, waterfront or attraction. Type II and III life jackets are most commonly used in these settings. In general, anyone who cannot swim well should wear a life jacket if they are going

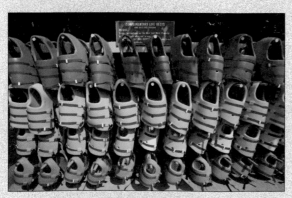

to be in or around the water at an aquatic facility; however, in some cases, such as on certain slides, life jackets are not permitted. In other cases, such as fast-moving winding rivers, life jackets are recommended or may be required. Life jackets may be available at a facility for rent or free of charge.

As a lifeguard, you may be tasked with:

- Ensuring that life jackets are U.S. Coast Guard approved. Inflatable toys and swim aids, such as water wings, swim rings and other flotation devices, are not designed to be used as substitutes for U.S. Coast Guard-approved life jackets or adult supervision.

- Ensuring that life jackets are in good condition. Buckles and straps should be in good working condition. There should be no rips, tears, holes or shrinkage of the buoyant materials.

- Helping patrons to select a properly sized life jacket. Life jackets are sized by weight. Check the U.S. Coast Guard label and be sure that it is matched to the weight range of the patron.

- Ensuring that life jackets are properly worn by patrons. A properly fitted life jacket should feel snug, keep the person's chin above the water and allow the person to breathe easily. The life jacket should not ride up on the patron's body in the water. Completely secure any straps, buckles or ties associated with the life jacket.

- Ensuring that patrons properly use life jackets. Correct any improper wearing or use of life jackets. Do not allow patrons to wear multiple life jackets or stack multiple life jackets on top of each other to be used as floats.

You should remove any extra empty life jackets from the water. An empty life jacket in the water should be a signal that something is wrong. Consistent enforcement of rules related to life jacket use can lead to appropriate behavior by all patrons.

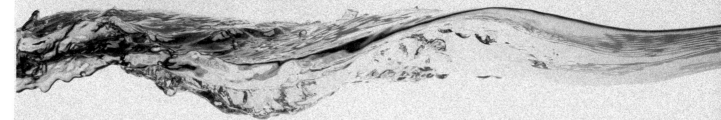

Type	Style	Typical Use	Features
I	Life jacket	Boating on offshore waters or rough water where rescue may be delayed	May help to turn an unconscious person from a face-down position to a vertical, face-up position, or to a face-up, slightly tipped-back position
II	Buoyant vest	Recreational boating on inland waters where a rescue is likely to occur quickly. Good for calm or inland water. Suitable for supervised use in pools and waterparks.	May help to turn an unconscious person from a face-down position to a vertical, face-up position, or to a face-up, slightly tipped-back position. Is less buoyant than a Type I life jacket
III	Flotation vest	Fishing or sailing on inland waters where a rescue is likely to occur quickly. Good for calm or inland water. Suitable for supervised use in pools and waterparks.	May help to keep a conscious person in a vertical, face-up position, or in a face-up, slightly tipped-back position; wearer may have to tilt the head back to avoid going face-down
IV	Throwable device, such as a buoyant cushion or ring buoy	Boating on inland waters with heavy boat traffic where help always is present	May be thrown to a victim in an emergency; does not take the place of wearing a life jacket or vest
V	Special use	Intended for specific activities, such as whitewater rafting and special offshore work environments	Acceptable only when used according to directions on its label

Guarding Wave Pools

Wave pools are popular attractions that produce waves of various heights, intervals and patterns. Wave pools vary in size, shape and depth (Figure 4-10). At one end is the head wall, where a mechanical system creates the waves. Lifeguards are stationed at various places around or in the pool and also may be stationed on the head wall for a better view of the pool (Figure 4-11). Wave pools operate on a cycle, such as 10 minutes with the waves on and 10 minutes with them off.

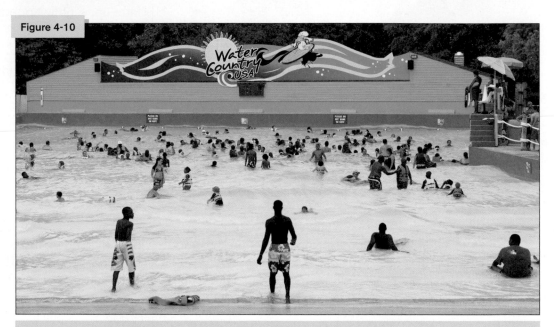

Figure 4-10

Wave pools are popular attractions at waterpark facilities.

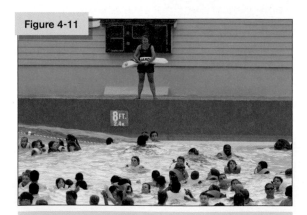

Figure 4-11

Lifeguards may be stationed along the head wall at a wave pool while performing patron surveillance.

When guarding a wave pool:

- Ensure that patrons enter only in the shallow end.
- When the waves are on, stand up to get a better view of patrons.
- Watch for swimmers who get knocked over by the waves or carried into deeper water by the undercurrent. Inexperienced swimmers may go to where the waves break because of the excitement.
- Do not let patrons dive into the waves or dive through inner tubes.
- Keep the areas around ladders and railings clear so that patrons can exit from the pool quickly.
- Keep other swimmers out of the pool during special activities, like surfing. The surfboards or boogie boards in the wave pool can present a hazard to others.
- Before performing an emergency rescue, turn the waves off using the emergency stop (E-stop) button at the lifeguard chair (Figure 4-12).
- Rotate positions only when the waves are off.

Guarding Organized Recreational Swim Groups

Groups of all sizes visit aquatic facilities for recreation. This includes groups from day-care centers, day camps and youth organizations as well as school groups, sports groups and groups visiting facilities for birthday parties. These groups may be based out of your facility and swim regularly or may visit one or more times as a field trip. Groups often are supervised by leaders, chaperones or camp counselors. These supervisors may assist with discipline but do not take the place of lifeguards. Group leaders may be in the water with the group, on the deck or shore, or a combination of both. Group leaders should know how to alert lifeguards in an emergency.

In some cases, most group members will have similar swimming abilities, such as a day-care center group composed of preschool-age nonswimmers. The swimming ability of other groups may vary widely, such as in a youth-camp group with a wider age range of children.

Sometimes, a group will reserve all or part of a facility for its own instructor to teach a class, lead a practice or conduct skill checks (Figure 4-13). These activities may include kayaking, SCUBA diving or swim team tryouts.

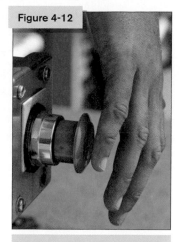

Figure 4-12

An emergency stop (E-stop) button can be pressed to turn off the waves in a wave pool when a rescue is required.

In general, when guarding groups, you should:

- Ensure that swimming areas are divided according to swimmers' abilities and are clearly marked.

- Ensure that patrons stay in the sections appropriate for their swimming abilities. Be aware that weak or nonswimmers, excited to be together enjoying a recreational activity, may attempt to venture into areas that are beyond their swimming ability.

- Provide U.S. Coast Guard-approved life jackets for weak or nonswimmers.

- Know how to identify group leaders or chaperones.

- Ensure that chaperones are actively supervising the members of their group and that the appropriate swimmer-to-chaperone ratio is met. If it appears that they are not doing so, alert your facility's manager.

- Signal for additional lifeguard coverage, such as a roving lifeguard, if you feel you cannot effectively guard your zone. You may need to do this at the beginning of the swim time while the group gets adjusted to the facility's rules or if large groups are concentrated in one area.

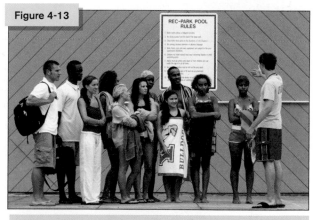

Figure 4-13

Groups sometimes reserve all or part of a facility for its own use.

For groups using buddy checks (see Guarding at Youth Camps, page 68), you may need to signal the buddy check, confirm that everyone is accounted for and count the individuals or buddy pairs, depending on the system being followed.

Regardless of a group's makeup or activities, as a lifeguard, you still are responsible for helping to ensure the safety of its members. To help groups remain safe and injury free, your facility's manager may develop plans and strategies in advance.

Strategies for Safe Group Visits

Facilities often implement additional strategies for injury prevention and swimmer management during group visits. Group leaders should meet in advance with managers at the facility to discuss appropriate plans and procedures. A copy of the facility rules as well as written expectations of group leaders should be provided in advance of the group visit, when possible. Strategies for ensuring safe group visits typically involve one or more of the following:

- **Booking procedure.** Before the visit, group leaders should provide the aquatic facility with information about how many group members and supervisors will be visiting. This is especially important with large camp groups, which require additional time to process through safety orientation, swimmer classification and identification procedures. Confirming the supervisor-to-swimmer ratios helps facility managers to plan appropriate staffing levels. Group leaders also should inform the facility about any special characteristics of the group, such as the percentage of swimmers and nonswimmers. Any staff who will be accompanying the group should be informed about how to help supervise group members around and in the water and how to help the lifeguards in an aquatic emergency.

- **Safety orientation.** Safety orientations are conducted when groups first arrive at the facility. The purpose is to educate all members of the visiting group on your facility's policies and rules and to point out key safety issues. You may be tasked with conducting these orientations.

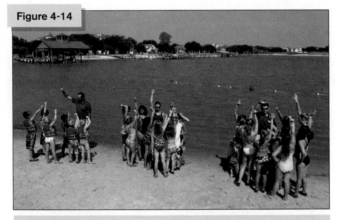

Figure 4-14

Color-coded wristbands are used to classify patrons by swimming ability.

- **Classification of swimming abilities.** Swim tests are administered to determine if a visitor has the minimum level of swimming ability required to participate safely in activities, such as swimming in water over his or her head or riding on certain slides. If your facility administers these tests, management may have developed a system for lifeguards to easily identify patrons' swim levels. For example, levels can be identified by color-coded wristbands or swim caps (Figure 4-14). A red armband might identify someone is a beginner who needs to stay in the shallow end; a green armband might identify someone who can go in deep water.

- **Designation of swimming areas.** Swimming areas should be clearly marked and defined according to swimmers' abilities and intended use. Buoyed ropes should divide shallow and deep water. Multi-use facilities often divide the water into sections for general recreation swim or lap swim, or divide areas for floatable features or play structures. In waterfront areas, the swimming area should be restricted from the nonswimming areas, and there should be some type of continuous barrier, such as buoyed lifelines, piers or decks, around the perimeter of areas set aside for weak or nonswimmers to prevent them from straying into deep water. All swimming areas should be explained to the group and its leaders during the safety orientation.

- **Identification of group leaders or adult chaperones.** Your facility should use an identification system so that lifeguards and other facility staff can easily locate group leaders or adult chaperones. For example, group leaders could wear a laminated lanyard or a brightly colored baseball cap or T-shirt to identify them as being responsible for that group.

- **Supplemental group strategies.** Other strategies, such as the buddy system and buddy checks, sometimes are used to provide an additional layer of protection. These are particularly helpful with camp groups, which can be large. For more details on the buddy system, see page 68.

How to Conduct a Safety Orientation

If you are tasked with providing a safety orientation to a visiting group, you will need to cover general water safety as well as information specific to your facility (Figure 4-15). When conducting a safety orientation:

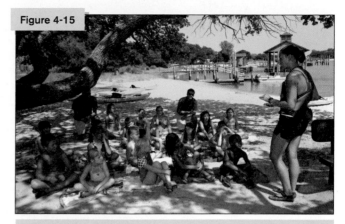

Figure 4-15

Welcome visiting groups to your facility by conducting a safety orientation.

- Ensure that group leaders or adult chaperones are present and that they can be clearly identified by all members of the facility staff.

- Make it fun and build rapport with the group. Ask questions rather than reading a list of rules. This allows you to become more familiar with what group members already know as well as gauge their level of understanding. Explain the reasons for any rules that group members do not understand.

- Identify areas where they can and cannot swim, if applicable.

- Point out where the lifeguards are stationed and inform the group how to get additional help if needed.

- Confirm the swimmer-to-supervisor ratio expected for group leaders and divide the group so that group leaders have a designated set of people to oversee.

- Issue any identification and/or swim classification items to group members and leaders, such as colored wristbands.

Safety topics typically covered during an orientation include general aquatic safety rules, swimming area sections, water depths, features or play structures, equipment, how to use approved floatation devices, rule signage locations and operational information, such as buddy checks or breaks.

How to Administer a Swim Test

Swim tests can be used to determine if a person has the minimum level of swimming ability required to participate safely in activities, such as swimming in deep water, riding a slide that empties into deep water or jumping off a diving board into deep water. There is no single set of swim-test criteria that best meets the needs of all facilities or organizations, nor is the following information intended to set a standard. If administering swim tests, each facility or organization should establish its own requirements based on the facility's design and features, the activities offered and common practices.

During your facility-specific training, you should be provided with standard procedures and criteria for conducting swim tests. Never administer a swim test while performing patron surveillance duty. When administering a swim test:

- Have the swimmer take the test in a safe area, such as near a wall, safety line or lap lane.

- Have the swimmer take the test in shallow water first. If successful, have the swimmer move to the deep water and take the test.

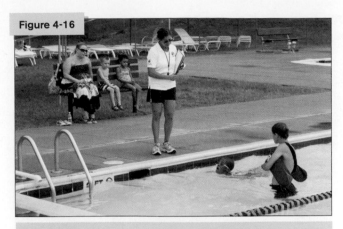

Figure 4-16

Have a lifeguard stationed near a patron during a swim test in case he or she needs assistance.

- Be prepared to assist a person who may struggle in the water while attempting the swim test. Swimmers may overestimate their abilities (Figure 4-16).
- Ensure that chaperone(s) are present during the test, if applicable.
- Ensure that the person has safely exited the water after the test is complete.

When the test is competed, tell the swimmer where he or she is permitted to swim.

To be eligible to swim in deep water, swimmers should be able to at least:

- Jump into the water, level off at the surface of the water and begin to swim.
- Swim at the surface of the water without using anything for support, such as touching the bottom, the wall or the safety line.
- Be able to swim a distance equal to the maximum width of the deep-water swimming area section of the facility.
- Demonstrate breath control—the ability to pick up or turn the head to get a breath while swimming.
- Exit the water independently.

After the initial test, additional swim tests should be conducted at intervals throughout a season to determine if swimming abilities have improved.

Guarding at Youth Camps

Some youth camps operate their own waterfront and pool facilities. If you are working at one of these camps, your area of responsibility and patron load may be smaller than those at a public facility because typically campers will be your only patrons. Some camps will supplement trained lifeguards with other staff who, after proper orientation, will serve as spotters or lookouts; however, these staff members never should take the place of lifeguards.

At the beginning of a camp session, all participants and staff who will be involved in aquatic activities should be given a swim test. After the initial test, additional swim tests should be conducted at intervals throughout the camp session to determine if participants' swimming abilities have improved. Participants who arrive after the initial test has been given also should be tested.

Youth camps with their own aquatic facilities often implement additional prevention strategies, including the buddy system, buddy boards and buddy checks.

Buddy Systems

The buddy system is used by camps to enhance safety for swimming groups. Under the buddy system, one participant is paired with another participant of similar swimming skills. The pair then is assigned to a specific swimming area. If buddies do not have similar swimming skills, the pair should remain in the swimming area suitable to the weakest swimmer's abilities.

Buddies must be instructed to stay together and be responsible for one another. They need to tell a lifeguard immediately if their buddy is in trouble or missing, at which time you should take immediate action.

The buddy system provides useful safeguards to help account for swimmers by having each buddy look out for the other; however, it does not replace lifeguard surveillance.

Buddy Boards

A buddy board helps to keep track of everyone in the swimming area (Figure 4-17). Typically it is a large, permanent structure mounted within the confines of the swimming area near the entrance.

Generally, a buddy board works as follows:

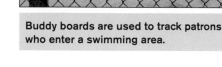

- Based on the initial swim test, each person gets a colored tag with his or her full name and group designation, such as a cabin or campsite number. Tags should be color-coded or labeled by swimming ability, such as "swimmer" or "nonswimmer."

- A lifeguard or other staff member is stationed at the buddy board to make sure that tags are placed correctly and that everyone who enters or leaves the swimming area moves his or her tag appropriately.

- Before buddies enter the water, they hang their tags on hooks on the section of the board that indicates the swimming area in which they will be swimming. The buddies' tags should be next to each other to indicate that they are a pair. Tags should be placed on separate hooks to facilitate a reliable count.

Buddy boards are used to track patrons who enter a swimming area.

- If buddies decide to move from one section to another, such as from the deep to the shallow area, they must first notify the person at the board and move their tags.

- When buddies leave the water, they move their tags to the "Out" section.

Buddy Checks

The primary purpose of buddy checks is to account for all swimmers and to teach buddies to continuously monitor their partners. Buddy checks often are set for specific timed intervals.

To initiate a buddy check, a lifeguard, lookout or supervisor gives a prearranged signal, such as a whistle blast. The buddies grasp each other's hands, raise their arms over their heads and hold still while the staff accounts for everyone (Figure 4-18). Buddies do not have to leave the water: those in shallow water may stand in place, those in deep water may move with their buddy to the side and those already on deck should remain there.

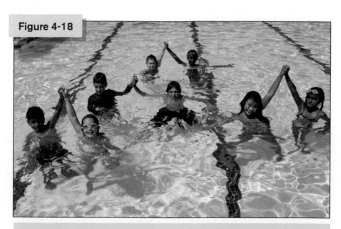

Buddy checks are used to account for each swimmer in a swim area.

Two methods commonly are used to confirm that the staff has accounted for everyone. Both use a buddy board or other tracking system.

- Method 1: Lifeguards count the swimmers in each area and relay those numbers to a monitor. The monitor checks the numbers against the total on the buddy board or other tracking device.
- Method 2: Each pair of buddies is given a number. The monitor calls off the numbers in order, and buddies respond when their number is called.

If everything matches, the buddy check is over. If a buddy check reveals a missing person, you should immediately suspect that the buddy is submerged and activate your facility's EAP.

Although the buddy system provides useful safeguards, buddy checks are not conducted frequently enough to substitute for normal surveillance. You should never depend on the buddy system as the only method of supervision. You must constantly scan your zone of responsibility, looking for the behaviors of swimmers in trouble.

WRAP-UP

As a lifeguard, one of your goals includes helping to ensure that serious injuries never happen. The more you know about how injuries occur, the better you will be able to prevent them. Good communication with patrons is vital in preventing injuries. You should inform patrons about the potential for injury and educate them about the consequences of risky behavior. It also is important to develop strategies for dealing with injury-prevention challenges at your facility.

Emergency Action Plans

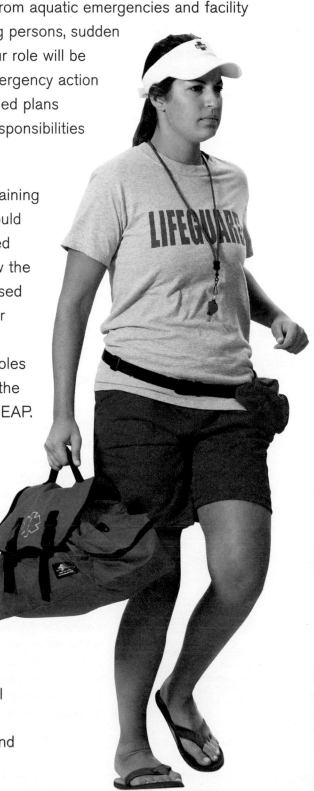

While on duty, you may need to respond to a variety of situations ranging from aquatic emergencies and facility problems to missing persons, sudden illness and severe weather. Your role will be spelled out in your facility's emergency action plan(s) (EAPs). EAPs are detailed plans describing the safety team's responsibilities in an emergency.

During orientation, in-service training and in simulation drills, you should learn and practice your assigned roles in EAPs. You should know the roles assigned to lifeguards based on where they are positioned or who is the primary rescuer and also become familiar with the roles assigned to other members of the safety team—all outlined in the EAP.

To be effective, lifeguard and safety teams should practice the EAPs regularly, using a variety of simulated emergency situations. Remember that in some emergencies, only a few minutes can make the difference between life and death. To give a drowning victim the greatest chance for survival and a normal outcome, you must be able to efficiently implement the EAP and provide resuscitative care. ■

TYPES OF EMERGENCY ACTION PLANS

Every aquatic facility has its own specific set of EAPs based on the unique characteristics at each facility. Factors such as the facility's layout, number of staff on duty at a time, location of back-up lifeguards and other safety team members, equipment used and typical response times of the local emergency medical services (EMS) system are included in the plan. EAPs should be practiced regularly and included in your facility's policies and procedures manual.

Aquatic facilities often have a general plan for water and land rescues, as well as additional plans designed to address specific situations. Examples of situation-based EAPs include:

- Water emergency—Drowning victim—active (Flowchart 5-1).
- Water emergency—Drowning victim—passive (Flowchart 5-2).
- Water emergency—Spinal injury victim.
- Water emergency—Missing person.
- Land emergency—Injury or illness.

Other situations requiring an EAP include evacuations, sheltering in place, severe weather, chemical spills or leaks, power failures and violence.

Along with detailing the role that you and your lifeguard team will play in an emergency, EAPs also identify the very important roles played by other members of the safety team.

Role of the Safety Team

As discussed in Chapter 1, the lifeguard team is part of a larger safety team—a network of people who prevent, prepare for, respond to and assist in an emergency at an aquatic facility (Figure 5-1).

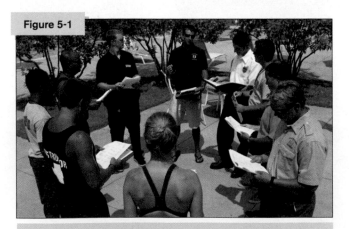

Figure 5-1

Safety teams consist of lifeguards; aquatics instructors; admissions personnel; retail, concession and administrative staff; maintenance, custodial and security personnel; supervisors and administrators.

Safety team members working on-site may include aquatics instructors; admissions personnel; retail, concession and administrative staff; maintenance, custodial and security personnel; supervisors and administrators. At parks, waterfronts and youth camps, other team members may include park rangers, game wardens, marine safety officers and EMS personnel stationed at on-site advanced first aid stations.

Additional members of the safety team may work off-site and often include upper-level management personnel. Members from a variety of departments within an organization, such as communications, public relations, risk management, legal counsel and executive leadership, may play a role. These team members often become involved as soon as possible after a serious injury or death.

Even if only one lifeguard is performing patron surveillance, other safety team members on-site should be in a position to see and/or hear your emergency signal(s) and immediately respond to help in an emergency.

Sample Emergency Action Plan Flow: Water Emergency

The following two flowcharts illustrate how an EAP could be implemented. The first example depicts a situation where no additional resuscitative care is needed after the victim has been removed from the water; the second illustrates a situation where additional resuscitative care is required. Your facility's EAPs will include decision points based on conditions found at the scene along with assigned roles and detailed instructions about how to proceed, which are based on specific circumstances and needs of the facility, such as staffing positions and levels and emergency response times.

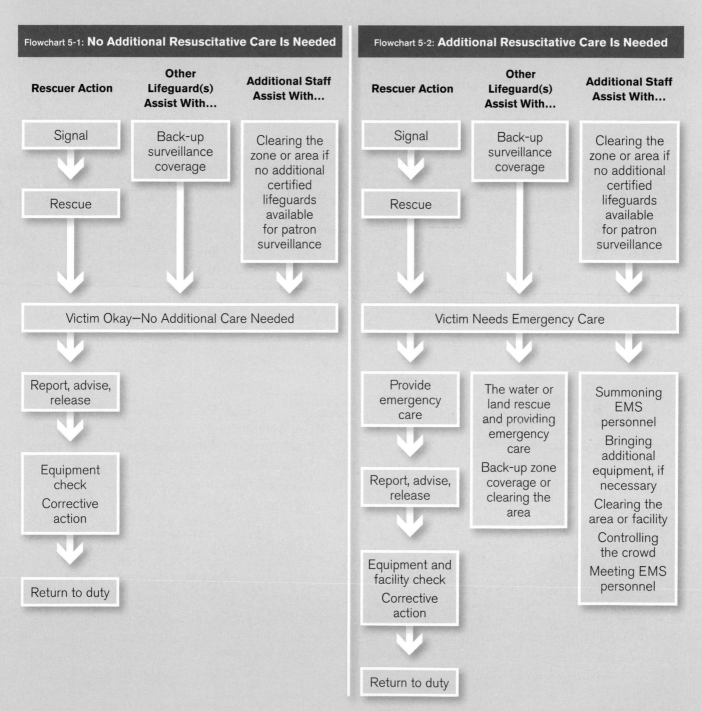

Flowchart 5-1: No Additional Resuscitative Care Is Needed

Rescuer Action · Other Lifeguard(s) Assist With... · Additional Staff Assist With...

Signal → Rescue → Victim Okay—No Additional Care Needed → Report, advise, release → Equipment check / Corrective action → Return to duty

Back-up surveillance coverage

Clearing the zone or area if no additional certified lifeguards available for patron surveillance

Flowchart 5-2: Additional Resuscitative Care Is Needed

Rescuer Action · Other Lifeguard(s) Assist With... · Additional Staff Assist With...

Signal → Rescue → Victim Needs Emergency Care → Provide emergency care → Report, advise, release → Equipment and facility check / Corrective action → Return to duty

Back-up surveillance coverage

The water or land rescue and providing emergency care / Back-up zone coverage or clearing the area

Clearing the zone or area if no additional certified lifeguards available for patron surveillance

Summoning EMS personnel / Bringing additional equipment, if necessary / Clearing the area or facility / Controlling the crowd / Meeting EMS personnel

---

If the victim was treated for serious injuries or illness, follow the facility EAP protocols for:

- Closing the facility.
- Contacting family members.
- Contacting the chain of command, such as supervisors or public relations personnel.
- Handling patrons and answering questions.
- Discussing the incident details.
- Operational debriefings.

Everyone needs to know his or her roles in an EAP. In a small facility, team members may be assigned several different roles, whereas in a large facility each person may have only one role.

Depending on the emergency, the number of staff available and procedures laid out in the EAP, other members of the safety team may support lifeguards by:

- Assisting with emergency rescues, if trained to do so.
- Summoning EMS personnel by calling 9-1-1 or the local emergency number.
- Bringing rescue equipment, such as a backboard or an automated external defibrillator (AED), to the scene.
- Clearing the swimming area and controlling bystanders.

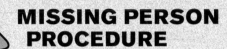

MISSING PERSON PROCEDURE

Every aquatic facility should include missing-person procedures in its EAP. All staff should be trained in these procedures during orientation.

Time is critical when a person is missing. For example, the missing person could be someone struggling in the water or a child who wandered off and cannot be found by his or her parent. Every missing-person report is serious.

During all missing-person search procedures, one person should be in charge to avoid confusion and wasting time. This may be the lifeguard supervisor or facility manager.

Lifeguards will begin the search, but if the missing person is not found immediately, they may ask other facility staff for help and call EMS personnel for back-up. You and other staff should continue the search until EMS personnel arrive on the scene to assist with the search. You can cancel the EMS response if you find the missing person and he or she does not need medical assistance.

The facility's EAP may include some or all of the following steps for a missing-person search:

- The lifeguard who takes the initial report should quickly alert other lifeguards about the situation. He or she then should find out the following from the patron who reported the person missing:
  - Where the person was last seen
  - How long the person has been missing
  - The person's age
  - The person's swimming ability
- The lifeguard should keep the reporting party with him or her until a positive identification of the missing person is made.
- A public address request for the missing person to report to a specific area may be made.
- All other lifeguards should clear the swimming areas and assist in the search, starting at the place where the missing person was last seen and expanding from there.
- If it is determined that the missing person is not in the water, lifeguards and other staff should meet in a designated location to begin an organized land search. The search should

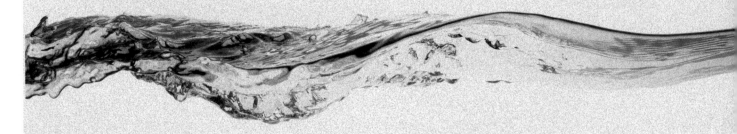

- Alerting additional safety team members.
- Securing and protecting the area or evacuating the facility.
- Notifying the chain of command, beginning with the lifeguard supervisor or facility manager, who then informs the appropriate individuals.
- Meeting and directing EMS responders to the scene.
- Collecting information for reports.
- Dealing with questions from patrons or the media.

All safety team members working on-site must know where equipment is stored, including the first aid kit, AED, backboard, resuscitation equipment and disposable gloves. Certification in CPR/AED and first aid is beneficial and often

include lawns, bathrooms, locker rooms, picnic areas and other play structures within the facility. Swimming areas should remain closed until it is determined that the missing person is not in the aquatic facility.

- A designated lifeguard or staff member should make an announcement over the public address system describing the missing person, if appropriate. (Follow the facility's policy as to whether or not you should describe a missing child.) Use a megaphone if necessary. Direct everyone to please stay calm and ask for volunteers, if they are needed. Ask the missing person to report to the main lifeguard area. In many cases, the person will not be aware that someone has reported him or her missing.
- If the missing person is not found in the aquatic facility, facility staff or EMS personnel should call the local police department, which will take over and expand the search.

EAPs for waterfront facilities also may include the following steps:

- One lifeguard should act as the lookout above the water level on a pier, raft or watercraft with rescue equipment.

- Lifeguards should look under piers, rafts, floating play structures and in other dangerous locations.
- Adult volunteers can help search shallow areas, but only lifeguards should search beyond chest-deep water. See Chapter 6, Water Rescue Skills, for information on sightings and cross bearings and line searches.

EAPs for camps also may include the following steps:

- Staff should quickly check the missing person's cabin or tent and other areas.
- All campers should be moved to a central location where a head count should be taken.
- Lifeguards should continue to search the entire waterfront until every person has been accounted for or until proper authorities take over.

EAPs for parks also may include the followings steps:

- Staff should search playgrounds, campsites and wooded areas.
- Park rangers, maintenance staff and volunteers can search land areas while lifeguards search the water.

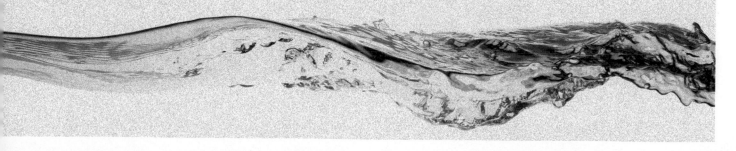

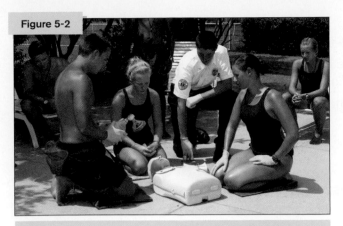

Figure 5-2

Safety team members should participate in emergency simulation drills.

is required for team members who may need to assist the lifeguard team. Safety team members also should practice with the lifeguard team by participating in emergency simulation drills (Figure 5-2).

In some situations, it may be necessary to solicit the assistance of bystanders. Although bystanders may not have the training required to handle emergencies, with direct communication and guidance they can help by controlling a crowd, relaying a message to other team members, getting equipment or summoning EMS personnel.

IMPLEMENTING AN EMERGENCY ACTION PLAN EAP

The following section describes a typical EAP designed for a general water or land emergency. In an actual emergency, the safety team member responsible for each task would be designated in the facility's specific EAP.

At the Onset of an Emergency

Recognize the Emergency

The first step in any EAP is recognition that an emergency is taking place in the water or on land and determine that someone needs immediate help.

Activate the EAP

Next, before leaving your station, activate the EAP by giving the prearranged signal, such as a long whistle blast, to alert other lifeguards and staff.

This step is critical. If your signal is not recognized, other lifeguards and safety team members will not realize that there is an emergency. Without their backup, your safety and the safety of patrons may be compromised.

The signals used to activate an EAP must be simple and clear. They will be predetermined based on the nature of the facility and the number of staff. One or more of the following signals are commonly used: whistles, your hands (for hand signals), public address systems, telephones, two-way radios, flags, horns, megaphones and electronic devices (buttons or switches) that must be triggered.

At a slide, the signal must alert the lifeguard stationed at the top to stop dispatching more riders. At a wave pool, pushing the emergency

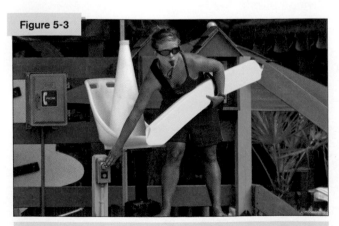

Figure 5-3

Pushing the emergency stop (E-stop) button stops waves at a wave pool.

stop (E-stop) button is required to stop the waves before attempting a rescue (Figure 5-3).

Perform a Water Rescue or Provide Emergency Care

Once you have given the signal, choose the appropriate rescue for the situation and provide care to the victim as necessary. Some rescues may require additional lifeguards to enter the water and assist with the water rescue.

CHOOSING WHERE TO WORK

It is very important that you choose your place of employment wisely. Before you accept a lifeguarding job, you should evaluate the potential working conditions. Are you going to be set up for success? Will you have the tools you need to perform your job? The best way to answer these questions is to "interview" potential employers. Just as they will ask you questions when they interview you, you should ask them questions about their facilities.

These questions should include:

- How many lifeguards will be on duty at one time?
- What is the length of lifeguard rotations?
- How many lifeguard stands are there?
- Are there scheduled meal breaks?
- Does the facility provide rescue equipment, such as rescue tubes, first aid kits and backboards?
- Does the facility provide uniforms, or are you required to purchase your own?
- Does the facility provide whistles, or are you required to provide your own?

- Has the facility established an emergency action plan (EAP)?
- Does the facility conduct new-employee orientations?
- Is there a staff manual outlining policies and procedures, and if so, is it available to you?

Single-Guard Facilities

Before accepting a job at a single-guard facility, take the time to evaluate how emergencies are handled at that site. Be sure to ask:

- Who will call EMS personnel in an emergency?
- Will another trained rescuer be available to assist you, such as to remove a passive victim from the water?

Lifeguards generally work together as a team to respond to emergency situations, so it is important for you to know how this would be accomplished with only one lifeguard on duty at a time.

You also should find out how the single-guard facility manages day-to-day activities, such as lifeguard rotations, meal breaks and general maintenance.

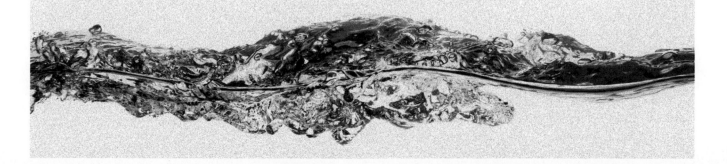

During the Emergency

Ensure Back-Up Zone Coverage

The lifeguard rotation should include back-up zone coverage plans that ensure back-up coverage is immediately available upon activating the EAP. For water rescues, the EAP may direct all lifeguards to stand in their chairs and adjust their zone coverage to include that of the lifeguard making the rescue. Alternatively, the plan may require lifeguards who are not on patron surveillance duty to take the rescuing lifeguard's place at the vacant lifeguard station.

Clear the Swimming Area

Sometimes an incident is serious enough to require clearing the swimming area. The lifeguard who is providing back-up coverage—or another member of the safety team identified in the EAP—makes this judgment and signals to patrons to leave the water. With the area cleared, other staff members are able to either assist with the rescue or provide additional care.

Summon EMS Personnel

If the incident involves a life-threatening emergency, someone must summon EMS personnel by immediately calling 9-1-1 or the local emergency number. A safety team member usually makes this call, but it might be made by a patron or other bystander; so, emergency numbers and other instructions, such as the facility's address, should be clearly displayed in the facility and at each phone (Table 5-1). In some facilities, a number, such as an 8 or 9, must be dialed first to place an outside call. This information also should be included in any instructions.

Some facilities and remote youth camps have on-site medical staff on their safety teams, such as emergency medical technicians (EMTs) or nurses. If this is the case, the facility's EAP may direct you to contact one of these members before or instead of calling 9-1-1.

When EMS personnel arrive, a member of the safety team meets them and directs them to the scene.

Table 5-1: **Sample Emergency Call Procedure: Ambulance, Fire, Police**

- Call 9-1-1 or the local emergency number.
- Identify yourself.
- Explain the situation briefly (e.g., unconscious child pulled from the water).
- Explain the purpose of the call (e.g., need an ambulance, need police).

Give the location.	Facility Name _____
	Physical Address _____
	_____
	Phone # _____

- Answer questions addressed to you.
- Do not hang up until the EMS call-taker tells you to do so.

Control Bystanders

You may need to control bystanders to prevent them from interfering with a rescue or emergency care. This may involve:

- Using a firm but calm voice to ask bystanders to move back so that care can be provided. Do not yell at patrons.
- Roping off areas or positioning chairs around the emergency site.
- Using the public address system to communicate with patrons.
- Repeating commands and requests as often as is necessary.
- Ensuring that EMS personnel have a clear path.
- Keeping bystanders and any children away from the rescue scene.

Any safety team member should be empowered to solicit aid from bystanders as appropriate, such as to summon EMS personnel or to help with crowd control. Always follow your facility's policies and procedures when seeking assistance from patrons. However, emergency plans should not rely on bystander aid in lieu of adequate staffing. Bystanders are not primary response personnel.

Evacuate the Facility

In certain circumstances, such as a fire or violent situation, you may need to evacuate the facility. To evacuate everyone safely:

- Give the predetermined signal and instruct patrons to clear the pool or waterfront area.
- Follow the facility's evacuation procedures to clear all areas of the facility, including locker rooms, lobby areas and staff rooms.
- Direct patrons to a position of safety.
- Ensure that patrons do not re-enter the facility until the facility is declared safe for re-entry. In emergency situations, EMS, fire or law enforcement personnel will inform facility staff when it is safe to re-enter.

After the Emergency

Report, Advise, Release

After the emergency has been resolved, you and other members of the safety team still have three important tasks to complete: report, advise and release.

Report the Incident

Staff members involved in the incident need to complete the appropriate incident report form as quickly as possible after providing care. Collect the required information about the victim, such as name, address and contact information, before you release the victim. After releasing the victim, you can continue filling out the information regarding the rescue. The person who made the rescue should fill out the form, recording only factual information of what was heard and seen and any action taken. Do not record personal opinions or information given to you by someone else. Depending on the circumstances, other lifeguards involved in the incident may sign your form as witnesses or fill out their own, separate forms.

TRAINING WITH EMERGENCY PERSONNEL

As a professional lifeguard, you may have the opportunity to train with local emergency medical services (EMS) personnel, including emergency medical technicians, paramedics, firefighters and law enforcement officers. These training sessions can be beneficial to both lifeguards and EMS personnel. In addition to fostering good relationships, training together gives lifeguards a better understanding of their role on the EMS team and familiarizes EMS personnel with the aquatic facility's emergency procedures.

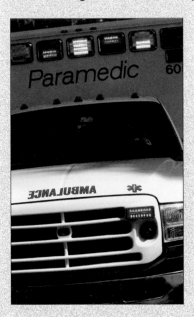

Your facility might offer a variety of joint in-service trainings including but not limited to:

- Medical emergency action plans and procedures.
- Emergency action plans for severe weather, and chemical and natural disasters.
- Threats to public safety and facility security.
- Types of equipment to be used during an emergency.

- Missing-person protocols for land and water.
- Public-indecency awareness.
- Demonstration of CPR/AED and lifeguarding skills.
- Practice and coordination of medical emergency action plans.
- Practice and coordination of missing person procedures.
- Practice and coordination of evacuation procedures for fire or other emergencies.
- Proper radio communications.
- Procedures for recognizing and handling suspicious behavior.

One of the benefits of these trainings is that you and your fellow lifeguards get a chance to see EMS responders in action and to practice interacting with them before an actual emergency occurs. For example, if your training session involves practicing how to transfer care to EMS personnel, you might discover that you may be expected to continue giving CPR even after EMS personnel arrive.

Likewise, EMS personnel may benefit from these training sessions by getting to see lifeguards carry out water rescues and provide emergency care. This gives EMS personnel the chance to become familiar with your skills and your facility's equipment.

Both EMS personnel and lifeguards benefit from trainings that cover emergency action plans. By practicing EAPs in advance, both have an opportunity to address potential problems. For example, while practicing an evacuation plan you may discover that the EMS stretcher does not fit in your facility's elevator.

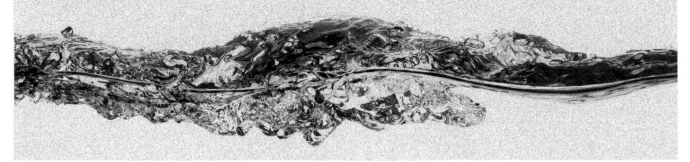

Sometimes you will be responsible for requesting witness statements from bystanders, although this usually is done by a lifeguard supervisor or manager. Witnesses should write their names, addresses phone numbers and statements on separate, dated forms, describing the incident in their own words. Do not tell witnesses what to put in their statements and separate witnesses when they are completing their statements; if they are allowed to be together, they may talk to each other, which may distort their perception of the emergency.

Remember that documentation is important for legal reasons as well as for tracking when, where and how often incidents occur. Reports provide valuable information for facilities to use when they assess safety protocols, such as staffing levels or placement of lifeguard stations.

Advise the Victim

Depending on the nature of the incident, your next step may be to advise the victim. For example, you might give the victim safety instructions to prevent a similar incident from recurring or recommend that the person follow up with a health care provider. In certain cases, you might advise the person not to return to the water for a period of time. In a serious or life-threatening emergency, it may be more appropriate to have EMS or medical personnel provide the advice. Always be certain to document your actions and any advice given to the victim on the incident report.

Release the Victim

A victim may be released only when the rescue and emergency care provided by you and your safety team is complete. In some cases, you will release the person under his or her own care or to a parent, guardian, camp counselor, group leader, instructor or other staff member. In other situations, you will release the victim to the care of advanced emergency care providers, such as EMS personnel. Always be sure to document that the victim was released.

Notify the Chain of Command

The facility's lifeguard supervisor or facility manager needs to be notified when emergencies occur. With a serious injury or death, the lifeguard supervisor or facility manager notifies the appropriate administrator(s) as soon as possible. The administrator works with responding agencies to determine who should contact the victim's family. Your chain of command also may offer advice and guidance on what needs to be done before reopening the facility.

Check the Equipment and the Facility

All equipment and supplies used in the rescue must be inspected. You or other safety team members must report and/or replace all damaged or missing items before returning to duty. Properly clean and disinfect any equipment or areas of the facility exposed to blood or other potentially infectious materials. Use biohazard bags to dispose of contaminated materials, such as used gloves and bandages. Place all soiled clothing in marked plastic bags for disposal or cleaning. If the facility was cleared or closed during the incident, put all required equipment back in place before reopening the facility.

Remove any equipment involved in the emergency, such as a tube, sled or mat, from rotation until it is cleared by the lifeguard supervisor or facility manager.

SAMPLE INCIDENT REPORT FORM

Date: _____ Time: _____ AM PM   Day: Mon Tue Wed Thur Fri Sat Sun

Facility Data:

Facility: _____   Phone Number: _____

Address: _____

City: _____   State: _____   Zip: _____

Patron Data: (complete a separate form for incidents involving more than one person)

Name: _____

Phone Number: (H): _____   (Cell): _____

Address: _____

City: _____   State: _____   Zip: _____

Family Contact: Name: : _____   Phone: _____

Date of birth: _____   Age: _____   Gender: Male Female

Incident Data:

Location of Incident: (describe the location below and mark an X on the facility diagram)

   Location: _____

   Water Depth, if a water rescue: _____

   Water Conditions: _____

   Facility Condition: _____

Description of Incident: (describe what happened and include any contributing factors such

as unaware of depth, medical reasons, etc.): _____

_____

_____

Did an injury occur? Yes No

If yes, describe the type of injury: _____

_____

Care Provided:

Did facility staff provide care? Yes No

Describe care provided in detail: _____

_____

_____

_____

_____

Patron Advised:

Describe any instructions provided to the patron: (cautioned to obey the rules, issued a

life jacket, etc.) _____

_____

Patron returned to activity?   Yes   No

Patron Released To:

Self   Parent/Guardian

EMS   Transported off-site   Medical Facility: _____

Staff Information:

Name and position title of staff that provided care: _____

Name(s) of assisting lifeguard(s) or staff involved in incident:

_____

_____

Report Prepared By:

Name: _____   Position: _____

Signature: _____   Date: _____

Witnesses (attach witness descriptions of incident)

Name: _____   Phone: _____

Address: _____

City: _____   State: _____   Zip: _____

Witnesses (attach witness descriptions of incident)

Name: _____   Phone: _____

Address: _____

City: _____   State: _____   Zip: _____

Refusal of Care:

Did victim refuse medical attention by staff?   Yes   No

If yes, victim (parent or guardian for a minor) signature: _____

Attachments:

Note any attachments such as EMS personnel report or follow-up conversations with the victim and/or parents or guardian.

If an injured victim was put on a backboard, EMS personnel usually will use that same backboard to transport the victim to a hospital. If this occurs, ask EMS personnel to temporarily exchange backboards with the facility; otherwise, immediately replace the backboard or close the facility until a backboard is available on site. Report any missing or damaged items to the lifeguard supervisor or facility manager.

Take Corrective Action

Before reopening the facility, you or another member of the safety team should correct any problems that contributed to the incident, such as tightening a loose step on a ladder. If a problem cannot be resolved, you may need to restrict access to the unsafe area.

Return to Duty

After completing your responsibilities for the rescue, return to surveillance duty at the appropriate lifeguard station. Follow the procedures for lifeguard rotations. Inform your supervisor if you need time to regroup or are too shaken by the incident to effectively focus on surveillance.

Reopen the Facility

During or after a significant incident, the lifeguard supervisor, facility manager or another individual as identified in the EAP decides whether to close the facility temporarily and then, when to reopen. The decision may depend on safety issues, such as whether enough lifeguards are ready to return to surveillance duty, all of the required equipment is in place or spills involving blood or other potentially infectious materials have been cleaned up.

Deal with Questions

Television or newspaper reporters, insurance company representatives and attorneys may ask questions about the emergency, as may people who are just curious. Do not give out any information about the incident or injured person. Only management or a designated spokesperson should talk to the media or others about an incident; your doing so may lead to legal action. The procedure for dealing with the media and others should be laid out in the policies and procedures manual and the EAP.

If people ask questions, let them know that you are not the appropriate person to speak to regarding the incident and refer them to the manager or spokesperson. Do not discuss the emergency with anyone who is not on the facility staff, except for safety team members who are there to assist staff. If the area where the incident happened is visible from public property, you cannot prevent people from taking pictures or filming from a public area. However, facility policy may state that permission from management is necessary before anyone is allowed to take photos or film inside the facility.

Attend the Operational Debriefing

The entire safety team may attend a meeting to talk about what happened before, during and after the emergency. Avoid assigning blame or criticizing anyone's actions or reactions. Goals of the debriefing are to:

- Examine what happened.
- Assess the effectiveness of the EAP.

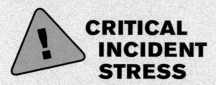

CRITICAL INCIDENT STRESS

In an emergency, a person may react both physically mentally. Physical reactions include muscles becoming more tense and the heart rate and breathing increasing. Mental and emotional stress may manifest as sleeplessness, anxiety, depression, exhaustion, restlessness, nausea or nightmares. Some effects may occur immediately, but others may appear days, weeks or even months after the incident. People react to stress in different ways, even with the same incident. Someone may not even recognize that he or she is suffering from stress or know its cause.

A critical incident may cause a strong emotional reaction and interfere with a lifeguard's ability to cope and function during and after the incident. For lifeguards, critical incidents include:

- A patron's death, especially the death of a child or a death following a prolonged rescue attempt.
- An event that endangers the rescuer's life or threatens someone important to the rescuer.
- The death of a co-worker on the job.
- Any powerful emotional event, especially one that receives media coverage.

These catastrophic events are especially stressful if the lifeguard believes that he or she did something incorrectly or failed to do something—even after doing exactly what he or she was trained to do. This stress is called *critical incident stress*. It is a normal reaction. Someone experiencing this usually needs help to recognize, understand and cope with the stress. If this type of stress is not identified and managed, it can disrupt a lifeguard's personal life and his or her effectiveness on the job. Facility management should help by contacting a licensed mental health professional.

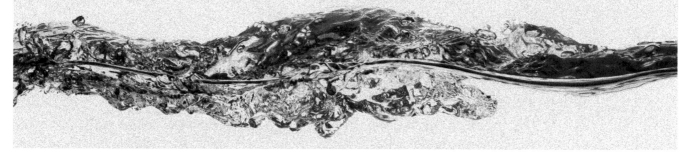

- Consider new ways to prevent similar incidents.
- Be alert for stress reactions after a critical incident. If the incident involved a serious injury or death and you need assistance in coping with the experience, a licensed mental health professional may help.

EMERGENCIES OUTSIDE OF YOUR ZONE

Emergencies sometimes occur away from the water in places such as locker rooms, concession areas, entrance and lobby areas, mechanical rooms, playgrounds and play areas and parking lots.

You must be prepared to respond to these emergencies even though they are outside of the immediate aquatic environment and not part of your zone of responsibility.

If you witness or are told about an emergency when you are *not* on surveillance duty, you should activate the predetermined EAP signal. If the signal cannot be heard

THE NEED FOR RESCUE DATA

Training agencies, such as the American Red Cross, can gain a great deal of useful information from reviewing aquatic facilities' rescue reports. Knowing the details about the emergencies to which lifeguards respond and the rescue methods that they use while on the job can help these agencies to determine what lifeguards and management need to know to be prepared and effective in an emergency.

As one example, the Department of Kinesiology at the University of North Carolina at Charlotte has developed a rescue reporting system to gather information for this purpose. The ultimate goal is to help the Red Cross and others learn more about what actually takes place when lifeguards are called upon to respond to an emergency. This includes details, such as:

- Environmental conditions at the time of the rescue.
- How lifeguards identified the emergency.
- Type of equipment used.

The information is gathered in a multiple-choice format and is completely anonymous. All emergencies, from a complex rescue to a simple reaching assist, can be reported. To access the survey, go to water-rescue.uncc.edu.

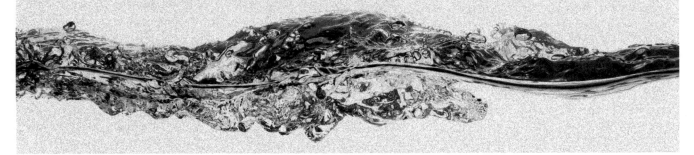

from your location, and you cannot or should not move the victim, you should send a patron to alert another staff member to initiate the facility's EAP. In the meantime, size up the scene, assess the victim's condition and give appropriate care.

You also could be summoned by other safety team members to respond to or assist with emergencies in other parts of your facility, such as a gymnasium, childcare area, cardio or weight room, sauna or park area. Whereas some of these areas might be supervised by facility staff trained in basic first aid, lifeguards might be called upon to respond in an emergency because they are trained at the professional level. Follow your facility EAPs for leaving your zone of responsibility to assist in these types of emergency situations.

WRAP-UP

EAPs are blueprints for handling emergencies. You need to know your EAP responsibilities and the roles given to all members of the safety team. Working as a team and practicing EAPs helps everyone know how to respond in an emergency and how to manage the stress it may cause.

Water Rescue Skills

You must always be prepared to enter the water to make rescues when on duty. This means that you have the proper equipment immediately available and are properly stationed to see your entire zone of responsibility. You should be scanning your zone, looking for signs indicating that someone may need help. If someone does need help, you must assess the victim's condition, perform an appropriate rescue, move the victim to safety and provide additional care as needed.

The skills discussed in this chapter will give you the tools needed to safely perform a rescue in most aquatic environments, although the steps may need to be modified, depending on the actual situation in the water. When performing a rescue, you should keep in mind the skill steps that you have learned, but focus on the ultimate objective—to safely rescue the victim and provide appropriate care. ■

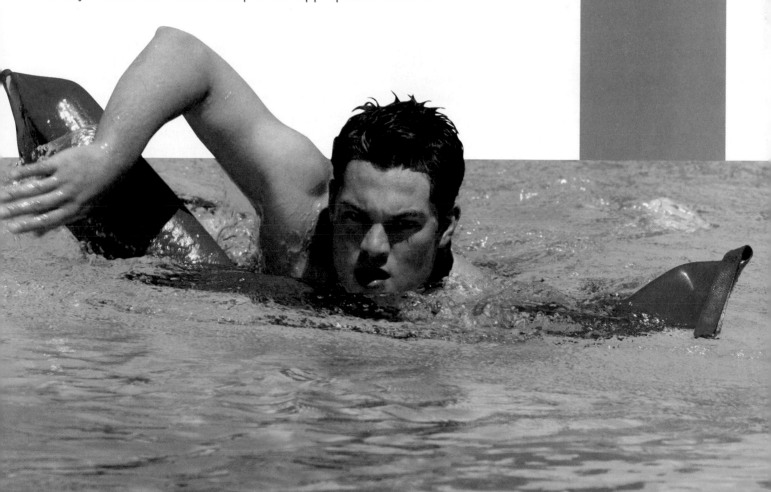

GENERAL PROCEDURES FOR A WATER EMERGENCY

In all situations involving a water rescue, follow these general procedures:

Activate the emergency action plan (EAP).

- Enter the water, if necessary.
- Perform an appropriate rescue.
- Move the victim to a safe exit point.
- Remove the victim from the water.
- Provide emergency care as needed.
- Report, advise and release.

Activate the Emergency Action Plan

As soon as you recognize an emergency situation, always immediately activate the EAP (Figure 6-1).

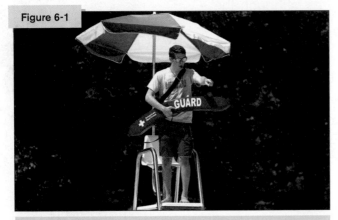

Figure 6-1

Immediately activate your facility's EAP when an emergency situation occurs.

Enter the Water, if Necessary

In some cases you will be able to use a reaching assist to pull a victim to safety from a deck or pier, such as a distressed swimmer at the surface. However, in most situations you will need to enter the water to perform a successful rescue.

You must quickly evaluate and consider many factors when choosing how to safely enter the water. Each time you rotate to a new station, keep in mind the following factors as you consider how to enter the water to perform a rescue: water depth, location and condition of the victim, location of other swimmers, design of the lifeguard station, your location, facility set-up and type of equipment used (rescue board, rescue buoy or rescue tube).

Perform an Appropriate Rescue

The type of water rescue you use will depend on the victim's condition. This includes whether the victim is active or passive, at or near the surface, submerged, or possibly has sustained an injury to the head, neck or spine. You should ensure that the victim's airway is above the surface of the water as you move the him or her to a safe exit point.

Begin your rescue by approaching the victim. Always keep the victim or the location where you last spotted the victim within your line of sight. When swimming, always travel with the rescue tube strapped on during your approach to the victim. An exception may be a waterfront setting where additional specialty rescue equipment may be used, such as a rescue board or watercraft. You may approach the victim by:

- Walking with a rescue tube to the victim in shallow water.
- Swimming with a rescue tube to the victim.

- Traveling on the deck or beach for a distance, then swimming with a rescue tube to the victim.
- Paddling on a rescue board.
- Navigating in a watercraft.

As you near a victim you need to maintain control and may need to reposition your rescue tube, rescue board or watercraft before making contact. For all assists and rescues when the victim is in distress or struggling, communicate directly with the person. Let the victim know that you are there to help and give any necessary instructions using short phrases. For example, say "I'm here to help. Grab the tube."

Be aware that the victim's condition and location can change between the time you notice the problem and when you complete your approach. For example, a victim who was struggling at the surface may begin to submerge as you approach, requiring you to use a different type of rescue than originally planned.

Move the Victim to a Safe Exit Point

After performing a water rescue, move the victim to a safe exit point. For some, this can be as simple as helping him or her to walk out of the water, such as in a simple assist. For others, it requires supporting the victim on the rescue tube while keeping his or her mouth and nose out of the water as you move to the safe exit point, such as in an active victim rear rescue.

Do not automatically return to the point where you entered; you may be able to reach another point faster. However, realize that the closest place on land may not be feasible for removing the victim: there may be limited deck space or lane ropes, or equipment or other features may block the way. Move quickly to the nearest point with appropriate access. Be sure that the chosen exit site has enough room to safely remove the victim from the water. You also will need enough space to provide any additional care needed, such as giving ventilations or CPR.

Remove the Victim from the Water

Safely remove the victim from the water. For conscious victims, this may involve simply assisting the victim out of the water. For victims who are unresponsive or victims suspected of having a head, neck or spinal injury, you will need to use a backboard or a rescue board.

Provide Emergency Care as Needed

The victim may need additional emergency care after the water rescue. This can range from helping the person regain composure to giving ventilations or performing CPR.

Report, Advise and Release

After an emergency, you and other members of the safety team must complete incident report forms, advise the victim on the next steps and release the victim to the appropriate parties. Every water rescue should have a written report. Documentation is important for legal reasons as well as for tracking when, where and how often incidents occur. After the victim is out of the water and care has been given, advise the person, as appropriate, by providing any safety instructions necessary to prevent the likelihood of the incident recurring. You then may release the victim to his or her own care or to a parent or guardian.

TRAIN TO THE STANDARD, MEET THE OBJECTIVE

In this course and throughout your ongoing training, you will be taught how to perform water rescues based on American Red Cross standards. You will learn these techniques in a specific manner. However, in the real world, no two aquatic emergencies are exactly alike. Actual rescue situations often are fast-moving and rapidly changing. You may not be able to follow each step exactly as you have learned and practiced. So, in an actual rescue, keep in mind the skill steps you have learned, but your primary focus should be on the overall objective—saving the victim's life.

During this course and on the job, you must make decisions and handle situations as they occur. Keep in mind these four core objectives in any rescue situation:

- Ensure the safety of the victim, yourself and others in the vicinity. This includes the entry, approach, rescue, removal and care provided.
- Use a rescue technique that is appropriate and effective for the situation.
- Provide an appropriate assessment, always treating life-threatening conditions first.
- Handle the rescue with a sense of urgency.

RESCUE SKILLS

This section contains summaries of water rescue skills that will be taught in this course, along with the objectives specific to each type of skill. Skill sheets describing the skill steps are located at the end of the chapter.

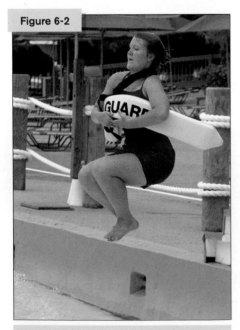

Figure 6-2

The compact jump can be used to enter water at least 5 feet deep from an elevated station.

Entries

The objective of entries is to get in the water quickly and safely, with rescue equipment, and begin approaching the victim (Figure 6-2). It may not be safe to enter the water from an elevated lifeguard stand if your zone is crowded or due to the design or position of the stand. You may need to climb down and travel along the deck or shore before entering the water. The type of entry used depends on:

- The depth of the water.
- The height and position of the lifeguard station (elevated or at ground level).
- Obstacles in the water, such as people, lane lines and safety lines.
- The location and condition of the victim.
- The type of rescue equipment.
- The design of the facility.

There are several ways to enter the water for a rescue:

- **Slide-in entry.** The slide-in entry is slower than other entries, but it is the safest in most conditions. This technique is useful in shallow water, crowded pools or when a victim with a head, neck or spinal injury is close to the side of the pool or pier.

- **Stride jump.** Use the stride jump only if the water is at least 5 feet deep and you are no more than 3 feet above the water.
- **Compact jump.** You can use the compact jump to enter water from the deck or from a height, depending on the depth of the water. If jumping from a height (when you are more than 3 feet above the water, such as on a lifeguard stand or pier), the water must be at least 5 feet deep.
- **Run-and-swim entry.** To enter the water from a gradual slope—zero-depth area, such as a shoreline or wave pool—use the run-and-swim entry.

Rescue Approaches

The objective of a rescue approach is to safely, quickly and effectively move toward the victim in the water while maintaining control of the rescue tube, keeping the victim in your line of sight. The best way to swim to the victim using a rescue tube is with a modified front crawl or breaststroke (Figure 6-3, A–B). With the rescue tube under your armpits or torso, swim toward the victim with your head up, keeping the rescue tube in control at all times. For long distances or if the rescue tube slips out from under your arms or torso while you are swimming, let the tube trail behind (Figure 6-4).

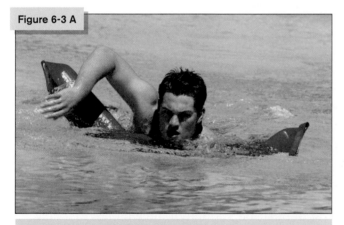

Figure 6-3 A

Modified front crawl approach

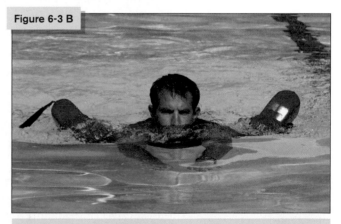

Figure 6-3 B

Modified breaststroke approach

If necessary, reposition the rescue tube in front of you before contacting the victim.

In shallow water, it may be quicker or easier to walk to the victim. Hold the rescue tube at your side and walk quickly toward the victim. If necessary, position the tube in front of you before contacting the victim.

Assists

The objective of an assist is to safely and effectively help a victim who is struggling in the water and move him or her to safety. Assists are the most common way that lifeguards help patrons who are in trouble in shallow water.

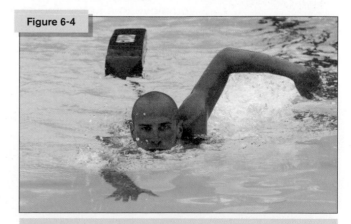

Figure 6-4

Allow the rescue tube to trail behind you when swimming long distances.

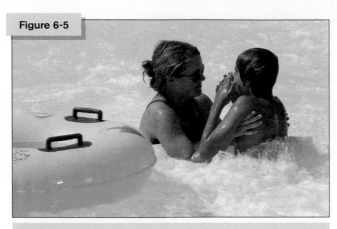

Figure 6-5

Simple assist

An assist may be required to help a patron:

- Stand up because he or she is small or has been thrown off balance, such as by landing at the bottom of a slide (Figure 6-5).
- Get to the surface when he or she is submerged in shallow water.
- Enter and exit an attraction.
- Get in or out of inner tubes or rafts.
- Reach shallow water or a ladder when he or she is tired.

You also may use an assist for a patron who is stuck on a slide or becomes frightened. In this instance, you should climb up the slide to reach the patron and talk to the patron to help calm him or her and provide direction.

If you are stationed in the water, such as when standing in a catch pool, assists can be performed quickly without interrupting patron surveillance. However, if a rescue is needed instead of an assist, activate the EAP.

The most common assists include the:

- **Simple assist.** A simple assist can be used in shallow water and may be merely helping a person to stand. The simple assist also may be used to rescue a victim who is submerged in shallow water and is within reach.
- **Reaching assist from the deck.** To assist a distressed swimmer who is close to the side of the pool or a pier, use a reaching assist from the deck by extending a rescue tube within the victim's grasp. A swimmer in distress usually is able to reach for a rescue device. However, a victim who is struggling to keep his or her mouth above the water's surface in order to breathe may not be able to grab a rescue tube. In this case, you may need to enter the water to rescue the victim using a front or rear victim rescue.

Rescuing a Victim at or Near the Surface

The objective of rescuing a victim at or near the surface of the water is to safely and confidently support the victim using the rescue tube before the victim submerges (Figure 6-6). The victim's airway should remain above the water while you move to a safe removal point, assess the victim's condition and then provide the appropriate care.

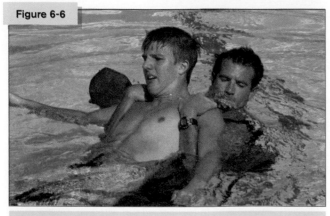

Figure 6-6

Active victim rear rescue

Use the following rescues for victims at or near the surface of the water:

- **Active victim front rescue:** for a drowning victim who is facing toward you
- **Active victim rear rescue:** for a drowning victim who is facing away from you
- **Passive victim rear rescue:** for a drowning victim is who is face-down at or near the surface in a vertical-to-horizontal position, seems unconscious and is not suspected of having a head, neck or spinal injury

Rescuing a Submerged Victim

Sometimes a drowning victim is below the surface. This could be in shallow water or in deep water beyond your reach. The objective in rescuing a submerged victim is to effectively and quickly go under water, make contact with the victim, bring him or her to the surface and support the victim on the rescue tube while maintaining an open airway (Figure 6-7, A–B). Continue to maintain an open airway while moving the victim to a safe exit point, remove the victim, assess the victim's condition and provide appropriate care.

Use the following rescues, based on the victim's position in the water:

■ **Submerged victim in shallow water:** for a victim who is passive, submerged in shallow water and beyond your reach

■ **Submerged victim in deep water:** for a victim who is submerged in deep water

An additional lifeguard may be necessary to provide assistance, especially for a deep water rescue. For example, the additional lifeguard may need to retrieve and position the rescue tube if you had to remove the strap to reach the victim.

In deep water, surface dives enable you to submerge to moderate depths to rescue or search for a submerged victim. When a victim is below the surface, you must be able to get under water or to the bottom using one of the following:

■ **Feet-first surface dive.**
■ **Head-first surface dive.**

Multiple-Victim Rescue

Sometimes two or more victims need to be rescued simultaneously. This may happen, for example, when a victim grabs a nearby swimmer to try to stay above the water (Figure 6-8) or when a parent attempts to rescue a child but is overcome by the child's strength. The objective for this rescue is the same as for any other active victim.

Several lifeguards should assist in a multiple-victim rescue, if possible. At least one lifeguard should check the bottom for possible submerged victims while other lifeguards rescue the victims at the surface.

Removal from Water

At this stage in the rescue, the objective is to safely and effectively remove the victim from the water, taking the victim's condition into account, and to provide the appropriate care. You must

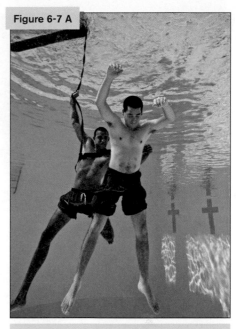
Figure 6-7 A

Rescuing a submerged victim.

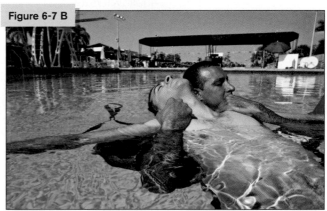
Figure 6-7 B

Bring the victim to the surface while supporting the victim on the rescue tube.

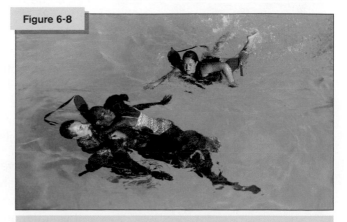
Figure 6-8

Multi-victim rescue

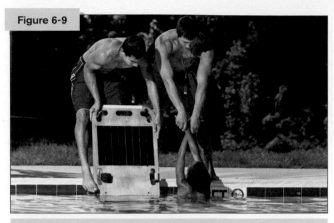

Figure 6-9

Two-person removal from the water using a backboard

keep the victim's airway above the water throughout the removal process (Figure 6-9).

Sometimes a victim is unconscious or too exhausted to climb out of the water, even on a ladder. The decision when and how to remove the victim should be made based on the victim's condition and size, how soon help is expected to arrive and whether a bystander can help. If a victim needs immediate first aid, such as ventilations or CPR, remove him or her from the water immediately and make sure that emergency medical services (EMS) personnel have been summoned. If you suspect that the victim has an injury to the head, neck or spine and the victim is breathing, special removal techniques are used to remove the victim (see Chapter 11, Caring for Head, Neck and Spinal Injuries).

Use one of the following techniques to remove a victim from the water:

- **Two-person removal from the water.** To perform the two-person removal from the water, use a backboard at the side of a pool or pier.
- **Walking assist.** Use the walking assist to help a conscious victim walk out of shallow water.
- **Beach drag.** On a gradual slope from a waterfront beach or zero-depth entry, the beach drag is a safe, easy way to remove someone who is unconscious or who cannot walk from the water. Do not use this technique if you suspect an injury to the head, neck or spine.
- **Front-and-back carry.** In a waterfront beach or zero-depth entry, two rescuers can use the front-and-back carry in shallow water if the person is unconscious or cannot get out of the water without help. Do not use this technique if you suspect an injury to the victim's head, neck or spine.

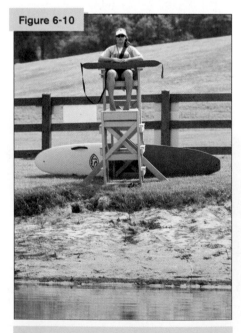

Figure 6-10

Have a rescue board ready for emergency use by the lifeguard stand.

ADDITIONAL RESCUE SKILLS FOR WATERFRONTS

Using a Rescue Board

At some waterfronts, a rescue board is used to patrol the outer boundaries of a swimming area. A rescue board also may be kept by the lifeguard stand, ready for emergency use (Figure 6-10). If the facility uses a rescue board, learn how to carry the board effectively, paddle quickly and maneuver the board in all conditions. Wind, water currents and waves affect how the you will be able to handle the board. Practice using a rescue board often to maintain your skills. Keep the board clean of suntan lotion and body oils, which can make it slippery.

The objective when using a rescue board is to reach the victim quickly, safely make contact, place the victim on the board and return to shore (Figure 6-11). If the victim is unconscious, loading the victim on the rescue board can be challenging. Depending on variables, including distance from shore, the rescue board may not be the most efficient method of rescue. Follow facility protocols for the use of the rescue board. When possible, multiple rescuers should assist in getting the victim to shore. Depending on variables, including distance from shore, the rescue board may not be the most efficient method of rescue. Follow facility protocols for the use of the rescue board.

Several skills are involved when using a rescue board:

- **Approaching a victim on a rescue board**
- **Rescuing an active victim with a rescue board**
- **Rescuing a passive victim with a rescue board**

Using Watercraft for Rescues

If your facility uses watercraft for rescues, you should practice to become skilled in managing them in all rescue situations and all weather conditions. The facility must train lifeguards in the use of the watercraft (Figure 6-12). Refer to the skill sheets at the end of this chapter for general guidelines on the use of various watercraft.

SPECIAL SITUATIONS AT WATERFRONTS

Sightings and Cross Bearings

When a drowning victim submerges at a waterfront, you must swim or paddle to his or her last-seen position. Take a *sighting* or a *cross bearing* to keep track of where the victim went underwater.

To take a sighting:

1. Note where the victim went underwater.
2. Line up this place with an object on the far shore, such as a piling, marker buoy, tree, building or anything that is identifiable. Ideally, the first object should be lined up with a second object on the shore (Figure 6-13). This will help you to maintain a consistent direction when swimming, especially if there is a current.
3. Note the victim's distance from the shore along that line.

With two lifeguards, a cross bearing can be used. To take a cross bearing:

1. Have each lifeguard take a sighting on the spot

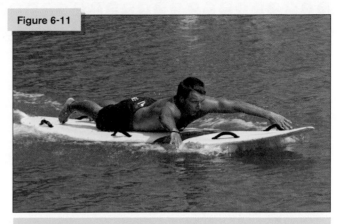

Figure 6-11

A rescue board can be used to rescue victims at a waterfront facility.

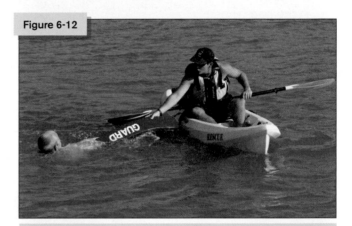

Figure 6-12

A rescue craft, such as a kayak, can be used to rescue victims at a waterfront facility.

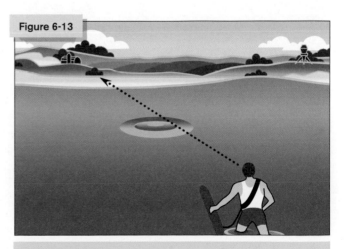

Figure 6-13

Taking a sighting

THROW BAGS

The throw bag, or rescue bag, is a throwing device often carried by paddlers, kayakers and swift-water rescue teams. It also may be used at swimming facilities, particularly in rescue watercraft. The throw bag is a nylon bag that holds a foam disk and coiled line inside. The disk gives the bag its shape and keeps it from sinking, but it does not provide floatation for someone in the water. Some bags have cord locks that are attached to hold the line in the bag. Those should be loosened before use.

To use a throw bag, you should hold the loop at the end of the line in one hand and throw the bag underhand with the other. Try to get the attention of the swimmer before you toss and throw the bag so that the line lands across the victim's shoulder

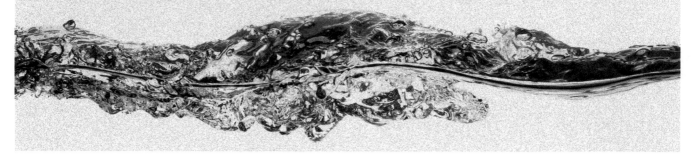

or slightly in front. The line plays out of the bag as it travels through the air. Tell the victim to grab onto the line and hold onto it. Pull the victim to safety. You may use an overhand toss for more distance or to throw over bushes along the shore. As with a ring buoy, always consider wind conditions and water current when using a throw bag.

A throw bag probably is the easiest way to throw a line. It has the advantage of being ready for use at all times. The line is unlikely to tangle during storage or transport. If the first toss misses, then the rope is used as a regular heaving line with weight provided by the bag partially filled with water. It is not easy to quickly re-stuff a wet line for a second throw. With all rescue equipment at a facility, you participate in the in-service training and practice to become proficient in the use of throw bags.

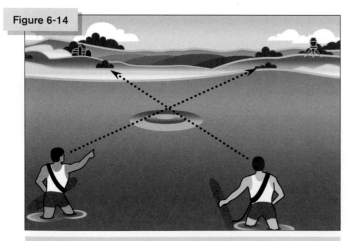

Figure 6-14

Taking a cross bearing

where the victim was last seen from a different angle (Figure 6-14).

2. Ask other people to help out as spotters from shore.

3. Have both lifeguards swim toward the victim along their sight lines.

4. Have both lifeguards check spotters on shore for directions. Spotters communicate with megaphones, whistles or hand signals.

5. Identify the point where the two sight lines cross. This is the approximate location where the victim went underwater.

If a person is reported as missing in or near the water, or you have attempted and are unable to locate a victim after submersion, a search is necessary.

Searching Shallow-Water Areas

To search shallow-water areas where the bottom cannot be seen:

1. Have a lifeguard oversee the search.

2. Ask adult volunteers and staff to link their arms and hold hands to form a line in the water. The shortest person should be in the shallowest water, and the tallest person should be in water no more than chest deep (Figure 6-15).

3. Have the whole line slowly move together across the area, starting where the missing person was last seen.

4. As the line moves forward, have searchers sweep their feet across the bottom with each step. If there is a current, walk downstream with the current. A typical search pattern is shown in Figure 6-16.

5. Have only trained lifeguards search deeper areas.

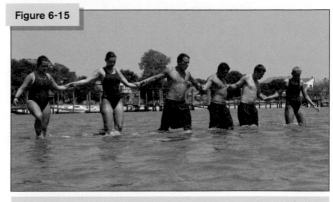

Figure 6-15

Lifeguards performing a shallow-water line search.

Searching Deep-Water Areas

Surface Dives

Feet-first and head-first surface dives enable lifeguards to submerge to moderate depths to search for a submerged victim.

Deep-Water Line Searches

The deep-water line search is used in water greater than chest deep when the bottom cannot be seen from the surface. The search should start at the point where the victim was last seen in the water. This point should be marked on the shoreline.

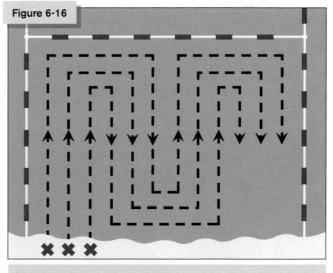

Figure 6-16

Search pattern

1. Wearing masks and fins, several lifeguards form a straight line an arm's length from each other (Figure 6-17).

2. One lifeguard should serve as the safety lookout above the water level on a pier, raft or watercraft with rescue equipment in case a searcher gets in trouble or the missing person is found.

3. On command from the lead lifeguard, all lifeguards perform the same type of surface dive (feet-first or head-first) to the bottom and swim forward a predetermined number of strokes—usually three. If the water is murky, searchers check the bottom by sweeping their hands back and forth in front of them, making sure to cover the entire area. To keep the water from becoming cloudier, try to avoid disturbing silt and dirt on the bottom. Be sure not to miss any areas on the bottom when diving and resurfacing.

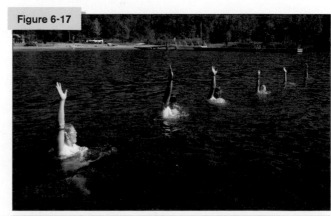

Figure 6-17

Lifeguards performing a deep-water line search.

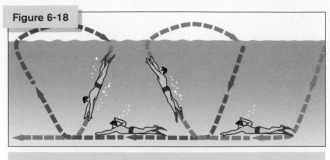

Figure 6-18

Deep-water search pattern

4. Lifeguards should return to the surface as straight up as possible.

5. The lead lifeguard accounts for all searchers, re-forms the line at the position of the person farthest back and backs up the line one body length. On command, the team dives again.

6. Lifeguards repeat this procedure until the victim is found or the entire area has been searched. Figure 6-18 shows one example of a search pattern: lifeguards move the line in one direction to the boundary of the search area, then turn at a 90-degree angle to the first line and repeat the sequence as necessary.

7. If the missing person is not found, lifeguards expand the search to nearby areas. Consider whether currents may have moved the victim.

8. Lifeguards continue to search until the person is found, emergency personnel take over or the search has been called off by officials.

9. If a lifeguard finds the victim, the lifeguard should bring the victim up by grasping the victim under the armpit and returning to the surface. Swim the victim to safety, keeping the victim on his or her back, with his or her face out of the water. A lifeguard with equipment should take over to maintain an open airway while moving the victim to safety. Remove the victim from the water, assess the victim's condition and provide appropriate care.

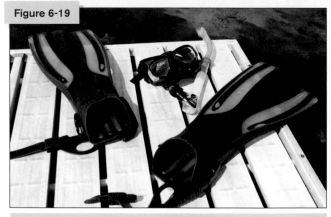

Figure 6-19

Mask and fins

Mask and Fins

A mask and fins should be used in an underwater search for a missing person at a waterfront (Figure 6-19). Use well-maintained equipment that is sized properly and fits you well.

Mask

A mask is made of soft, flexible material, with non-tinted, tempered safety glass and a head strap that is easily adjusted. Choose a mask that allows blocking or squeezing of the nose to equalize pressure. Some masks have additional features, such as molded nosepieces or purge valves. Regardless of the design, a proper fit is essential: a good fit prevents water from leaking into the mask. Each lifeguard at a waterfront facility should have a mask that fits his or her face.

To check that a mask fits properly:

1. Place the mask against your face without using the strap. Keep hair out of the way.

2. Inhale slightly through your nose to create a slight suction inside the mask. This suction should keep the mask in place without being held.

3. Adjust the strap so that the mask is comfortable. The strap should be placed on the crown of the head for a proper fit. If it is too tight or too loose, the mask may not seal properly.

4. Try the mask in the water. If it leaks a little, adjust how the strap sits on the back of your head and tighten the strap if needed. If the mask continues to leak, check it again with suction. A different size may be needed if the leaking persists.

To prevent the mask from fogging, rub saliva on the inside of the face plate and rinse the mask before putting it on. Commercial defoggers also can be used.

If your mask starts to fill with water while you are submerged, you can remove the water by pressing the palm of one hand against the top of your mask, which loosens the bottom seal. At the same time, blow air out of your nose and tilt your head slightly to push the water out. Alternatively, you can pull the bottom of the mask away from your face to break the seal, ensuring that the top part still is firm against your face, and blow air out of your nose. If your mask has a purge valve, blow air out of your nose and excess water exits via the purge valve.

Fins

Fins provide more speed and allow users to cover greater distances with less effort. A good fit is important for efficient movement. Fins come in different sizes to fit the foot; the blades also differ in size. Fins with larger blades enable the person to swim faster but require more leg strength. Fins should match your strength and swimming ability. Each lifeguard at a waterfront facility should have fins that fit his or her feet.

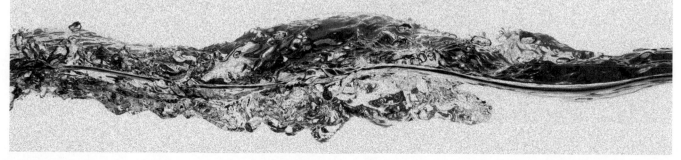

EQUALIZING PRESSURE UNDERWATER

As you descend into deep water, water pressure increases and presses against the empty spaces in your skull, especially those inside your ears. This can cause pain or even injury. To relieve this pressure, you need to force more air into the empty spaces so that the air pressure matches the water pressure. This is called "equalizing." Be sure that you equalize early and often by taking the following steps:

1. Place your thumb and finger on your nose or on the nosepiece of your mask if you are wearing one.

2. Pinch your nose and keep your mouth shut. Try to exhale gently through your nose until the pressure is relieved.

3. Repeat this as needed to relieve ear pressure. If your ears hurt, do not attempt to go deeper until successfully equalizing the pressure.

4. If you are using a mask when descending, the increased water pressure will cause the mask to squeeze your face. To relieve the squeezing, exhale a small amount of air through your nose into the mask.

If you are unable to equalize the pressure because of a head cold or sinus problem, you should return to the surface rather than risk an injury.

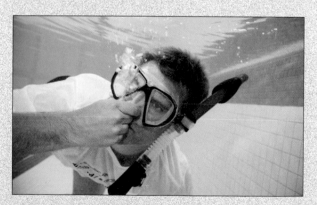

Wetting your feet and the fins first makes it easier to put them on. Do not pull the fins on by the heels or straps of the fins. This can cause a break or tear. Push your foot into the fin, and then slide the fin's back or strap up over your heel.

Use a modified flutter kick when swimming with fins. The kicking action is deeper and slower, with a little more knee bend, than the usual flutter kick. Swimming underwater is easier if you use your legs only, not your arms; keep your arms relaxed at your side. In murky water, hold your arms out in front to protect your head and feel for the victim.

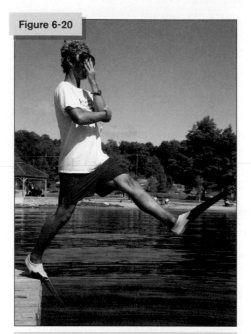

Figure 6-20

Stepping out with a long stride to enter the water when using a mask and fins.

Entering the Water with Mask and Fins

It is important to learn how to enter the water safely while wearing equipment. You should enter using a slide-in entry or with a stride jump when entering from a height of less than 3 feet. Never enter head-first wearing a mask and fins. If entering the water from a sloping beach, carry the fins until you are thigh-deep in the water and then put them on.

To do a stride jump with mask and fins:

1. Put one hand over the mask to hold it in place, keeping your elbow close to your chest. Keep your other hand at your side.

2. Make sure no swimmers or other objects are below.

3. Step out with a long stride over the water but do not lean forward (Figure 6-20). The fins will slow your downward motion as you enter the water.

4. Swim keeping your arms at the side and face in the water or hold your arms out in front to protect your head if visibility underwater is poor.

WHEN THINGS DO NOT GO AS PRACTICED

Even with the best preparations and practice, circumstances sometimes may require you to deviate from your facility's EAP during an emergency. The skills in this section are designed to help you deal with some of those situations that may affect your safety or could significantly delay life saving care. Your facility must determine under what circumstances these additional emergency skills can be used. Skill sheets are located at the end of the chapter.

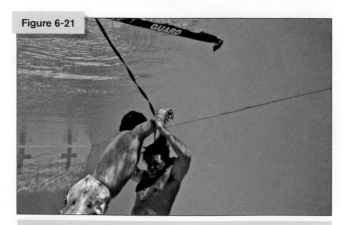

Figure 6-21

Front head-hold escape

Escapes

A drowning victim may grab you if your technique is faulty or if the rescue tube slips out of position (Figure 6-21). You should always hold onto the rescue tube because it helps both you and the victim stay afloat. However, if you lose control of the tube and a victim grabs you, use one of the following skills to escape:

- **Front head-hold escape:** when the victim grabs you from the front.

- **Rear head-hold escape:** when the victim grabs you from behind.

COLD WATER

A serious concern at many waterfront facilities is someone suddenly entering into cold water—water that is 70 [or 77]° F (21 [or 25]° C) or lower. This usually happens in one of two ways: a person falls in accidentally, or a person enters intentionally without proper protection. In some cases, a swimmer may be underwater in warmer water and suddenly enter a *thermocline*, a sharp change in temperature from one layer of water to another.

As a general rule, if the water feels cold, consider it to be cold. Cold water can have a serious effect on a victim and on the lifeguard making the rescue.

Sudden entry into cold water may cause the following negative reactions:

- A *gasp reflex*, a sudden involuntary attempt to "catch one's breath," may cause the victim to inhale water into the lungs if the face is underwater.

- If the person's face is not underwater, he or she may begin to hyperventilate. This can cause unconsciousness and lead to breathing water into the lungs.

- An increased heart rate and blood pressure can cause cardiac arrest.

- A victim who remains in the cold water may develop *hypothermia*, (below-normal body temperature), which can cause unconsciousness.

However, the body has several natural mechanisms that may help to increase the person's chances of survival. In cold water, body temperature begins to drop almost as soon as the person enters the water. If cold water is swallowed, the cooling is accelerated. When a person remains in cold water, the body's core temperature drops and body functions slow almost to a standstill, sharply decreasing the need for oxygen. Any oxygen in the blood is diverted to the brain and heart to maintain minimal functioning of these vital organs. Because of this response, some victims have been successfully resuscitated after being submerged in cold water for an extended period.

Rescues in Cold Water

It is important to locate and remove a victim from cold water as quickly as possible. Because you also will be affected by cold water, you should attempt the rescue without entering the water, if possible.

You can extend a rescue tube to reach the victim, but the victim might not be able to maintain a hold on the equipment because his or her hands and arms are numb from the cold.

If you must enter the water, take a rescue tube attached to a towline. A *line-and-reel*, which is a buoyant piece of rope or cord attached to rescue equipment, may be used to tow the lifeguard and the victim to safety. Wear body protection, such as a wetsuit, gloves, booties and hood, if possible.

When the victim is out of the water, assess his or her condition. Victims who have been submerged in cold water still may be alive even with:

- A decreased or undetectable pulse rate.
- No detectable breathing.
- Bluish skin that is cold to the touch.
- Muscle rigidity.

Begin giving ventilations or CPR, as needed, and provide first aid for hypothermia as soon as possible. The sooner the victim receives advanced medical care, the better the chances are for survival.

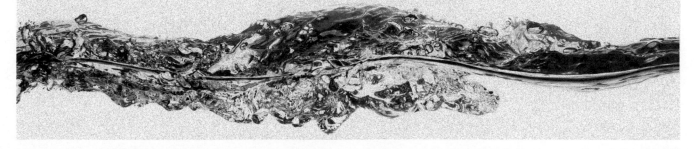

In-Water Ventilations

Always remove a victim who is not breathing from the water as soon as possible to provide care. However, if you cannot immediately remove the victim or if doing so will delay care, then perform in-water ventilations (Figure 6-22). Once conditions allow you to remove the victim from the water, stop ventilations, remove the victim and then resume care immediately.

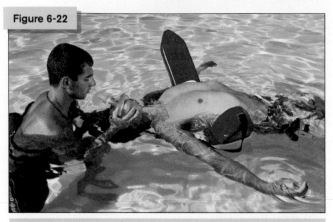

Figure 6-22

Perform in-water ventilations if the victim cannot be removed immediately or if doing so will delay care.

Quick Removal from Shallow Water for a Small Victim

If you have rescued a passive or unconscious person who is smaller than you and a backboard is not immediately available, you may be able to lift the victim out of the water. Simply place the victim on the side, get yourself out of the water and begin providing care. Do not use this technique if you suspect a spinal injury but the victim is breathing and a backboard is on the way.

WRAP-UP

You must learn and practice water rescue skills so you will be able to effectively respond to aquatic emergencies. However, it is just as important that you to know how to adapt these skills to the actual circumstances encountered during a real-world situation. Emergencies can happen quickly, and conditions can change in an instant. In an emergency, you should perform the rescue, bring the victim to a safe exit point, remove the victim from the water and provide the appropriate care. Never jeopardize your own safety, always use rescue equipment (such as a rescue tube) and keep your eye on the ultimate objective—saving the victim's life.

ENTRIES

Slide-In Entry

1 Sit down on the edge facing the water. Place the rescue tube next to you or in the water.

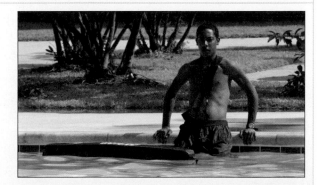

2 Lower your body into the water feet-first.

3 Retrieve the rescue tube.

4 Place the rescue tube across your chest with the tube under your armpits, focus on the victim and begin the approach.

Stride Jump

1 Squeeze the rescue tube high against your chest with the tube under your armpits.

2 Hold the excess line to keep the line from getting caught on something when jumping into the water.

3 Leap into the water with one leg forward and the other leg back.

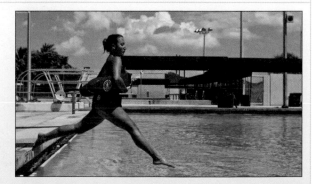

4 Lean slightly forward, with your chest ahead of your hips, and focus on the victim when you enter the water.

Continued on Next Page ▶

ENTRIES *continued*

Stride Jump *continued*

| 5 | Squeeze or scissor your legs together right after they make contact with the water for upward thrust. |

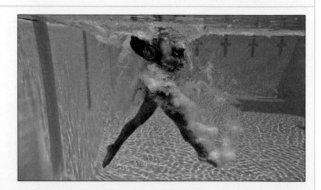

| 6 | Focus on the victim and begin the approach. |

Note: *Use the stride jump only if the water is more than 5 feet deep and you are no more than 3 feet above the water. You may need to climb down from an elevated lifeguard station and travel on land before entering the water.*

Compact Jump

| 1 | Squeeze the rescue tube high against your chest with the tube under your armpits. |

| 2 | Hold the excess line to keep it from getting caught in the lifeguard chair or other equipment when jumping into the water. |

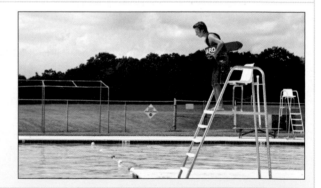

| 3 | Jump out and away from the lifeguard chair, pool deck or pier. In a wave pool, time the jump to land on the crest (top) of a wave. |

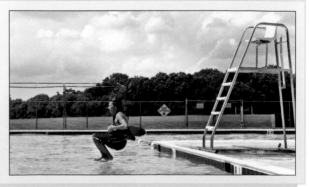

4 Bend your knees and keep your feet together and flat to absorb the shock if you hit the bottom. Do not point your toes or keep your legs straight or stiff.

5 Let the buoyancy of the rescue tube bring you back to the surface.

6 Focus on the victim when surfacing and begin the approach.

Note: *If you are more than 3 feet above the water, the water must be at least 5 feet deep. It may not be safe to enter the water from an elevated lifeguard stand if your zone is crowded or as a result of the design or position of the stand. You may need to climb down before entering the water.*

Run-and-Swim Entry

1 Hold the rescue tube and the excess line and run into the water, lifting your knees high to avoid falling.

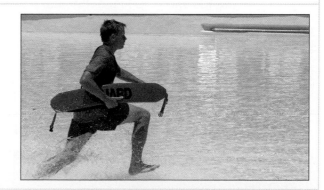

2 When you can no longer run, either put the rescue tube across your chest and lean forward or drop the tube to the side and start swimming, letting the rescue tube trail behind. Do not dive or plunge head-first into the water; this could cause a serious head, neck or spinal injury.

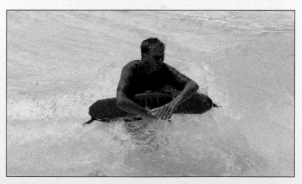

ASSISTS

Simple Assist

1 Approach the person who needs help while keeping the rescue tube between you and that person.

2 Reach across the tube and grasp the person at the armpit to help the person maintain his or her balance.

- If the person is underwater, grasp the person under the armpits with both hands and help him or her stand up.

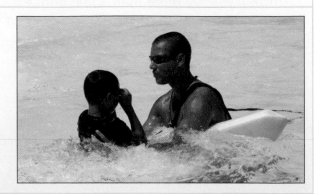

3 Assist the person to the exit point, if necessary.

Reaching Assist from the Deck

1 Extend the tube to the victim, keeping your body weight on your back foot and crouching to avoid being pulled into the water.

- Remove the rescue tube strap from your shoulder if necessary to reach the victim and hold the shoulder strap in one hand and extend the tube to the victim with the other hand.

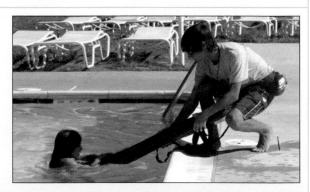

2 Tell the victim to grab the rescue tube.

3 Slowly pull the victim to safety.

Note: *A swimmer in distress generally is able to reach for a rescue device. However, a victim who is struggling to keep his or her mouth above the water's surface to breathe may not be able to grab a rescue tube. In those cases, you may need to enter the water to rescue the victim using a front or rear victim rescue.*

RESCUES AT OR NEAR THE SURFACE OF THE WATER

Active Victim Front Rescue

1 Approach the victim from the front.

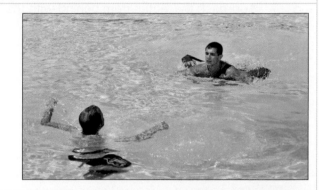

2 As you near the victim, grab the rescue tube from under your arms with both hands and begin to push the tube out in front of you. Continue kicking to maintain momentum.

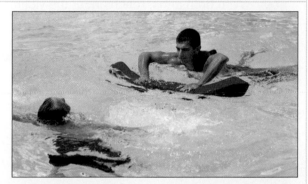

3 Thrust the rescue tube slightly under water and into the victim's chest, keeping the tube between you and the victim. Encourage the victim to grab the rescue tube and hold onto it.

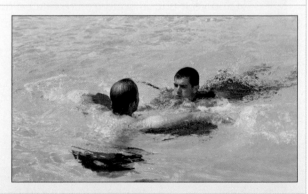

4 Keep kicking, fully extend your arms and move the victim to a safe exit point. Change direction, if needed.

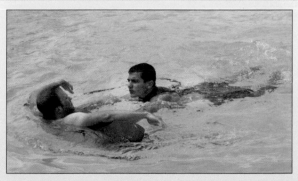

RESCUES AT OR NEAR THE SURFACE OF THE WATER *continued*

Active Victim Rear Rescue

1 Approach the victim from behind with the rescue tube across your chest.

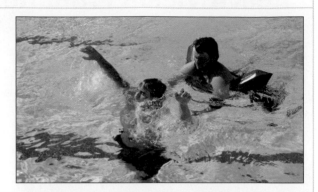

2 With both arms, reach under the victim's armpits and grasp the shoulders firmly. Tell the victim that you are there to help and continue to reassure the victim throughout the rescue.

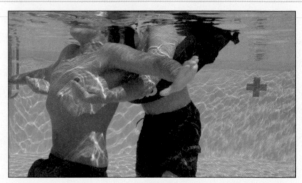

3 Using your chest, squeeze the rescue tube between your chest and the victim's back.

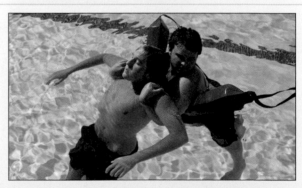

4 Keep your head to one side to avoid being hit by the victim's head if it moves backwards.

5 Lean back and pull the victim onto the rescue tub.

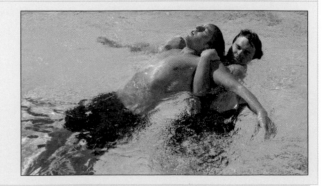

6 | Use the rescue tube to support the victim so that the victim's mouth and nose are out of the water.

7 | Tow the victim to a safe exit point.

Passive Victim Rear Rescue

1 | Approach a face-down victim from behind with the rescue tube across your chest.

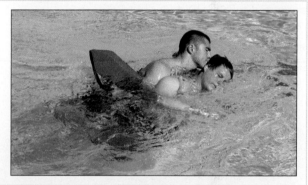

2 | With both arms, reach under the victim's armpits and grasp the shoulders firmly. You may be high on the victim's back when doing this.

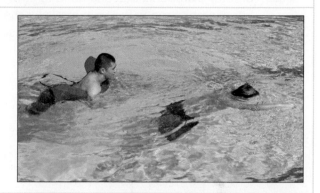

3 | Using your chest, squeeze the rescue tube between your chest and the victim's back.

4 | Keep your head to one side to avoid being hit by the victim's head if it moves backwards.

5 | Roll the victim over by dipping your shoulder and rolling onto your back so that the victim is face-up on top of the rescue tube. Keep the victim's mouth and nose out of the water. Place the tube under the victim below the shoulders so that the victim's head naturally falls back to an open-airway position.

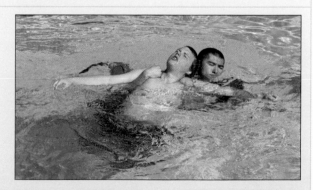

Continued on Next Page

RESCUES AT OR NEAR THE SURFACE OF THE WATER *continued*

Passive Victim Rear Rescue *continued*

6 Tow the victim to a safe exit point. For greater distances, use one hand to stroke. For example, reach the right arm over the victim's right shoulder and grasp the rescue tube. Then use the left hand to stroke.

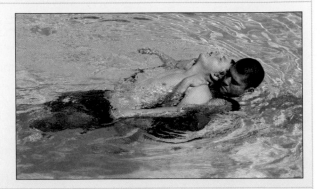

7 Remove the victim from the water, assess the victim's condition and provide appropriate care.

MULTIPLE-VICTIM RESCUE

If you are the only lifeguard rescuing two victims who are clutching each other:

1 Approach one victim from behind.

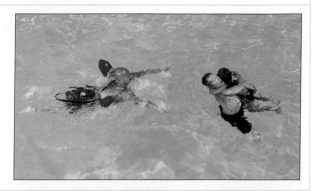

2 With both arms, reach under the victim's armpits and grasp the shoulders. Squeeze the rescue tube between your chest and the victim's back, keeping your head to one side of the victim's head.

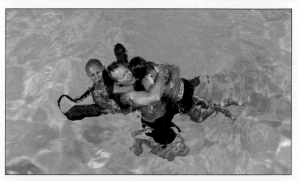

3 Use the rescue tube to support both victims with their mouths and noses out of the water. Talk to the victims to help reassure them.

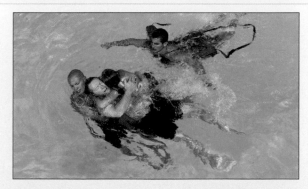

4 Support both victims until other lifeguards arrive or the victims become calm enough to assist with moving to a safe exit point.

Note: *Whenever possible, more than one rescuer should assist with a multiple-victim rescue.*

RESCUING A SUBMERGED VICTIM

Submerged Victim in Shallow Water

1 Swim or quickly walk to the victim's side. Let go of the rescue tube but keep the strap around your shoulders.

2 Submerge and reach down to grab the victim under the armpits.

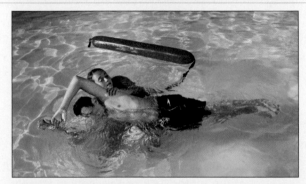

3 Simultaneously pick up the victim, move forward and roll the victim face-up once surfaced.

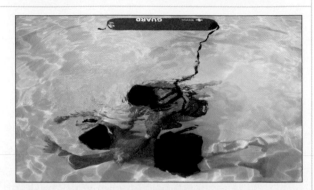

4 Grab the rescue tube and position it under the victim's shoulders. The victim's head should fall back naturally into an open-airway position. If an assisting lifeguard is there with the backboard, skip this step and proceed to remove the victim from the water.

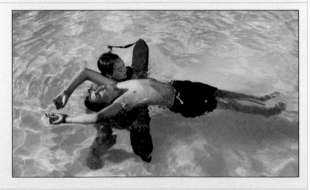

5 Move the victim to a safe exit point, remove the victim from the water, assess the victim's condition and provide appropriate care.

Tip: *If the water depth is shallow enough, you can use the simple assist to lift the victim to the surface, then position him or her on the rescue tube, if needed, to complete the rescue.*

Feet-First Surface Dive

1 Swim to a point near the victim. Release the rescue tube but keep the strap around your shoulders.

2 Position your body vertically, then at the same time press both hands down to your sides and kick strongly to raise your body out of the water.

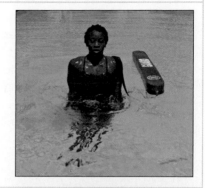

3 Take a breath, then let your body sink underwater as you begin to extend your arms outward with palms upward, pushing against the water to help you move downward. Keep your legs straight and together with toes pointed. Tuck your chin and turn your face to look down toward the bottom.

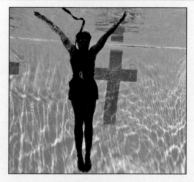

4 As downward momentum slows, repeat the motion of extending your arms outward and sweeping your hands and arms upward and overhead to go deeper.

5 Repeat this arm movement until you are deep enough to reach the victim.

Tips:

- *Do not release all of the air in your lungs while you are submerging; instead, exhale gently. Save some air for your return to the surface.*
- *As you descend into deep water, be sure to equalize pressure early and often.*

RESCUING A SUBMERGED VICTIM *continued*

Feet-First Surface Dive *continued*

If you must swim underwater, such as for a deep-water line search, also perform the following steps:

1 When deep enough to reach the victim, tuck your body and roll to a horizontal position.

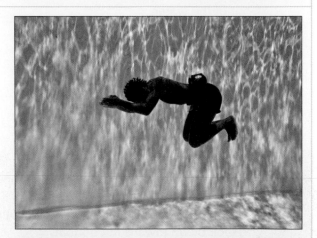

2 Extend your arms and legs and swim underwater.

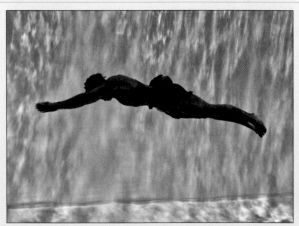

Head-First Surface Dive

1 Swim to a point near the victim and release the rescue tube.

2 Gain momentum using a swimming stroke.

3 Take a breath, sweep your arms backwards to your thighs and turn them palms-down.

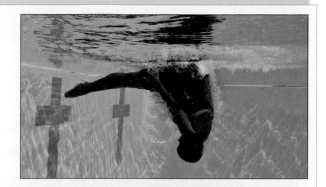

4 Tuck your chin to your chest and flex at the hip sharply while your arms reach downward toward the bottom.

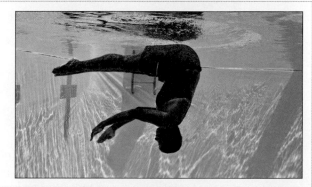

5 Lift your legs upward, straight and together so that their weight above the water helps the descent. Get in a fully extended, streamlined body position that is almost vertical.

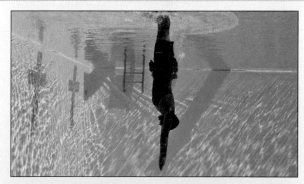

6 If you need to go deeper, such as for a deep-water line search, do a simultaneous arm pull with both arms to go deeper, then level out and swim forward underwater.

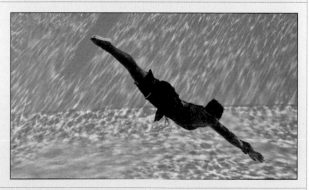

Tips:

■ *If the depth of the water is unknown or the water is murky, hold one or both arms extended over the head toward the bottom or use a feet-first surface dive.*

■ *As you descend into deep water, be sure to equalize pressure early and often.*

RESCUING A SUBMERGED VICTIM *continued*

Submerged Victim in Deep Water

1 Perform a feet-first surface dive, and position yourself behind the victim.

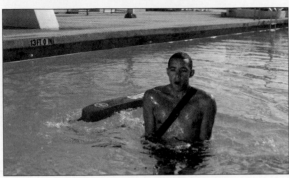
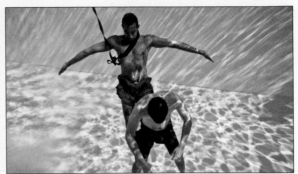

2 Reach one arm under the victim's arm (right arm to right side or left arm to left side) and across the victim's chest. Hold firmly onto the victim's opposite side.

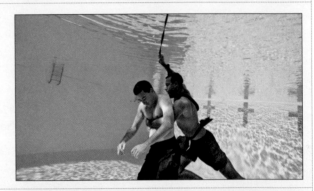

3 Once you have hold of the victim, reach up with your free hand and grasp the towline. Pull it down and place it in the same hand that is holding the victim. Keep pulling the towline this way until nearing the surface.

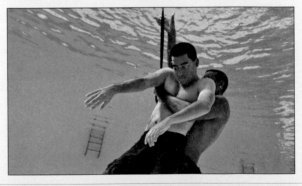

4 As you surface, tilt the victim back so that he or she is face-up. Grasp and position the rescue tube so that it is squeezed between your chest and the victim's back. If a victim is passive, place the tube below the victim's shoulders so the victim's head naturally falls back into an open-airway position. However, if the victim is active and begins to struggle, you will need to grasp tighter.

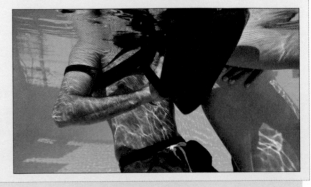

5 Reach your free arm over the tube and under the victim's armpit. Grasp his or her shoulder firmly (right arm to right shoulder or left arm to left shoulder).

6 Move your other arm from across the victim's chest and grasp the victim's shoulder firmly.

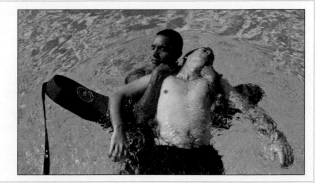

7 Tow the victim to a safe exit point. Remove the victim from the water, assess the victim's condition and provide appropriate care.

Tip: *Depending on the depth of the water, use one of the following techniques:*

- *If you must remove the strap from your shoulder to descend and reach the victim, continue to hold onto the strap so that the rescue tube can be used to help bring the victim to the surface.*

- *If the victim is deeper than the length of the strap and towline, release the strap and towline, grasp the victim, push off the bottom (if possible) and kick to the surface. Once at the surface, place the rescue tube in position behind the victim and continue the rescue.*

- *If you have released the strap of the rescue tube, it might not be within reach when you return to the surface. An additional lifeguard responding to your EAP signal should assist by placing the rescue tube in position so that you can continue the rescue. If this is not possible, you may need to move to safety without the rescue tube.*

REMOVAL FROM THE WATER

Two-Person Removal from the Water Using a Backboard

1 The primary lifeguard brings the victim to the side and turns him or her to face the wall. Another lifeguard brings a backboard with the head immobilizer and the straps removed, if possible.

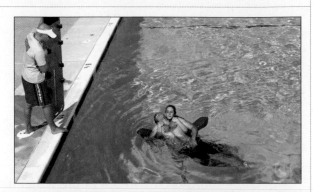

2 The lifeguard on land crosses his or her hands to grab the victim's wrists and pulls the victim up slightly to keep the head above the water and away from the wall. Support the victim's head so that the head does not fall forward.

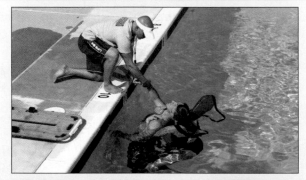

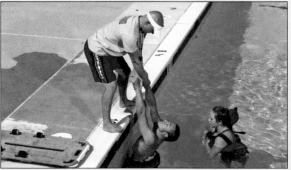

3 The primary lifeguard ensures that the victim's face is out of the water and climbs out of the water, removes the rescue tube and gets the backboard.

4 The primary lifeguard guides the backboard, foot-end first, down into the water along the wall next to the victim. The second lifeguard then turns the victim onto the backboard. Each lifeguard then quickly grasps one of the victim's wrists and one of the handholds of the backboard.

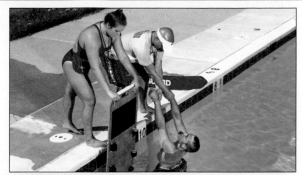

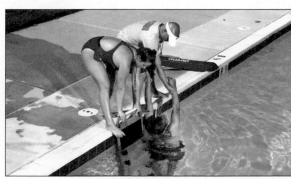

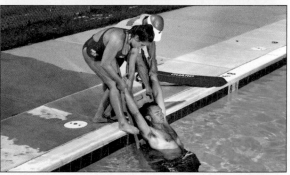

5 When the primary lifeguard gives the signal, both lifeguards pull the backboard and victim onto land, resting the underside of the board against the edge. (Remember to lift with the legs and not with the back.) The lifeguards step backward and then carefully lower the backboard onto the ground. If other lifeguards or additional help is available, they can provide assistance by pulling or pushing the backboard.

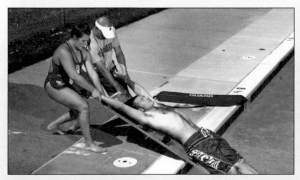

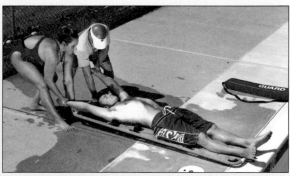

6 Lifeguards provide immediate and appropriate care based on the victim's condition. Continue care until EMS personnel arrive and assume control over the victim's care.

Tips:

- *It may be easier to submerge the board initially if the board is angled, foot-end first, toward the wall.*

- *As soon as the board is submerged, turn the victim onto the board then allow the board to float up beneath the victim.*

- *Once the board is submerged, the second lifeguard can help to stabilize the board against the wall, placing his or her foot against the backboard, if necessary.*

REMOVAL FROM THE WATER *continued*

Walking Assist

1 Place one of the victim's arms around your neck and across your shoulder.

2 Grasp the wrist of the arm that is across your shoulder. Wrap your free arm around the victim's back or waist to provide support.

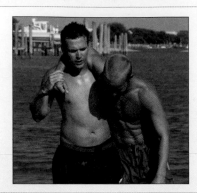

3 Hold the victim firmly and assist him or her in walking out of the water.

4 Have the victim sit or lie down while you monitor his or her condition.

Beach Drag

1 Stand behind the victim and grasp him or her under the armpits, supporting the victim's head as much as possible with your forearms. Let the rescue tube trail behind, being careful not to trip on the tube or line. If another lifeguard is available to assist, each of you should grasp the victim under an armpit and support the head.

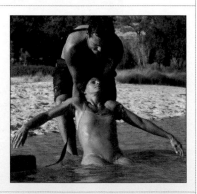

2 Walk backward and drag the victim to the shore. Use your legs, not your back.

3 Remove the victim completely from the water, then assess the victim's condition and provide appropriate care.

Front-and-Back Carry

1 From behind the victim, one lifeguard reaches under the victim's armpits. This lifeguard grasps the victim's right wrist with his or her right hand, and the victim's left wrist with his or her left hand. The lifeguard then crosses the victim's arms across the his or her chest.

2 The second lifeguard stands between the victim's legs, facing the victim's feet. This lifeguard bends down and grasps the victim under the knees. On signal, both lifeguards lift the victim and carry him or her out of the water while walking forward.

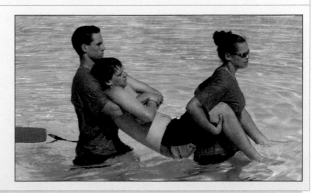

USING A RESCUE BOARD

Approaching a Victim on a Rescue Board

1 Hold onto the sides of the board, about mid-board when entering the water.

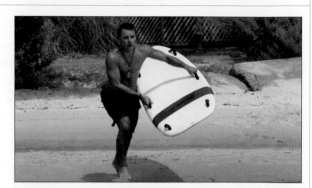

2 When the water is knee-deep, lay the rescue board on the water and push it forward. Climb on just behind the middle and lie down in the prone position. If needed, place your foot into the water to help steer. For better balance, place a foot on either side of the rescue board in the water.

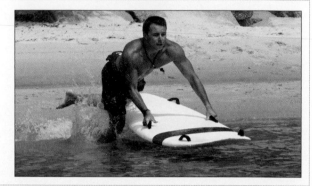

3 Paddle with the front of the board toward the victim using either a front-crawl or a butterfly arm stroke. If you need to change to a kneeling position to better see the victim, paddle a few strokes before moving on the board.

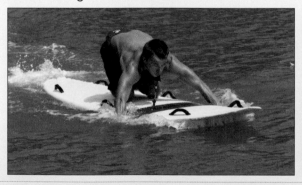

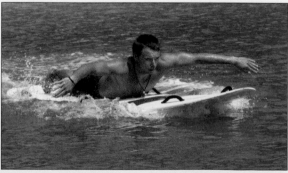

4 Continue paddling with your head up and the victim in your sight until you reach the victim.

Rescuing an Active Victim with a Rescue Board

1 Approach the victim from the side so that the side of the rescue board is next to the victim.

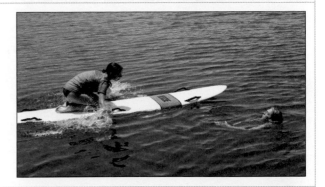

2 Grasp the victim's wrist and slide off of the rescue board on the opposite side.

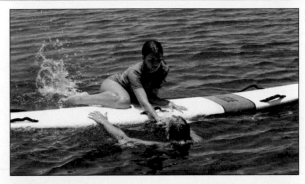

3 Help the victim to reach his or her arms across the rescue board. Encourage the victim to relax while you kick to turn the board toward shore.

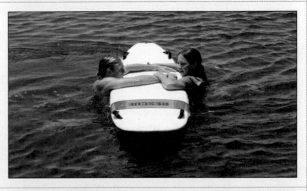

4 Stabilize the rescue board and help the victim onto the board.

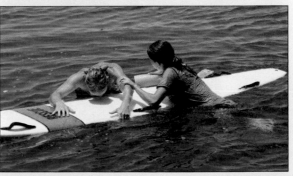

5 Tell the victim to lie on his or her stomach, facing the front of the board.

Continued on Next Page

USING A RESCUE BOARD *continued*

Rescuing an Active Victim with a Rescue Board *continued*

6 Carefully climb onto the board from the back with your chest between the victim's legs. Take care to avoid tipping the rescue board and keep your legs in the water for stability.

7 Paddle the rescue board to shore.

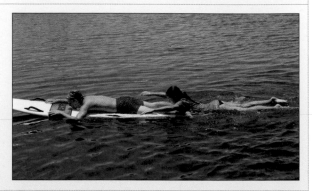

8 Slide off of the board and help the victim off of the board onto shore with a walking assist.

Rescuing a Passive Victim with a Rescue Board

To rescue someone who is unconscious or cannot hold onto or climb onto the rescue board:

1 Approach the victim from the side. Position the rescue board so that the victim is slightly forward of the middle of the rescue board.

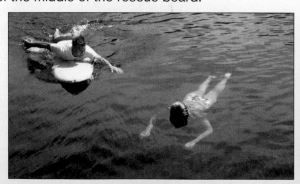
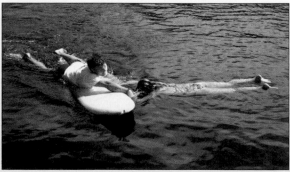

2 Grasp the victim's hand or wrist and slide off of the board on the opposite side, flipping the rescue board over toward you. Hold the victim's arm across the board with the victim's chest and armpits against the far edge of the board.

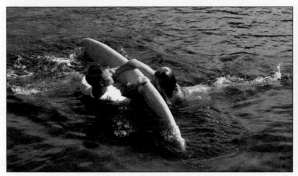
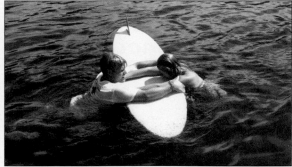

3 Grasp the far edge of the rescue board with the other hand.

4 Kneel on the edge of the rescue board using your own body weight to flip the board toward you again. Catch the victim's head as the rescue board comes down.

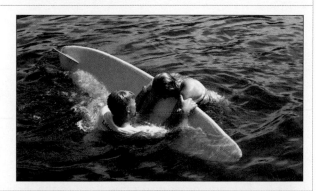

5 Position the victim lying down lengthwise in the middle of the rescue board with the victim's head toward the front of the rescue board.

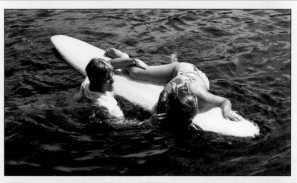

6 Kick to turn the board toward shore. Carefully climb onto the board from the back with your chest between the victim's legs. Be careful not to tip the rescue board and keep your legs in the water for stability.

7 Paddle the rescue board to shore.

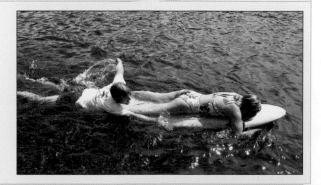

Continued on Next Page

USING A RESCUE BOARD *continued*

Rescuing a Passive Victim with a Rescue Board *continued*

8	Help the victim to safety with the beach drag or other removal technique.

Tips:

- *Make sure that the victim's armpits are along the edges of the board before flipping the board.*
- *Use caution when flipping the board to ensure that the victim's armpits, and not the upper arms, remain along the edge of the board during the flip.*

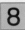 # USING WATERCRAFT FOR RESCUES

Using a Square Stern Rowboat for Rescues

1	Extend an oar or rescue tube to the victim and pull him or her to the center of the stern (rear) of the craft. This is the most stable area on which to hold.	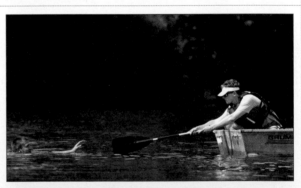
2	If the victim cannot hold the oar or rescue tube, move the stern close to the victim and grasp the victim's wrist or hand and pull him or her to the stern.	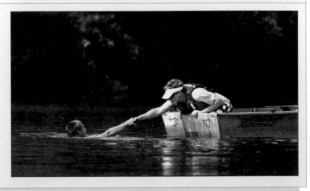

3 Have the victim hold onto the stern while you move the watercraft to safety. Be sure that his or her mouth and nose remains above water.

4 If the victim needs to be brought onto the craft, help the victim over the stern and move the watercraft to safety.

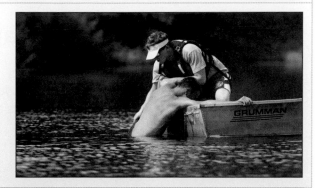

Using a Motorized Watercraft for Rescues

1 Always approach the victim from downwind and downstream.

2 Shut off the engine about three boat-lengths from the victim and coast or paddle to the victim.

3 Bring the victim on board before restarting the engine.

Using a Kayak for Rescues

1 Extend the rescue tube to a distressed swimmer or active victim.

2 Instruct the victim to hold onto the rescue tube while you paddle to shore.

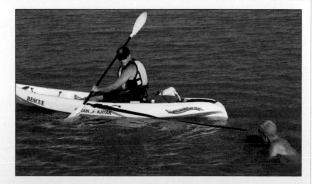

3 Ensure that the victim continues to hold the tube and that his or her mouth and nose remain above water as you paddle.

WHEN THINGS DO NOT GO AS PRACTICED

Front Head-Hold Escape

1 As soon as the victim grabs hold, take a quick breath, tuck your chin down, turn your head to either side, raise your shoulders and submerge with the victim.

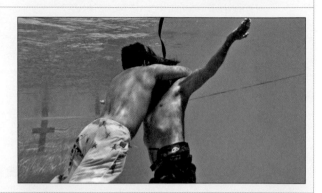

2 Once underwater, grasp the victim's elbows or the undersides of the victim's arms just above the elbows. Forcefully push up and away. Keep your chin tucked, your arms fully extended and your shoulders raised until you are free.

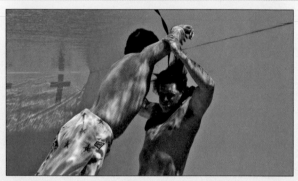

3 Quickly swim underwater, out of the victim's reach. Surface and reposition the rescue tube and try the rescue again.

Rear Head-Hold Escape

1 Take a quick breath, tuck your chin down, turn your head to either side, raise your shoulders and submerge with the victim.

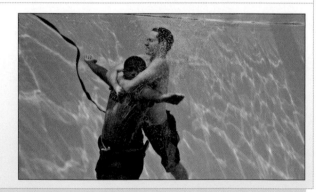

2 Once underwater, grasp the victim's elbows or the undersides of the victim's arms just above the elbows. Forcefully push up and away while twisting your head and shoulders. Keep your chin tucked, your arms fully extended and your shoulders raised until you are free.

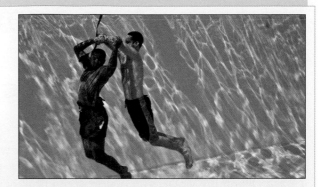

3 Quickly swim underwater, out of the victim's reach. Surface and reposition the rescue tube and try the rescue again.

In-Water Ventilations

1 Ensure that the rescue tube is placed under the victim so that his or her airway falls into an open position.

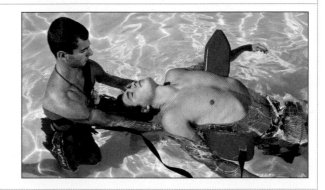

2 From behind the victim's head, position the assembled resuscitation mask.

■ If you are in deep water, perform the skill with support from the rescue tube.

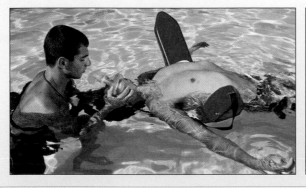 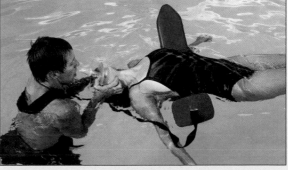

3 Give ventilations.

4 Remove the victim from the water as soon as conditions allow, then immediately resume providing care.

WHEN THINGS DO NOT GO AS PRACTICED
continued

Quick Removal from Shallow Water for a Small Victim

To remove a small passive victim from shallow water if a backboard is not immediately available:

1 Bring the victim to the side of the pool or pier into shallow water.

2 Maintain contact with the victim by rotating the victim on his or her back into the crook of your arm. Be sure to support the head above the surface of the water. Place your other arm under the victim's knees.

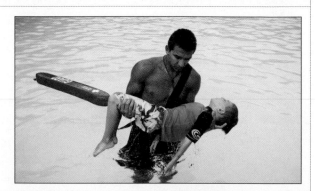

3 Lift the victim carefully and place him or her on the pool deck, pier or dock.

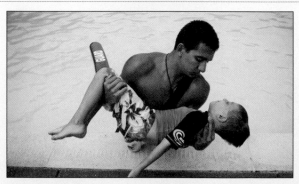

4 Exit the water, assess the victim's condition and provide the appropriate care.

Notes:

- *If the victim must be moved to provide further care, place the victim on a backboard with the assistance of another rescuer.*

- *Do not use this technique if you suspect a spinal injury, the victim is breathing and a backboard is on the way.*

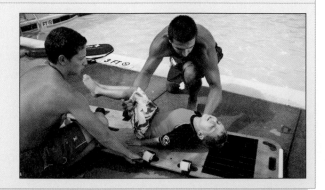

Before Providing Care and Victim Assessment

A fter you rescue a victim from the water, your next steps are to identify any life-threatening conditions by performing a primary assessment and providing care. You also will need to perform a primary assessment if a victim is injured or becomes ill on land. While caring for a victim, it is crucial that you protect yourself and others from the transmission of infectious disease.

In this chapter, you will learn how infectious diseases occur and how you can prevent them from spreading. This chapter also covers the general procedures for responding to sudden illness and injury on land. ■

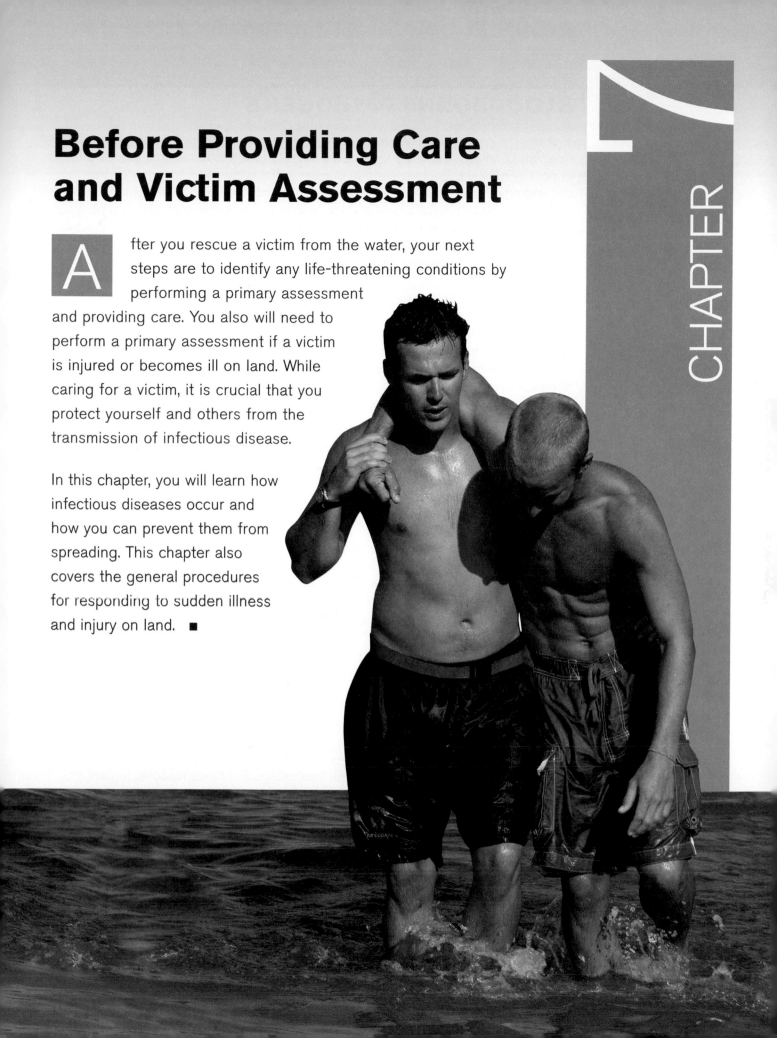

BLOODBORNE PATHOGENS

Bloodborne pathogens, such as bacteria and viruses, are present in blood and body fluids and can cause disease in humans. Pathogens are found almost everywhere in our environment. Bacteria can live outside of the body and commonly do not depend on other organisms for life. If a person is infected by bacteria, antibiotics and other medications often are used to treat the infection. Viruses depend on other organisms to live. Once viruses are in the body, they are difficult to kill. This is why prevention is critical. The bloodborne pathogens of primary concern to lifeguards are the hepatitis B virus, hepatitis C virus and HIV (Table 7-1).

Hepatitis B

Hepatitis B is a liver infection caused by the hepatitis B virus. Hepatitis B may be severe or even fatal; the hepatitis B virus can live in the body for up to 6 months before symptoms appear. These may include flu-like symptoms such as fatigue, abdominal pain, loss of appetite, nausea, vomiting and joint pain. *Jaundice* (yellowing of the skin and eyes) is a symptom that occurs in the later stage of the disease.

Medications are available to treat chronic hepatitis B infection, but they do not work for everyone. The most effective means of prevention is the hepatitis B vaccine. This vaccine, which is given in a series of three doses, provides immunity to the disease. Scientific data show that hepatitis B vaccines are safe for adults, children and infants. Currently, no evidence exists indicating that hepatitis B vaccine causes chronic illnesses.

Your employer must make the hepatitis B vaccination series available to you because you could be exposed to the virus at work. The vaccination must be made available within 10 working days of initial assignment, after appropriate training has been completed. However, you can choose to decline the vaccination series. If you decide not to be vaccinated, you must sign a form affirming your decision.

Hepatitis C

Hepatitis C is a liver disease caused by the hepatitis C virus. Hepatitis C is the most common chronic bloodborne infection in the United States. The symptoms are similar to those for hepatitis B infection and include fatigue, abdominal pain, loss of appetite, nausea, vomiting and jaundice. Currently, no vaccine exists against hepatitis C and no treatment is available to prevent infection after exposure. Hepatitis C is the leading cause of liver transplants. For these reasons, hepatitis C is considered to be more serious than hepatitis B.

HIV

HIV is the virus that causes AIDS. HIV attacks white blood cells and destroys the body's ability to fight infection. This weakens the body's immune system. The infections that strike people whose immune systems are weakened by HIV are called *opportunistic infections.* Some opportunistic infections include severe pneumonia, tuberculosis, Kaposi's sarcoma and other unusual cancers.

People infected with HIV may not feel or look sick initially. A blood test, however, can detect the HIV antibody. When an infected person has a significant drop in a certain type of white blood cells or shows signs of having certain infections or cancers, he or she may be diagnosed as having AIDS. These infections can cause fever, fatigue, diarrhea, skin rashes, night sweats, loss of appetite, swollen lymph glands and significant weight loss. In the advanced stages, AIDS is a very serious condition. People with AIDS eventually develop life-threatening infections and can die from these infections. Currently, there is no vaccine against HIV.

There are many other illnesses, viruses and infections to which you may be exposed. Keep immunizations current, have regular physical check-ups and be knowledgeable about other pathogens. For more information on the illnesses listed above and other diseases and illnesses of concern, contact the Centers for Disease Control and Prevention (CDC) at 800-342-2437 or go to cdc.gov.

Table 7-1: How Bloodborne Pathogens Are Transmitted

Disease	Signs and Symptoms	Mode of Transmission	Infectious Material
Hepatitis B	Fatigue, abdominal pain, loss of appetite, nausea, vomiting, joint pain, jaundice	Direct and indirect contact	Blood, saliva, vomitus, semen
Hepatitis C	Fatigue, dark urine, abdominal pain, loss of appetite, nausea, jaundice	Direct and indirect contact	Blood, saliva, vomitus, semen
HIV	Symptoms may or may not appear in the early stage; late-contact-stage symptoms may include fever, fatigue, diarrhea, skin rashes, night sweats, loss of appetite, swollen lymph glands, significant weight loss, white spots in the mouth or vaginal discharge (signs of yeast infection) and memory or movement problems	Direct and possibly indirect contact	Blood, saliva, vomitus, semen, vaginal fluid, breast milk

HOW PATHOGENS SPREAD

Exposures to blood and other body fluids occur across a wide variety of occupations. Lifeguards, health care providers, emergency medical services (EMS) personnel, public safety personnel and other workers can be exposed to blood through injuries from needles and other sharps devices, as well as by direct and indirect contact with skin and mucous membranes. For any disease to be spread, including bloodborne diseases, all four of the following conditions must be met:

- A pathogen is present.
- A sufficient quantity of the pathogen is present to cause disease.
- A person is susceptible to the pathogen.
- The pathogen passes through the correct entry site (e.g., eyes, mouth and other mucous membranes, non-intact skin, or skin pierced by needlesticks, animal and human bites, cuts, abrasions and other means).

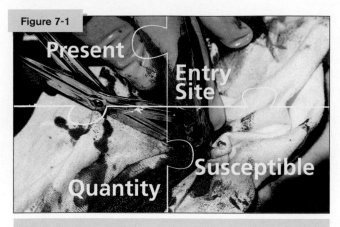

How pathogens spread

To understand how infections occur, think of these four conditions as pieces of a puzzle (Figure 7-1). All of the pieces must be in place for the picture to be complete. If any one of these conditions is missing, an infection cannot occur.

At the workplace, bloodborne pathogens, such as hepatitis B virus, hepatitis C virus and HIV, are spread primarily through direct or indirect contact with infected blood or other body fluids. These viruses are not spread by food or water or by casual contact, such as hugging or shaking hands. The highest risk of transmission while at work is unprotected direct or indirect contact with infected blood.

Direct Contact

Direct contact transmission occurs when infected blood or body fluids from one person enters another person's body. For example, direct contact transmission can occur through infected blood splashing in the eye or from directly touching the body fluids of an infected person with a hand that has an open sore (Figure 7-2).

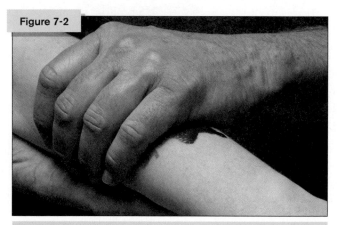

Direct contact

Indirect Contact

Some bloodborne pathogens also can be transmitted by indirect contact (Figure 7-3). *Indirect contact transmission* can occur when a person touches an object that contains the blood or other body fluid of an infected person and that infected blood or other body fluid enters the body through a correct entry site. These objects include soiled dressings, equipment and work surfaces that have been contaminated with an infected person's blood or other body fluids. For example, indirect contact can occur when a person picks up blood-soaked bandages with a bare hand, and the pathogens enter through a break in the skin on the hand.

Droplet and Vector-Borne Transmission

Other pathogens, such as the flu virus, can enter the body through *droplet transmission*. This occurs when a person inhales droplets from an infected person's cough or sneeze (Figure 7-4). *Vector-borne transmission* of diseases occurs when the body's skin is penetrated by an infectious source, such as an animal or insect bite or sting (Figure 7-5). Examples of diseases spread through vector-borne transmission include malaria and West Nile virus.

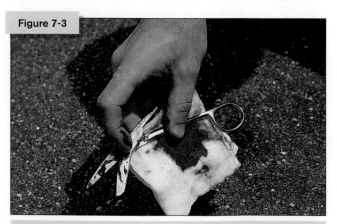

Indirect contact

Risk of Transmission

Hepatitis B, hepatitis C and HIV share a common mode of transmission—direct or indirect contact with infected blood or other body fluids—but they differ in the risk of transmission. Individuals who have received the hepatitis B vaccine and have developed immunity to the virus have virtually no risk for infection by the hepatitis B virus. For an unvaccinated person, the risk for infection from hepatitis B-infected blood from a needlestick or cut exposure can be as high as 30 percent, depending on several factors. In contrast, the risk for infection from hepatitis C-infected blood after a needlestick or cut exposure is about 2 percent, and the risk of infection from HIV-infected blood after a needlestick or cut exposure is less than 1 percent.

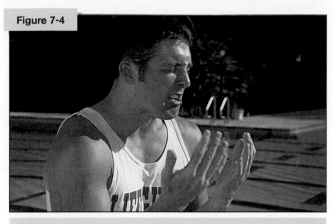

Figure 7-4

Droplet transmission

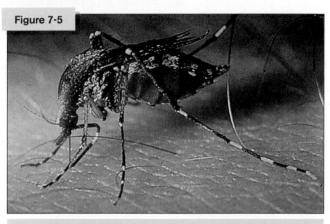

Figure 7-5

Vector-borne transmission

PREVENTING THE SPREAD OF BLOODBORNE PATHOGENS

OSHA Regulations

The federal Occupational Safety and Health Administration (OSHA) issued regulations about on-the-job exposure to bloodborne pathogens. OSHA determined that employees are at risk when they are exposed to blood or other body fluids. Employers should follow OSHA requirements regarding job-related exposure to bloodborne pathogens, which are designed to protect you from disease transmission. This includes reducing or removing hazards from the workplace that may place employees in contact with infectious materials, including how to safely dispose of needles.

OSHA regulations and guidelines apply to employees who may come into contact with blood or other body substances that could cause an infection. These regulations apply to lifeguards because, as professional rescuers, lifeguards are expected to provide emergency care as part of their job. These guidelines can help lifeguards and their employers meet the OSHA bloodborne pathogens standard to prevent transmission of serious diseases. For more information about the OSHA Bloodborne Pathogens Standard 29 CFR 1910.1030 and the Needlestick Safety and Prevention Act, go to osha.gov.

Exposure Control Plan

OSHA regulations require employers to have an exposure control plan. This is a written program outlining the protective measures that employers will take to eliminate or minimize employee exposure incidents. The plan also should detail how the employer will meet other OSHA requirements, such as recordkeeping. The exposure control plan guidelines should be made available to lifeguards and should specifically explain what they need to do to prevent the spread of infectious diseases.

Standard Precautions

Standard precautions are safety measures that combine universal precautions and body substance isolation (BSI) precautions and are based on the assumption that all body fluids may be infectious. Standard precautions can be applied though the use of:

- Personal protective equipment (PPE).
- Good hand hygiene.
- Engineering controls.
- Work practice controls.
- Proper equipment cleaning.
- Spill clean-up procedures.

EMPLOYERS' RESPONSIBILITIES

OSHA's regulations on bloodborne pathogens require employers to protect employees in specific ways including:

- Identifying positions or tasks covered by the standard.
- Creating an exposure control plan to minimize the possibility of exposure and making the plan easily accessible to employees.
- Developing and putting into action a written schedule for cleaning and decontaminating the workplace.
- Creating a system for easy identification of soiled material and its proper disposal.
- Developing a system of annual training for all covered employees.
- Offering the opportunity for employees to get the hepatitis B vaccination at no cost to them.

- Establishing clear procedures to follow for reporting an exposure.
- Creating a system of recordkeeping.
- In workplaces where there is potential exposure to injuries from contaminated sharps, soliciting input from nonmanagerial employees with potential exposure regarding the identification, evaluation and selection of effective engineering and work practice controls.
- If a needlestick injury occurs, recording the appropriate information in the sharps injury log, including:
  o Type and brand of device involved in the incident.
  o Location of the incident.
  o Description of the incident.
- Maintaining a sharps injury log in a way that protects the privacy of employees.
- Ensuring confidentiality of employees' medical records and exposure incidents.

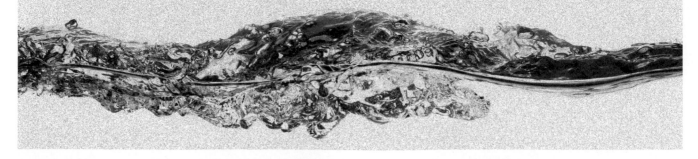

Personal Protective Equipment

PPE appropriate for your job duties should be available at your workplace and should be identified in the exposure control plan. PPE includes all specialized clothing, equipment and supplies that prevent direct contact with infected materials (Figure 7-6). These include, but are not limited to, breathing barriers, non-latex disposable (single-use) gloves, gowns, masks, shields and protective eyewear (Table 7-2).

Table 7-2: **Recommended Personal Protective Equipment Against Hepatitis B, Hepatitis C and HIV Transmission in Prehospital Settings**				
Task or Activity	**Disposable Gloves**	**Gown**	**Mask**	**Protective Eyewear**
Bleeding control with spurting blood	Yes	Yes	Yes	Yes
Bleeding control with minimal bleeding	Yes	No	No	No
Emergency childbirth	Yes	Yes	Yes	Yes
Oral/nasal suctioning; manually clearing airway	Yes	No	No, unless splashing is likely	No, unless splashing is likely
Handling and cleaning contaminated equipment and clothing	Yes	No, unless soiling is likely	No	No

U.S. Department of Health and Human Services, Public Health Services, 1989. A curriculum guide for public safety and emergency response workers: Prevention of transmission of acquired immunodeficiency virus and hepatitis B virus. Atlanta: U.S. Department of Health and Human Services, Centers for Disease Control and Prevention. With modifications from Nixon, Robert G., 1999. Communicable diseases and infection control for EMS, Prentice Hall.

Guidelines for using PPE to prevent infection include the following:

- Avoid contact with blood and other body fluids.
- Use CPR breathing barriers when giving ventilations to a victim.
- Wear disposable gloves when providing care, particularly if there is a risk of coming into contact with blood or other body fluids.
  - Do not use gloves that are discolored, torn or punctured. Do not clean or reuse disposable gloves.
  - Cover any cuts, scrapes or sores and remove jewelry, including rings, before wearing disposable gloves.
  - Avoid handling items such as pens, combs or radios when wearing soiled gloves.
  - Change gloves before providing care to a different victim.

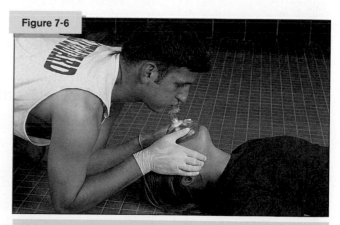

Figure 7-6

Personal protectice equipment includes breathing barriers and gloves.

■ In addition to gloves, wear protective coverings, such as a mask, eyewear and a gown, when there is a likelihood of coming in contact with blood or other body fluids that may splash.

■ Remove disposable gloves without contacting the soiled part of the gloves and dispose of them in a proper container. See the skill sheet located at the end of the chapter for steps to removing gloves properly.

Tip: *To put gloves on with wet hands if near the pool, fill the gloves with water and place your hand inside the glove.*

Hand Hygiene

Hand washing is the most effective measure to prevent the spread of infection. Wash your hands before providing care, if possible, so that they do not pass pathogens to the victim. Wash your hands frequently, such as before and after eating, after using the restroom and every time you have provided care. By washing hands often, you can wash away disease-causing germs that have been picked up from other people, animals or contaminated surfaces.

To wash your hands correctly, follow these steps:

1. Wet your hands with warm water.
2. Apply liquid soap to your hands.
   o Rub your hands vigorously for at least **15** seconds, covering all surfaces of your hands and fingers, giving added attention to fingernails and jewelry.
3. Rinse your hands with warm, running water.
4. Dry your hands thoroughly with a disposable towel.
5. Turn off the faucet using the disposable towel.

Alcohol-based hand sanitizers and lotions allow you to cleanse your hands when soap and water are not readily available and your hands are not visibly soiled. If your hands contain visible matter, use soap and water instead. When using an alcohol-based hand sanitizer:

■ Apply the product to the palm of one hand.

■ Rub your hands together.

■ Rub the product over all surfaces of your hands, including nail areas and between fingers, until the product dries.

■ Wash your hands with antibacterial hand soap and water as soon as they are available.

In addition to washing your hands frequently, it is a good idea to keep your fingernails shorter than ¼ inch and avoid wearing artificial nails.

Engineering Controls and Work Practice Controls

Engineering controls are objects used in the workplace that isolate or remove a hazard, thereby reducing the risk of exposure. Examples of engineering controls include:

■ Biohazard bags and labels.

■ PPE.

■ Sharps disposal containers (Figure 7-7).

■ Self-sheathing needles.

Figure 7-7

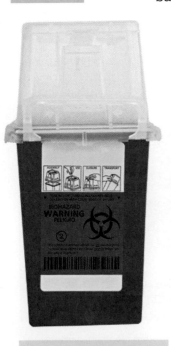

Sharps disposal container

- Safer medical devices, such as sharps with engineered injury protections or needleless systems.

Work practice controls are methods of working that reduce the likelihood of an exposure incident by changing the way a task is carried out. Examples of work practice controls include:

- Disposing of sharp items (e.g., broken glass) in puncture-resistant, leak-proof, labeled containers.

- Avoiding splashing, spraying and splattering droplets of blood or other potentially infectious materials when performing all procedures.

- Removing and disposing of soiled protective clothing as soon as possible.

- Cleaning and disinfecting all equipment and work surfaces soiled by blood or other body fluids.

- Using good hand hygiene.

- Not eating, drinking, smoking, applying cosmetics or lip balm, handling contact lenses, or touching the eyes, mouth or nose when in an area where exposure to infectious materials is possible.

- Isolating contaminated areas so other employees or people do not walk through and become exposed.

Be aware of any areas, equipment or containers that may be contaminated. Biohazard warning labels are required on any container holding contaminated materials, such as used gloves, bandages or trauma dressings. Signs should be posted at entrances to work areas where infectious materials may be present.

Equipment Cleaning and Spill Clean-Up

After providing care, you should clean and disinfect the equipment and surfaces. In some cases, you will need to properly dispose of certain equipment. Handle all soiled equipment, supplies and other materials with care until they are properly cleaned and disinfected (Figure 7-8). Place all used disposable items in labeled containers. Place all soiled clothing in marked plastic bags for disposal or washing (Figure 7-9). Commercial blood spill kits are available.

Take the following steps to clean up spills:

- Wear disposable gloves and other PPE.

- Clean up spills immediately or as soon as possible after the spill occurs.

- Rope off or place cones around the area so others do not accidentally get exposed by walking through the spill.

- If the spill is mixed with sharp objects, such as broken glass and needles, do not pick these

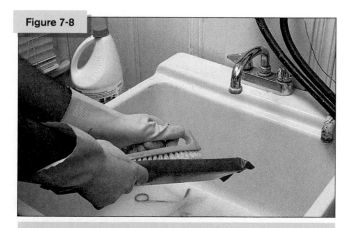

Figure 7-8

Clean and disinfect all equipment after use.

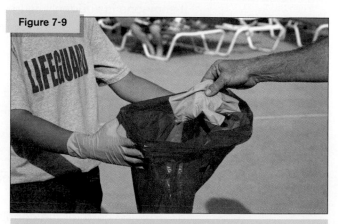

Figure 7-9

Use a biozhazard bag to dispose of soiled materials.

up with your hands. Use tongs, a broom and dustpan or two pieces of cardboard.

- Flood the area with a fresh disinfectant solution of approximately 1½ cups of liquid chlorine bleach to 1 gallon of water (1 part bleach per 9 parts water, or about a 10 percent solution), and allow it to stand for at least 10 minutes.

- Use appropriate material to absorb the solution and dispose of it in a labeled biohazard container.

- Scrub soiled boots, leather shoes and other leather goods, such as belts, with soap, a brush and hot water. If you wear a uniform to work, wash and dry it according to the manufacturer's instructions.

IF YOU ARE EXPOSED

If you are exposed to a bloodborne pathogen, take the following steps immediately:

- Clean the contaminated area thoroughly with soap and water. Wash needlestick injuries, cuts and exposed skin.

- If you are splashed with blood or other potentially infectious material around your mouth or nose, flush the area with water.

- If your eyes are involved, irrigate them with clean water, saline or sterile irrigants for 20 minutes.

Following any exposure incident:

- Report the exposure incident to the appropriate supervisor immediately and to the EMS personnel when they take over the care of the victim. This step can be critical to receive appropriate post-exposure treatment.

- Document what happened. Include the time and date of the exposure as well as the circumstances of the exposure, any actions taken after the exposure and any other information required by your employer.

- Seek immediate follow-up care as identified in your facility exposure control plan.

GENERAL PROCEDURES FOR INJURY OR SUDDEN ILLNESS ON LAND

If someone is suddenly injured or becomes ill, activate the facility's emergency action plan (EAP). Use appropriate first aid equipment and supplies and follow these general procedures:

1. Size up the scene.
   o Move the victim only if necessary for his or her safety.
2. Perform a primary assessment.
   o Obtain consent if the victim is conscious.
3. Summon EMS, if needed.
4. Perform a secondary assessment, if no life-threatening conditions are found.
5. Provide care for the conditions found.
6. Report, advise and release.

Size-Up the Scene

When you size-up the scene, your goal is to determine if the scene is safe for you, other lifeguards, EMS personnel, the victim(s) and any bystanders. You should:

- Use your senses to check for hazards that could present a danger to you or the victim, such as unusual odors that would indicate a gas leak or fire, sights that would indicate anything out of the ordinary or sounds, such as an explosion.
- Determine what caused the injury or the nature of the illness.
- Determine the number of injured or ill victims.
- Determine what additional help may be needed.
- Put on the appropriate PPE.

If the scene appears to be unsafe, move to a safe distance, notify additional members of the safety team and wait for their arrival.

Moving a Victim

When an emergency occurs in the water, you must remove the victim from the water so that you can provide care. However, for emergencies on land, you should care for the victim where he or she is found.

Ideally, when a victim is on land, you should move him or her only after you have conducted an assessment and provided care. Moving a victim needlessly can lead to further pain and injury. Move an injured victim on land only if:

- You are faced with immediate danger.
- You need to get to other victims who have more serious injuries or illnesses.
- It is necessary to provide appropriate care (e.g., moving a victim to the top or bottom of a flight of stairs to perform CPR).

If you must leave a scene to ensure your personal safety, you must make all attempts to move the victim to safety as well.

Your safety is of the utmost importance. Lifting and moving a victim requires physical strength and a high level of fitness. If you improperly lift a victim, you can permanently injure yourself.

When moving a victim, consider the victim's height and weight; your physical strength; obstacles, such as stairs and narrow passages; distance to be moved; availability of others to assist; victim's condition; and the availability of transport aids.

To improve your chances of successfully moving a victim without injuring yourself or the victim:

- Lift with your legs, not your back. Keep your legs shoulder-width apart, head up, back straight and shoulders square.
- Avoid twisting or bending anyone who has a possible head, neck or spinal injury.
- Do not move a victim who is too large for you to move comfortably.
- Walk forward when possible, taking small steps and looking where you are going.

There are several ways to move a victim. Non-emergency moves include:

- **Walking assist.** Either one or two responders can use the walking assist for a conscious person who simply needs assistance to walk to safety.

- **Two-person seat carry.** The two-person seat carry requires a second responder. This carry can be used for any person who is conscious and not seriously injured.

Emergency moves include:

- **Clothes drag.** The clothes drag can be used to move a conscious or unconscious person suspected of having a head, neck or spinal injury. This move helps to keep the person's head, neck and back stabilized.
- **Pack-strap carry.** The pack-strap carry can be used with conscious and unconscious people. Using this carry with an unconscious person requires a second responder to help position the injured or ill person on your back.
- **Ankle drag.** Use the ankle drag (also known as the foot drag) to move a person who is too large to carry or move in any other way.

Perform a Primary Assessment

Conduct a primary assessment to determine if the victim has any life-threatening conditions and, if so, summon EMS personnel. The primary assessment includes checking the victim for responsiveness, breathing and a pulse, and scanning for severe bleeding.

Check the Victim for Responsiveness

A person who can speak is conscious. Remember, if a person is conscious, you must obtain consent before providing care. Document any refusal of care by the victim on an incident or rescue report. If a witness is available, have him or her listen, and document in writing, any refusal of care.

If an adult or child appears to be unresponsive, tap the victim on the shoulder and shout, "Are you okay?" If an infant appears to be unresponsive, tap the infant's shoulder and shout or flick the bottom of the infant's foot to see if he or she responds.

Summon EMS Personnel

If you are unsure of the victim's condition or notice that the condition is worsening, summon EMS personnel. As a general rule, summon EMS personnel for any of the following conditions:

- Unconsciousness or altered level of consciousness (LOC), such as drowsiness or confusion
- Breathing problems (difficulty breathing or no breathing)
- Any victim recovered from underwater who may have inhaled water
- Chest pain, discomfort or pressure lasting more than a few minutes or that goes away and comes back or that radiates to the shoulder, arm, neck, jaw, stomach or back
- Persistent abdominal pain or pressure
- No pulse
- Severe external bleeding (bleeding that spurts or gushes steadily from a wound)
- Vomiting blood or passing blood
- Severe (critical) burns
- Suspected poisoning

- Seizures in the water
- Seizures on land, unless the person is known to have periodic seizures. If not, summon EMS personnel for a seizure on land if:
  - ○ The seizure lasts more than 5 minutes.
  - ○ The person has repeated seizures with no sign of slowing down.
  - ○ The person appears to be injured.
  - ○ The cause of the seizure is unknown.
  - ○ The person is pregnant.
  - ○ The person is known to have diabetes.
  - ○ The person fails to regain consciousness after the seizure.
  - ○ The person is elderly and may have had a stroke.
  - ○ This is the person's first seizure.
- Suspected or obvious injuries to the head, neck or spine
- Stroke
- Painful, swollen, deformed areas (suspected broken bone) or an open fracture
- Victim's physical condition is unclear or is worsening

Open the Airway and Check for Breathing and Pulse

You must open the victim's airway and quickly check for breathing and a pulse for no more than **10** seconds (Figure 7-10). Perform these tasks concurrently. If a victim is able to speak, the airway is functional and he or she is breathing. However, even if a victim can speak, you must continue to assess breathing because breathing status, rate and quality can change suddenly.

Figure 7-10

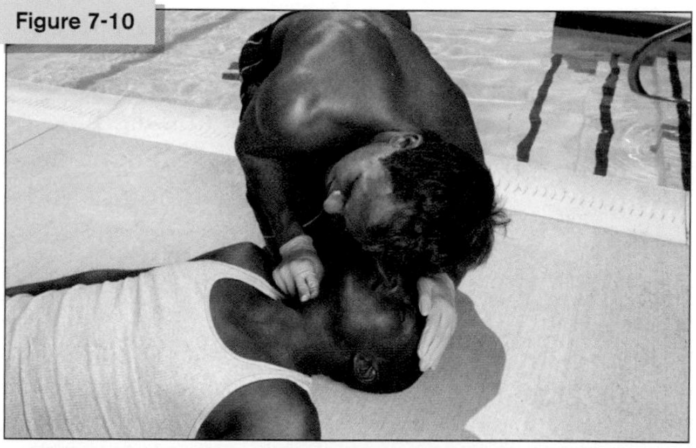

When conducting a primary assessment, first open the victim's airway and check for breathing and a pulse for no more than 10 seconds.

Opening the Airway

When a victim is unconscious, the tongue relaxes and can block the flow of air through the airway, especially if the victim is lying on his or her back. To check for breathing and give ventilations, you must manually tilt the head or thrust the jaw to move the tongue away from the back of the throat. The method used to open the airway depends on the number of rescuers responding, the position of the rescuer to the victim, and whether you suspect the victim has an injury to the head, neck or spine. The three methods for opening the airway are the:

- **Head-tilt/chin-lift:** used when the rescuer is positioned at the victim's side
- **Jaw-thrust maneuver (with head extension):** used when the rescuer is positioned above the victim's head
- **Jaw-thrust maneuver (without head extension):** used when the victim is suspected of having an injury to the head, neck or spine

For a child, tilt the head slightly past the neutral position, but not as far as you would for an adult. For an infant, tilt the head to the neutral position (Table 7-3).

Table 7-3: Head Positions for Giving Ventilations to an Adult, a Child and an Infant

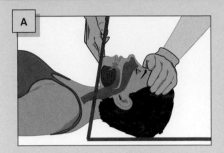 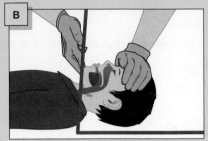 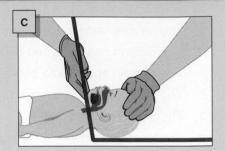

Correct head position using the head-tilt/chin-lift technique for (A) an adult, (B) a child and (C) an infant

Checking for Breathing

To check for breathing, position your ear over the mouth and nose so that you can hear and feel air as it escapes while you look for the chest to rise and fall. Normal, effective breathing is regular, quiet and effortless. Isolated or infrequent gasping in the absence of other breathing in an unconscious person may be *agonal gasps*, which can occur even after the heart has stopped beating. Be aware that this is not breathing. In this situation, care for the victim as though he or she is not breathing at all. If there is foam (white or pinkish in color) in the airways and exuding from the mouth and nostrils, wipe it away.

Checking for a Pulse

With every heartbeat, a wave of blood moves through the blood vessels. This creates a beat called the pulse. You can feel it with your fingertips in the arteries near the skin. Sometimes the pulse may be difficult to find, since it may be slow or weak. If you do not find a pulse within 10 seconds, do not waste any more time attempting to find one. Assume that there is no pulse and begin care immediately.

To check for a pulse:

- For an adult or child, feel for a carotid pulse by placing two fingers in the middle of the victim's throat and then sliding them into the groove at the side of the victim's neck closest to you. Press in lightly; pressing too hard can compress the artery.

- For an infant, feel for the brachial pulse on the inside of the upper arm between the infant's elbow and shoulder. Press in lightly; pressing too hard can compress the artery.

Give 2 Ventilations if Appropriate

For victims of cardiac arrest (witnessed sudden collapse), it is necessary to immediately begin CPR chest compressions. However, in certain situations, such as drowning or another respiratory event, giving ventilations before beginning CPR is important because children and infants, as well as adult victims of hypoxia, are more likely to experience respiratory emergencies.

For adults:

- If you find an adult who is unconscious and not breathing as a result of drowning, hypoxia or another respiratory problem, you should give the victim

2 ventilations before starting compressions (see Chapter 8, Breathing Emergencies, for further information on breathing emergencies).

- However, if an adult is not breathing and does not have a pulse, you should assume that the problem is a cardiac emergency. In this case, skip the 2 ventilations and begin CPR chest compressions (see Chapter 9, Cardiac Emergencies, for more on cardiac emergencies).

For a child or infant:

- If you find that a child or an infant is unconscious and not breathing, you should give the victim 2 ventilations. The only exception to this rule is if you witness a child or an infant suddenly collapse. In this case, it is assumed that it is a cardiac emergency, in which case you should skip the 2 ventilations and begin CPR chest compressions.

Using a Resuscitation Mask to Give Ventilations

You should always use a resuscitation mask when giving ventilations (Figure 7-11). To ensure that you are giving adequate ventilations, the mask must be properly placed and sealed over the victim's mouth and nose. Each ventilation should last about 1 second and make the victim's chest clearly rise and fall.

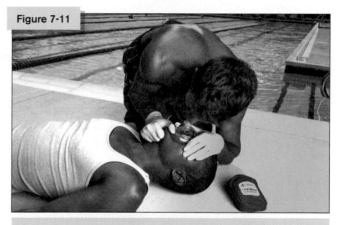

Figure 7-11

Use a resuscitation mask when giving ventilations.

To use a resuscitation mask to give ventilations:

- Position yourself at the victim's head, either on the victim's side or above the head.

- Position the mask over the victim's mouth and nose. Use both hands to hold the mask in place to create an airtight seal.

- If you are on the victim's side, tilt the victim's head back while lifting the chin. If you are behind the victim's head, lift the jaw. For a victim with a suspected head, neck or spinal injury, use the jaw-thrust (without head extension) maneuver.

- Blow into the one-way valve, ensuring that you can see the chest clearly rise and fall. Each ventilation should last about 1 second, with a brief pause between breaths to let the exhaled breath escape.

Scan for Severe Bleeding

As you move into place to begin providing care based on the conditions that you find, you should do a quick visual scan of the victim for severe bleeding. Be sure to scan the victim's entire body from head to toe. Breathing and cardiac emergencies are the most critical conditions and should be handled first. If the victim is bleeding severely, additional lifeguards should assist by controlling the bleeding.

Recovery Positions

In most cases, you should leave the victim in a face-up position and maintain an open airway if he or she is unconscious but breathing. This is particularly important if you suspect the victim has a spinal injury. However, there are a few situations in which you should move a victim into a modified high arm in endangered spine (H.A.IN.E.S) recovery position to keep the airway open and clear even if a spinal injury is suspected. Examples of these situations include if you are alone and have to leave the victim (e.g., to call for help), or you cannot maintain an open and clear airway because of fluids or vomit. Placing a victim in this position will help keep the airway open and clear.

Perform a Secondary Assessment

If you are certain that the victim does not have any life-threatening conditions, you should perform a secondary assessment to identify any additional problems. The secondary assessment provides additional information about injuries or conditions that may require care and could become life-threatening if not addressed. See Chapter 10, First Aid, for more information on injuries, illnesses and performing a secondary assessment.

Provide Care for the Conditions Found

Provide care for the conditions found during the primary and/or secondary assessments. Always treat life-threatening situations first. Other lifeguards and/or safety team members should assist as outlined in the EAP, by getting equipment and summoning EMS personnel or in the actual delivery of care, such as giving two-person CPR or using an AED. Care should be continued until EMS personnel take over, if needed.

Report, Advise and Release

Once appropriate care is given, be sure to complete incident report forms, advise the victim on next steps and release the victim to the appropriate parties.

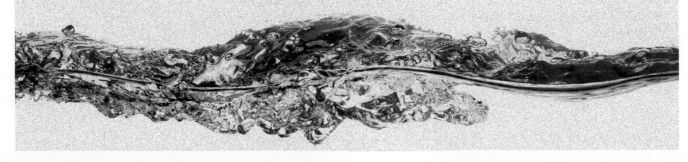

ONE AGE DOES NOT FIT ALL

For the purpose of the skills in this manual:

- Anyone approximately 12 years of age or older is an adult.
- Anyone age 1 year to about 12 years is a child.
- An infant is anyone younger than 1 year.

However, for the purpose of operating an AED:

- Anyone 1 to 8 years of age or weighing less than 55 pounds is a child.

If precise age or weight is not known, use your best judgment and do not delay care while determining age.

CALL FIRST OR CARE FIRST?

If you are alone when responding to someone who is ill, you must decide whether to Call First or Care First.

If you are ALONE:

- Call First (call 9-1-1 or the local emergency number before providing care) for:
  - Any adult or child about 12 years of age or older who is unconscious.
  - A child or an infant who you witnessed suddenly collapse.
  - An unconscious child or infant known to have heart problems.

- Care First (provide **2** minutes of care, then call 9-1-1 or the local emergency number) for:
  - An unconscious child (younger than about age 12) who you did not see collapse.
  - Any victim of a nonfatal drowning.

Call First situations are likely to be cardiac emergencies in which time is a critical factor. In Care First situations, the conditions often are related to breathing emergencies.

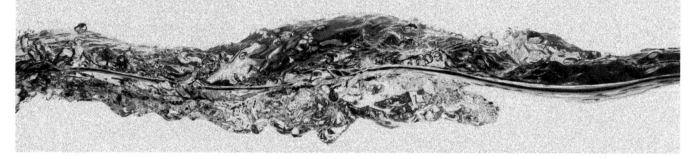

WRAP-UP

As a professional lifeguard, you are an important link in the EMS system and have a duty to act and to meet professional standards. One of these standards is taking appropriate precautions to protect yourself and others against the transmission of infectious diseases. You also should be familiar with and always follow the general procedures for responding to injury or sudden illness on land. These include the following: activating the EAP, sizing up the scene, performing an initial assessment, summoning EMS personnel by calling 9-1-1 or the local emergency number, and after caring for any life-threatening injuries, performing a secondary assessment.

REMOVING DISPOSABLE GLOVES

Note: *To remove gloves without spreading germs, never touch your bare skin with the outside of either glove.*

1 Pinch the glove.

- Pinch the palm side of one glove near your wrist.
- Carefully pull the glove off so that it is inside out.

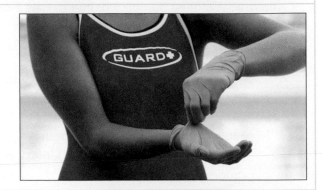

2 Slip two fingers under the glove.

- Hold the glove in the palm of your gloved hand.
- Slip two fingers under the glove at the wrist of the remaining gloved hand.

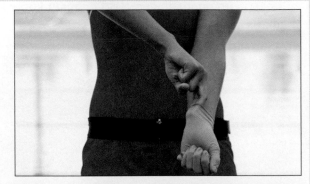

3 Pull the glove off.

- Pull the glove until it comes off, inside out.
- The first glove should end up inside the glove you just removed.

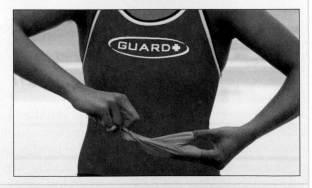

4 Dispose of gloves and wash hands.

- Dispose of gloves and other PPE in a proper biohazard container.
- Wash your hands thoroughly with soap and running water, if available. Otherwise, rub hands thoroughly with an alcohol-based sanitizer if hands are not visibly soiled.

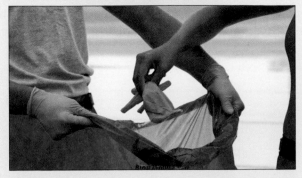

USING A RESUSCITATION MASK

Note: *Activate the EAP, size-up the scene for safety and then perform a primary assessment. Always select the properly sized mask for the victim.*

Head-Tilt/Chin-Lift

1 Kneel to the side of the victim's head.

2 Position the mask.
- Place the rim of the mask between the victim's lower lip and chin.
- Lower the mask until it covers the victim's mouth and nose.

3 Seal the mask.
- Place the thumb and fingers of one hand around the top of the mask.
- Place the thumb of your other hand on the bottom of the mask and slide your first two fingers onto the bony part of the victim's chin.
- Press downward on the mask with your top hand and the thumb of your lower hand to seal the top and bottom of the mask.

4 Tilt the victim's head back and lift the chin to open the airway.

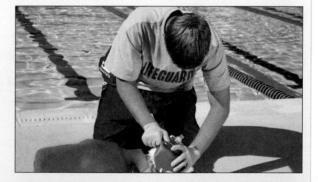

5 Blow into the mask.
- Each ventilation should last about 1 second and make the chest clearly rise. The chest should fall before the next ventilation is given.

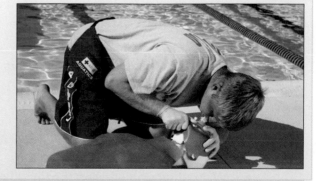

USING A RESUSCITATION MASK *continued*

Jaw-Thrust (With Head Extension) Maneuver

1 Position the mask.

- Kneel above the victim's head.
- Place the rim of the mask between the lower lip and chin.
- Lower the resuscitation mask until it covers the victim's mouth and nose.

2 To seal the mask and open the airway:

- Using the elbows for support, place your thumbs and index fingers along each side of the resuscitation mask to create a "C."
- Slide your 3rd, 4th and 5th fingers into position to create an "E" on both sides of the victim's jawbone.
- Hold the mask in place while you tilt the head back and lift the jaw into the mask.

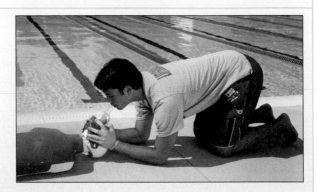

3 Blow into the mask.

- Each ventilation should last about 1 second and make the chest clearly rise. The chest should fall before the next ventilation is given.

Jaw-Thrust (Without Head Extension) Maneuver

Position the mask.

1
- Kneel above the victim's head.
- Place the rim of the mask between the lower lip and chin.
- Lower the resuscitation mask until it covers the victim's mouth and nose.

To seal the mask and open the airway:

2
- Place your thumbs and index fingers along each side of the resuscitation mask to create a "C."
- Slide your 3rd, 4th and 5th fingers into position to create an "E" on both sides of the victim's jawbone.
- Without moving or tilting the head back, lift the lower jaw up with your fingers along the jawbone to seal the mask to the face.

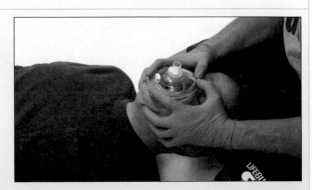

3 Blow into the mask.

- Each ventilation should last about **1** second and make the chest clearly rise. The chest should fall before the next ventilation is given.

 ## PRIMARY ASSESSMENT—**ADULT**

Note: *Always follow standard precautions when providing care. Activate the EAP and get an AED on the scene as soon as possible.*

Size-up the scene for safety and then:

1 Check for responsiveness .

- Tap the shoulder and ask, "Are you okay?"

2 If no response, summon EMS personnel.

- If the victim is face-down, roll the victim onto his or her back while supporting the head, neck and back.

3 Open the airway and quickly check for breathing and a pulse for no more than **10** seconds.

- To open the airway:
  - From the side, use the head-tilt/ chin-lift technique.
  - From above the victim's head, use the jaw-thrust (with head extension) maneuver.
  - If a head, neck or spinal injury is suspected, use the jaw-thrust (without head extension) maneuver.

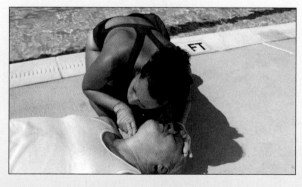

- Look, listen and feel for breathing.
- Feel for a carotid pulse by placing two fingers in the middle of the victim's throat and then sliding them into the groove at the side of the neck closest to you. Press lightly.

Note: *For a breathing emergency (e.g., drowning, hypoxia), give 2 ventilations before scanning for severe bleeding. If at any time the chest does not rise, the airway might be blocked. Provide care for an unconscious choking victim.*

Continued on Next Page

PRIMARY ASSESSMENT—**ADULT** *continued*

4 Quickly scan for severe bleeding.

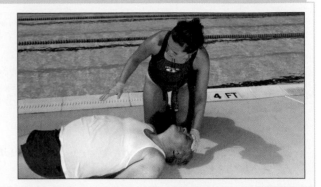

5 Provide care as needed.

- If no breathing or pulse, perform CPR.
- If no breathing but there is a pulse, give **1** ventilation about every **5** seconds.
- If there is severe bleeding and the victim is breathing, provide first aid care for the bleeding.
- If unconscious but breathing, leave the victim in a face-up position. Place in a modified H.A.IN.E.S. recovery position only if you:
  - ○ Are alone and must leave the victim (e.g., to call for help).
  - ○ Cannot maintain an open and clear airway because of fluids or vomit.

 # PRIMARY ASSESSMENT—**CHILD AND INFANT**

Note: *Always follow standard precautions when providing care. Activate the EAP and get an AED on the scene as soon as possible.*

Size-up the scene for safety and then:

1 Check for responsiveness.

- For a child, tap the shoulder and shout, "Are you okay?"
- For an infant, tap the shoulder or flick the underside of the foot and shout.

2 If no response, summon EMS personnel.

- If the victim is face-down, roll the victim onto his or her back while supporting the head, neck and back.

Open the airway and check for breathing and a pulse for no more than **10** seconds.

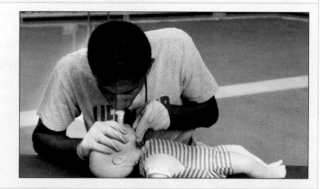

- To open the airway:
  - From the side, use the head-tilt/chin-lift technique.
  - From above the victim's head, use the jaw-thrust (with head extension) maneuver.
  - If you suspect a head, neck or spinal injury, use the jaw-thrust (without head extension) maneuver.
- Look, listen and feel for breathing.
- Check for a pulse.
  - For a child, feel for a carotid pulse by placing two fingers in the middle of the victim's throat and then sliding them into the groove at the side of the neck closest to you. Press in lightly; pressing too hard can compress the artery.
  - For an infant, feel for the brachial pulse on the inside of the upper arm between the infant's elbow and shoulder. Press lightly.

Note: *If you witnessed a child or an infant suddenly collapse, skip step 4.*

 If no breathing, give **2** ventilations. Each ventilation should last about 1 second and make the chest clearly rise.

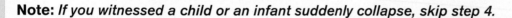

- The chest should fall before the next ventilation is given.

Note: *If at any time the chest does* **not** *rise during Step 4, the airway might be blocked. Provide care for an unconscious choking victim.*

 Quickly scan for severe bleeding.

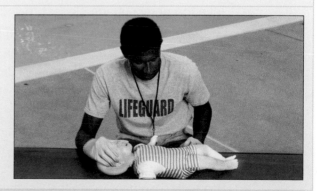

Continued on Next Page

PRIMARY ASSESSMENT—**CHILD AND INFANT** *continued*

6 Provide care as needed.

- If no breathing or pulse, perform CPR.
- If no breathing but there is a pulse, give **1** ventilation about every **3** seconds.
- If there is severe bleeding and the victim is breathing, provide first aid care for the bleeding.
- If unconscious but breathing, leave the victim in a face-up position. Place in a modified H.A.IN.E.S recovery position only if you:
  o Are alone and have to leave the victim (e.g., to call for help).
  o Cannot maintain an open and clear airway because of fluids or vomit.

 ## RECOVERY POSITIONS

Note: *If the victim is unconscious but breathing, leave him or her in a face-up position. Place in a modified H.A.IN.E.S. recovery position only if you:*

- *Are alone and must leave the victim (e.g., to call for help).*
- *Cannot maintain an open and clear airway because of fluids or vomit.*

To place a victim in the modified H.A.IN.E.S. recovery position:

1 Kneel at the victim's side.

2 Roll the victim away from you.

- Reach across the victim's body, lift up the arm farthest from you and place it next to the head with the palm facing up.
- Take the person's arm closest to you and place it next to his or her side.
- Grasp the leg farthest from you and bend it up.
- Using your hand that is closest to the victim's head, cup the base of the victim's skull in the palm of your hand and carefully slide your forearm under the victim's shoulder closest to you. Do not lift or push the head or neck.
- Place your other hand under the arm and hip closest to you.
- Using a smooth motion, roll the victim away from you by lifting with your hand and forearm. Keep the victim's head in contact with his or her extended arm and be sure to support the head and neck with your hand.
- Stop all movement when the victim is on his or her side.

3 Place the top leg on the other leg so that both knees are in a bent position.

4 Make sure the arm on top is in line with the upper body.

- If you must leave the person to get help, place the hand of the upper arm palm side down with the fingers under the armpit of the extended lower arm.

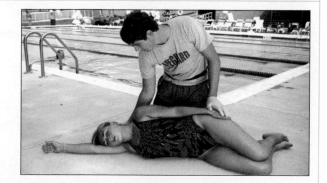

Another option for a recovery position for an infant is to:

1 Carefully position the infant face-down along your forearm.

2 Support the infant's head and neck with your other hand while keeping the infant's mouth and nose clear.

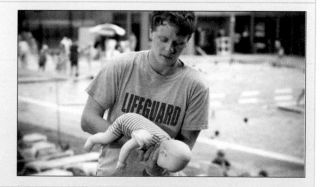

MOVING A VICTIM—**NON-EMERGENCY MOVES**

Note: *Do not use these non-emergency moves for a victim suspected of having a head, neck or spinal injury.*

Walking Assist

Note: *Either one or two lifeguards can use this method with a conscious victim.*

To help a victim who needs assistance walking to safety:

1 Stand at one side of the victim, place the victim's arm across your shoulders and hold it in place with one hand.

2 Support the victim with your other hand around the victim's waist.

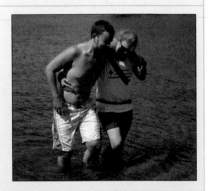

3 Walk the victim to safety.

Two-Person Seat Carry

The two-person seat carry requires a second rescuer. To perform the carry:

1 Put one arm under the victim's thighs and the other across the victim's back.

2 Interlock your arms with those of a second rescuer under the victim's legs and across the victim's back.

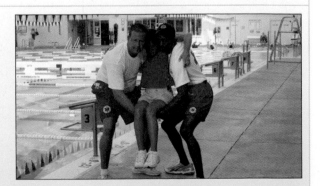

3	Have the victim place his or her arms over both rescuers' shoulders.

4	Lift the victim in the "seat" formed by the rescuers' arms and carry the victim to safety.

 # MOVING A VICTIM—**EMERGENCY MOVES**

Pack-Strap Carry

Note: *This move is not safe for a victim suspected of having a head, neck or spinal injury.*

To move either a conscious or an unconscious victim with no suspected head, neck or spinal injury:

1	Have the victim stand or have a second rescuer support the victim in a standing position.

2	Position yourself with your back to the victim. Keep your back straight and knees bent so that your shoulders fit into the victim's armpits.

3	Cross the victim's arms in front of you and grasp the victim's wrists.

4	Lean forward slightly and pull the victim up and onto your back.

5	Stand up and walk to safety.

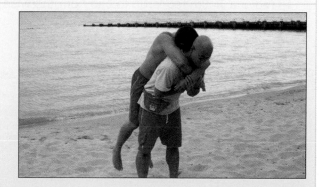

MOVING A VICTIM—**EMERGENCY MOVES** *continued*

Clothes Drag

Note: *The clothes drag is an appropriate emergency move for a victim suspected of having a head, neck or spinal injury.*

1 Position the victim on his or her back.

2 Kneel behind the victim's head and gather the victim's clothing behind his or her neck.

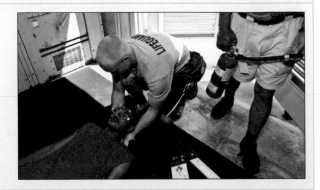

3 Pull the victim to safety, cradling the victim's head with his or her clothes and your hands.

Ankle Drag

Note: *This move is not safe for a victim suspected of having a head, neck or spinal injury.*

To move a victim too large to carry or otherwise move:

1 Stand at the victim's feet, firmly grasp the victim's ankles and carefully move backward. Keep your back as straight as possible; do not twist.

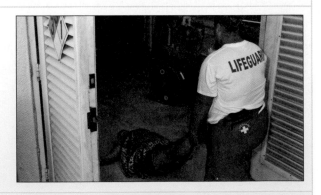

2 Pull the victim in a straight line being careful not to bump the victim's head.

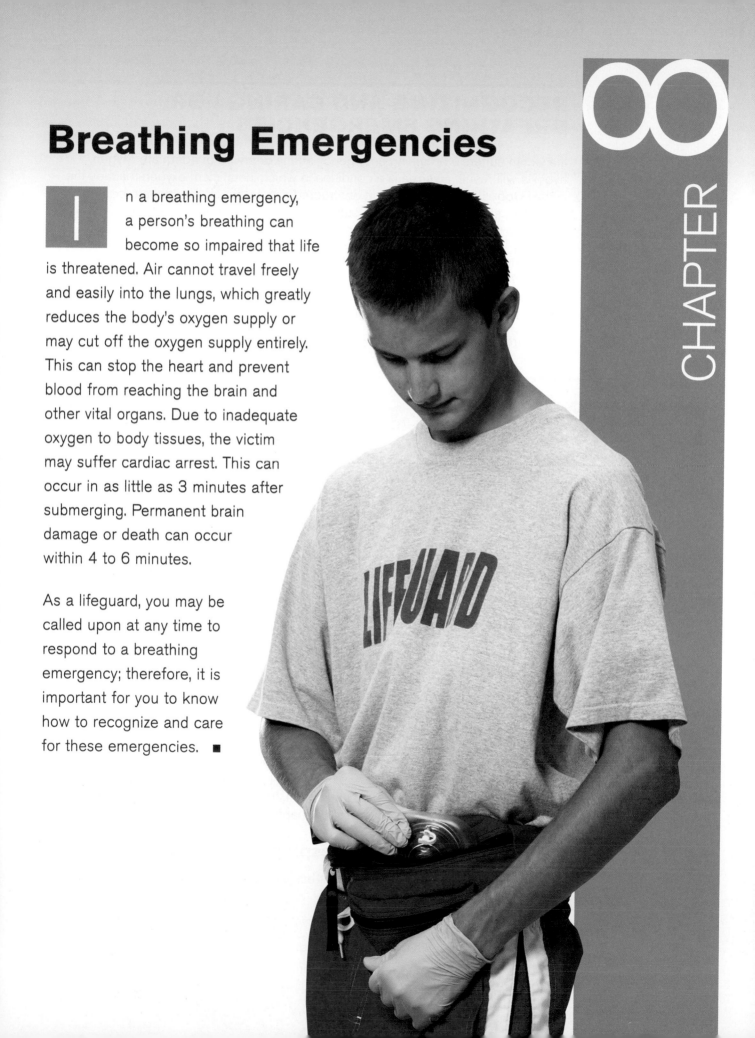

Breathing Emergencies

I n a breathing emergency, a person's breathing can become so impaired that life is threatened. Air cannot travel freely and easily into the lungs, which greatly reduces the body's oxygen supply or may cut off the oxygen supply entirely. This can stop the heart and prevent blood from reaching the brain and other vital organs. Due to inadequate oxygen to body tissues, the victim may suffer cardiac arrest. This can occur in as little as 3 minutes after submerging. Permanent brain damage or death can occur within 4 to 6 minutes.

As a lifeguard, you may be called upon at any time to respond to a breathing emergency; therefore, it is important for you to know how to recognize and care for these emergencies. ■

RECOGNIZING AND CARING FOR BREATHING EMERGENCIES

If a victim suffers a breathing emergency and is deprived of adequate oxygen, hypoxia will result. *Hypoxia* is a condition in which insufficient oxygen reaches the cells. Hypoxia may result from an obstructed airway, shock, inadequate breathing, drowning, strangulation, choking, suffocation, cardiac arrest, head trauma, carbon monoxide poisoning or anaphylactic shock.

Signs and symptoms of hypoxia include increased breathing and heart rates, *cyanosis* (a condition that develops when tissues do not get enough oxygen and turn blue, particularly in the lips and nail beds), changes in level of consciousness (LOC), restlessness and chest pain.

There are two types of breathing (also referred to as respiratory) emergencies: *respiratory distress*, a condition in which breathing becomes difficult, and *respiratory arrest*, a condition in which breathing stops. Respiratory distress can lead to *respiratory failure*, which occurs when the respiratory system is beginning to shut down, which in turn can lead to respiratory arrest.

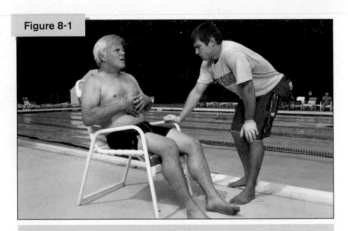

Figure 8-1

Watch and listen for breathing problems in a conscious victim. Ask the victim how he or she feels.

Breathing problems can be identified by watching and listening to a conscious victim's breathing and by asking the victim how he or she feels (Figure 8-1). Because oxygen is vital to life, always ensure that the victim has an open airway and is breathing. Without an open airway, a victim cannot breathe and will die. A victim who can speak or cry is conscious, has an open airway, is breathing and has a pulse.

Respiratory Distress

A victim who is having difficulty breathing is experiencing respiratory distress.

Causes of Respiratory Distress

Respiratory distress can be caused by a partially obstructed airway; illness; chronic conditions, such as asthma and emphysema; electrocution, including lightning strikes; heart attack; injury to the head, chest, lungs or abdomen; allergic reactions; drugs; poisoning; emotional distress; or anaphylactic shock.

Signs and Symptoms of Respiratory Distress

Signs and symptoms of respiratory distress include:

- Slow or rapid breathing.
- Unusually deep or shallow breathing.
- Shortness of breath or noisy breathing.
- Dizziness, drowsiness or light-headedness.
- Changes in LOC.

ASTHMA

Asthma is an ongoing illness in which the airways swell. An asthma attack happens when an asthma trigger, such as dust or exercise, affects the airways, causing them to suddenly swell and narrow. This makes breathing difficult, which can be frightening.

Recognizing an Asthma Attack

You can often tell when a person is having an asthma attack by the hoarse whistling sound made when inhaling and/or exhaling. This sound, known as *wheezing*, occurs because airways have narrowed or become obstructed.

Signs and symptoms of an asthma attack include coughing or wheezing; coughing that occurs after exercise, crying or laughing; difficulty breathing; shortness of breath; rapid, shallow breathing; sweating; tightness in the chest; inability to talk without stopping frequently for a breath; bent posture with shoulders elevated and lips pursed to make breathing easier; and feelings of fear or confusion.

Caring for an Asthma Attack

You may need to assist a person with asthma in using an inhaler. Before doing so, obtain consent and then follow these general guidelines, if local protocols allow:

1. Help the person sit up and rest in a position comfortable for breathing.

2. If the person has prescribed asthma medication, help him or her take it.

3. Shake the inhaler and then remove the cover from the mouthpiece. Position the spacer if you are using one.

4. Have the person breathe out fully through the mouth and then place the lips tightly around the inhaler mouthpiece.

5. Have the person inhale deeply and slowly as you or the person depresses the inhaler canister to release the medication, which he or she then inhales into the lungs.

6. Have the person hold his or her breath for a count of 10. If using a spacer, have the person take 5 to 6 deep breaths with the spacer still in the mouth, without holding his or her breath.

7. Once the inhalation is complete, have the person rinse his or her mouth with water to reduce side effects.

8. Monitor the person's condition.

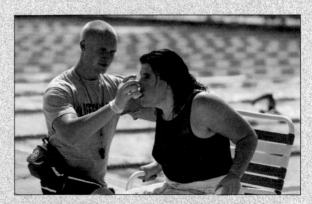

Assist a victim with using an asthma inhaler if local protocols allow.

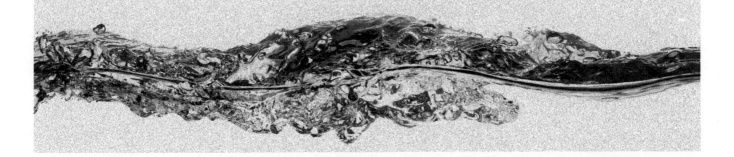

- Increased heart rate.
- Chest pain or discomfort.
- Skin that is flushed, pale, ashen or bluish.
- Unusually moist or cool skin.
- Gasping for breath.
- Wheezing, gurgling or high-pitched noises.
- Inability to speak in full sentences.
- Tingling in the hands, feet or lips.
- Feelings of apprehension or fear.

Caring for Respiratory Distress

You do not need to know the cause of respiratory distress to provide care. When you find a victim experiencing difficulty breathing, activate the emergency action plan (EAP) and:

- Maintain an open airway.
- Summon emergency medical services (EMS) personnel.
- Help the victim to rest in a comfortable position that makes breathing easier.
- Reassure and comfort the victim.
- Assist the victim with any of his or her prescribed medication.
- Keep the victim from getting chilled or overheated.
- Administer emergency oxygen, if available and you are trained to do so.

Someone with asthma or emphysema who is in respiratory distress may try to do pursed-lip breathing. To assist with this, have the person assume a position of comfort. After he or she inhales, have the person slowly exhale through the lips, pursed as though blowing out candles. This creates back pressure, which can help to open airways slightly until EMS personnel arrive and take over.

Respiratory Arrest

A victim who has stopped breathing is in respiratory arrest.

Causes of Respiratory Arrest

Respiratory arrest may develop from respiratory distress, respiratory failure or other causes including drowning; obstructed airway (choking); injury to the head, chest, lungs or abdomen; illness, such as pneumonia; respiratory conditions, such as emphysema or asthma; heart attack; coronary heart disease (such as angina); allergic reactions (food or insect stings); electrocution, including lightning strikes; shock; poisoning; drugs; and emotional distress.

Caring for Respiratory Arrest

Although respiratory arrest may have many causes, you do not need to know the exact cause to provide care. Begin by following the general procedures for injury or sudden illness on land.

To check to see if someone is breathing, look to see if the victim's chest clearly rises and falls (Figure 8-2). Listen for escaping air and feel for air against the side of your face when checking for breathing and a pulse during the primary assessment. The normal breathing rate for an adult is between 12 and 20 breaths per minute; however, some people breathe slightly slower or faster. You usually can observe the chest rising and falling.

Normal, effective breathing is regular, quiet and effortless. In an unconscious person, you may detect isolated or infrequent gasping in the absence of other breathing. These are called *agonal gasps,* which can occur even after the heart has stopped beating. Agonal gasps are not breathing—care for the victim as though he or she is not breathing at all.

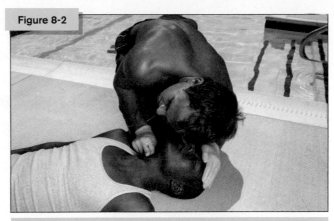

Figure 8-2

Check breathing by watching if the victim's chest clearly rises and falls.

Drowning Victims

Anyone who experiences respiratory impairment from submersion in water is a drowning victim. Drowning may or may not result in death. Victims who have been pulled from the water and are not breathing are in immediate need of ventilations. In general, if the victim is rescued quickly enough, giving ventilations may resuscitate the victim. Without oxygen, a victim's heart will stop and death will result. Your objective is to get the victim's mouth and nose out of the water, open the airway and give ventilations as quickly as possible.

Always ensure that victims who have been involved in a drowning incident are taken to the hospital, even if you think the danger has passed. Complications can develop as long as 72 hours after the incident and may be fatal.

GIVING VENTILATIONS

Giving ventilations is a technique for breathing air into a victim to provide the oxygen necessary to survive. The air you exhale contains enough oxygen to keep a person alive.

Each ventilation should last about 1 second and make the chest clearly rise. The chest should fall before you give the next ventilation. Give 1 ventilation every 5 seconds for an adult. Give 1 ventilation about every 3 seconds for a child or an infant.

When giving ventilations to a victim:

- Maintain an open airway by keeping the head tilted back in the proper position.
- Seal the mask over the victim's mouth and nose.
- Give ventilations for about 2 minutes, then reassess for breathing and a pulse.
- If the victim has a pulse but is not breathing, continue giving ventilations.

Continue giving ventilations until:

- The victim begins to breathe on his or her own.
- Another trained rescuer takes over.
- More advanced medical personnel, such as EMS personnel, take over.
- You are too exhausted to continue.

- The victim has no pulse, in which case you should begin CPR or use an AED if one is available and ready to use.
- The scene becomes unsafe.

CPR Breathing Barriers

CPR breathing barriers help to protect you against disease transmission when giving ventilations or performing CPR. CPR breathing barriers include resuscitation masks and bag-valve-mask resuscitators (BVMs). A resuscitation mask should be in your hip pack.

Figure 8-3

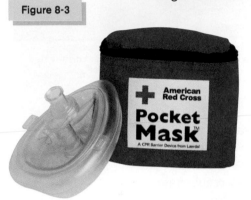

Resuscitation mask

Resuscitation Masks

A resuscitation mask allows you to breathe air (with or without emergency oxygen) into a victim without making mouth-to-mouth contact.

Resuscitation masks have several benefits. They help to get air quickly to the victim through both the mouth and nose; create a seal over the victim's mouth and nose; can be connected to emergency oxygen, if equipped with an oxygen inlet; and protect against disease transmission.

A resuscitation mask should have the following characteristics (Figure 8-3):

Figure 8-4

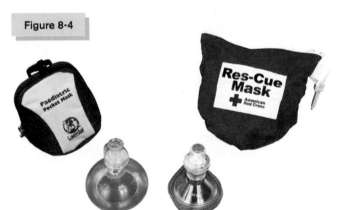

Pediatric resuscitation masks

- Be easy to assemble and use
- Be made of transparent, pliable material that allows you to make a tight seal over the victim's mouth and nose
- Have a one-way valve for releasing exhaled air
- Have a standard 15- or 22-mm coupling assembly (the size of the opening for the one-way valve)
- Have an inlet for delivering emergency oxygen (if facility protocols include administering emergency oxygen)
- Work well under different environmental conditions, such as extreme heat or cold or in the water

Pediatric resuscitation masks are available and should be used to care for children and infants (Figure 8-4). You should not use adult resuscitation masks on children or infants in an emergency situation unless a pediatric resuscitation mask is not available and EMS personnel advise you to do so. Always use the appropriate equipment matched to the size of the victim.

Figure 8-5

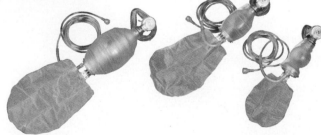

BVMs come in a variety of sizes for use with adults, children and infants.

Bag-Valve-Mask Resuscitators

A BVM has three parts: a bag, a valve and a mask (Figure 8-5). By placing the mask on the victim's face and squeezing the bag, you open the one-way valve, forcing air into the victim's lungs. When you release the bag, the valve closes and air from the surrounding environment refills the bag. Because it is necessary to maintain a tight seal on the mask, two rescuers should operate a BVM. (One rescuer positions and seals the mask, while the second rescuer squeezes the bag.)

BVMs have several advantages in that they:

- Increase oxygen levels in the blood by using the air in the surrounding environment instead of the air exhaled by a rescuer.
- Can be connected to emergency oxygen.
- Are more effective for giving ventilations than a resuscitation mask when used correctly by two rescuers.
- Protect against disease transmission and inhalation hazards if the victim has been exposed to a hazardous gas.
- May be used with advanced airway adjuncts.

BVMs come in various sizes to fit adults, children and infants; you should use the appropriately sized BVM for the size of the victim. Using an adult BVM on an infant has the potential to cause harm, and they should *not* be used unless a pediatric BVM is not available *and* more advanced medical personnel advise you to do so.

Giving Ventilations–Special Considerations

Frothing

A white or pinkish froth or foam may be coming out of the mouth and/or nose of victims of fatal and nonfatal drownings. This froth results from a mix of mucous, air and water during respiration. If you see froth, clear the victim's mouth with a finger sweep before giving ventilations. If an unconscious victim's chest does not clearly rise after you give a ventilation, retilt the head and then reattempt ventilations. If the ventilations still do not make the chest clearly rise, assume that the airway is blocked and begin care for an unconscious choking victim.

Vomiting

When you give ventilations, the victim may vomit. Many victims who have been submerged vomit because water has entered the stomach or air has been forced into the stomach during ventilations. If this occurs, quickly turn the victim onto his or her side to keep the vomit from blocking the airway and entering the lungs (Figure 8-6). Support the head and neck, and turn the body as a unit. After vomiting stops, clear the victim's airway by wiping the victim's mouth out using a finger sweep and suction if necessary, turn the victim onto his or her back and continue with ventilations.

You can use a finger sweep to clear the airway of an unconscious victim when the blockage is visible, but when available, you should use a

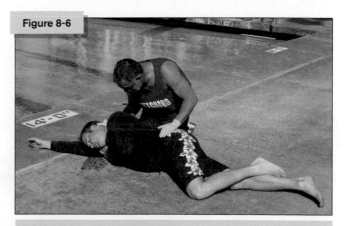

Figure 8-6

If a victim vomits, turn him on his side to keep the vomit from entering the victim's airway and entering the lungs.

ANAPHYLAXIS

Anaphylactic shock, also known as *anaphylaxis*, is a severe allergic reaction that can cause air passages to swell and restrict breathing. In susceptible people, triggers can include insect bites or stings, certain food and food additives, medication and chemicals.

Anaphylactic shock is a life-threatening condition and requires immediate care.

Anyone at risk should wear a medical identification tag, bracelet or necklace.

Recognizing Anaphylaxis

Some possible signs and symptoms of anaphylaxis include swelling of the face, neck, hands, throat, tongue or other body part; itching of the tongue, armpits, groin or any body part; rash or hives; weakness, dizziness or confusion; redness or welts on the skin; red watery eyes; nausea, abdominal pain or vomiting; rapid heart rate; wheezing, difficulty breathing or shortness of breath; difficulty swallowing; tight feeling in the chest and throat; low blood pressure; and shock.

Caring for Anaphylaxis

If you suspect that someone is experiencing anaphylaxis, you should immediately:

- Summon EMS personnel.
- Provide emergency care.
- Remove the victim from the source of the allergy.
- Assist with the person's prescribed

epinephrine auto-injector, if local protocols allow. (*Epinephrine* is a form of adrenaline medication prescribed to treat the symptoms of severe allergic reactions.)

- Administer emergency oxygen, if it is available and you are trained to do so.

Before assisting with an epinephrine auto-injector:

- Determine whether the person already has taken epinephrine or antihistamine. If so, DO NOT administer another dose, unless directed to do so by more advanced medical personnel.
- Check the label to confirm that the prescription of the auto-injector is for the person.
- Check the expiration date of the auto-injector. If it has expired, DO NOT use it.
- Confirm that the liquid is clear and not cloudy, if the medication is visible. If it is cloudy, DO NOT use it.
- Leave the safety cap on until the auto-injector is ready to use. Carefully avoid accidental injection when assisting a person by *never* touching the needle end of the device.

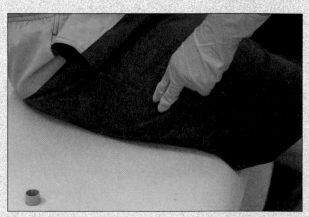

Locate the injection site.

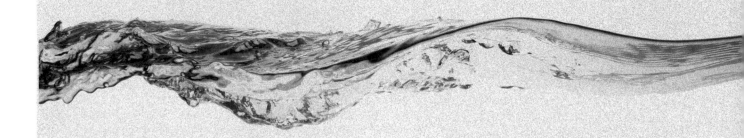

Two injectable epinephrine systems are available commercially, by prescription only, in spring-loaded syringes that function when pressed into the thigh. They are the EpiPen® (which includes one dose) and Twinject® (which includes two doses).

To assist with administering epinephrine:

1. Locate the outside middle of one thigh to use as the injection site, ensuring that there are no obstructions to the skin, such as keys, coins or seams.

2. Grasp the auto-injector firmly in your fist and pull off the safety cap with your other hand.

3. Hold the (black) tip (needle end) near the person's outer thigh so that the auto-injector is at a 90-degree angle to the thigh.

4. Quickly and firmly push the tip straight into the outer thigh. You will hear a click.

5. Hold the auto-injector firmly in place for 10 seconds, then remove it from the thigh and massage the injection site with a gloved hand for several seconds.

If using Twinject:

1. Remove the device from the hard case.

2. Remove the green cap, labeled "1." You will see a red tip. Do not put your thumb, finger or hand over the red tip.

3. Remove the green cap, labeled "2."

4. Place the red tip against the middle of the outer thigh, press down hard until the needle enters the thigh (it will go through light clothing), and hold for a count of 10.

5. Remove the Twinject from the thigh. Check the rounded, red tip. If the needle is exposed, the dose was given.

6. Continue to monitor the person's condition and observe the person's response to the epinephrine.

7. Place the used auto-injector in a proper sharps container and give it to more advanced medical personnel when they arrive.

Only the victim should self-administer the second dose included with the Twinject injector.

Check state and local regulations regarding use of prescription and over-the-counter medications.

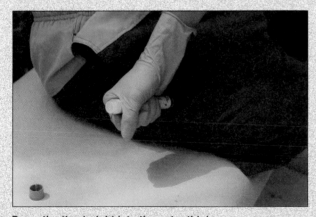

Press the tip straight into the outer thigh.

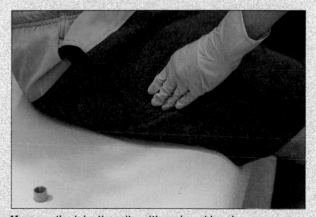

Massage the injection site with a gloved hand.

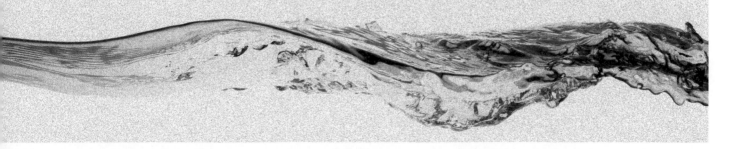

manual suction device to suction the airway clear. *Suctioning* is the process of removing foreign matter from the upper airway by means of a manual device.

When using a manual suction device:

- Remove the protective cap from the tip of the suction catheter.
- Measure and check the suction tip to prevent inserting the suction tip too deeply.
- Suction for no more than 15 seconds at a time for an adult, 10 seconds for a child and 5 seconds for an infant.

Air in the Stomach

When giving ventilations, blow slowly, with just enough air to make the victim's chest clearly rise. The chest should fall before you give the next ventilation. If you blow too much air into the victim, air may enter the stomach, causing gastric distention. The victim then will likely vomit, which can obstruct the airway and complicate resuscitation efforts.

Suspected Head, Neck or Spinal Injury

If you suspect that an unconscious victim has a head, neck or spinal injury, always take care of the airway and breathing first. Open the airway by using the jaw-thrust (without head extension) maneuver to check for breathing or to give ventilations (Figure 8-7). If the jaw-thrust (without head extension) maneuver does not open the airway, use the head-tilt/chin-lift technique. See Chapter 11, Caring for Head, Neck and Spinal Injuries, for more information on injuries to the head, neck or spine.

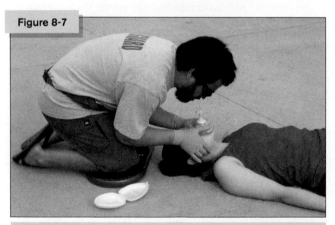

Figure 8-7

Jaw-thrust (without head extension) maneuver

If the victim vomits, quickly roll the victim onto his or her side to prevent aspiration or choking. You can do this even if the victim is immobilized on a backboard. Simply turn the board and victim, ensuring that the head is securely fastened to the board. After vomiting stops, remove vomit from the victim's mouth using a finger sweep or suction device if necessary, turn the victim onto the back and continue with ventilations.

Dentures

If the victim is wearing dentures, leave them in place unless they become loose and block the airway. Dentures help to support the victim's mouth and cheeks, making it easier to seal the mask when giving ventilations.

Mask-to-Nose Ventilations

If the victim's mouth is injured, you may need to give ventilations through the nose. To give mask-to-nose ventilations using a resuscitation mask:

- Open the airway using a head-tilt/chin-lift technique.
- Place the resuscitation mask over the victim's mouth and nose.
- Use both of your hands to keep the victim's mouth closed.

- Seal the resuscitation mask with both of your hands.
- Give ventilations.

Mask-to-Stoma Ventilations

Some victims may breath through a stoma—an opening in the neck as a result of surgery. If so, keep the airway in a neutral position as you look, listen and feel for breathing with your ear over the stoma. To give ventilations, make an airtight seal with a round pediatric resuscitation mask around the stoma or tracheostomy tube and blow into the mask.

Table 8-1: Giving Ventilations—Adult, Child and Infant

	Giving Ventilations
Adult	- 1 ventilation every 5 seconds - Each ventilation should last about 1 second and make the chest clearly rise. - The chest should fall before you give the next ventilation.
Child and Infant	- 1 ventilation every 3 seconds - Each ventilation should last about 1 second and make the chest clearly rise. - The chest should fall before you give the next ventilation.

When giving ventilations:

- Maintain an open airway by keeping the head tilted back in the proper position.
- Seal the mask over the victim's mouth and nose.
- Give ventilations for about 2 minutes, then reassess for breathing and a pulse.
- If the chest does not clearly rise, the airway could be blocked. Retilt the head and attempt another ventilation. If the chest still does not clearly rise, provide care for an unconscious victim.
- If the victim vomits, roll the victim onto the side and clear the victims' mouth using a finger sweep and suction, if necessary. Turn the victim onto the back and continue giving ventilations.
- If the victim has a pulse but is not breathing, continue giving ventilations.

Continue ventilation cycles until:

- The victim begins to breathe on his or her own.
- The victim has no pulse, in which case you should begin CPR or use an AED if one is available and ready to use.

AIRWAY OBSTRUCTION

An airway obstruction is the most common cause of breathing emergencies. A victim whose airway is blocked can quickly stop breathing, lose consciousness and die. A partial airway obstruction can move some air to and from the lungs, often while wheezing.

There are two types of airway obstruction: mechanical and anatomical. Any foreign body lodged in the airway is a *mechanical obstruction* and requires immediate attention. An *anatomical airway obstruction* is caused by the body itself, most commonly the tongue. An unconscious victim loses muscle tone, which may cause the tongue to fall back and block the airway.

Causes of Airway Obstructions

Common causes of choking include:

- Swallowing poorly chewed food.
- Drinking alcohol before or during meals. (Alcohol dulls the nerves that aid swallowing, making choking on food more likely.)
- Eating too fast or talking or laughing while eating.
- Walking, playing or running with food or small objects, such as toy parts or balloons, in the mouth.
- Wearing dentures. (Dentures make it difficult to sense whether food is fully chewed before it is swallowed.)

Caring for Airway Obstructions

A conscious person who is clutching the throat is showing what is commonly called the *universal sign of choking*. This person's airway may be partially or completely obstructed.

Complete airway obstruction occurs when the person cannot cough, speak, cry or breathe and requires *immediate* action. The objective in this case is to clear the obstruction before the person becomes unconscious.

Protocols for caring for a conscious choking victim may vary, but abdominal thrusts, back blows and chest thrusts each have been proven to effectively clear an obstructed airway in conscious victims. Frequently, a combination of more than one technique may be needed to expel an object and clear the airway.

Conscious Choking

You must get consent before helping a conscious choking person (Figure 8-8). If the person is a child or infant, get consent from a parent or guardian, if present. If no parent or guardian is present, consent is implied. If you suspect a person is choking, ask the victim, "Are you choking?" Then, identify yourself and ask if you can help. If the victim is coughing, encourage continued coughing. If the victim cannot cough, speak or breathe, activate the EAP and have another person summon EMS personnel.

When caring for a conscious choking adult, perform a combination of 5 back blows followed by 5 abdominal thrusts. Each back blow and abdominal thrust should be a separate and distinct attempt to dislodge the object. For a conscious child, use a combination of 5 back

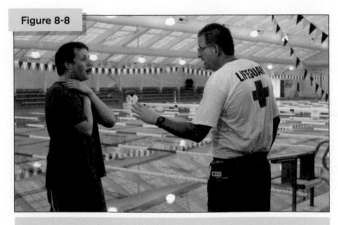

Figure 8-8

Obtain consent before providing care.

Table 8-2: **Providing Care for Obstructed Airway–Adult, Child and Infant**		
	Conscious Choking	**Unconscious Choking**
Adult and Child	■ 5 back blows ■ 5 abdominal thrusts (Use chest thrusts if you cannot reach around the victim or the victim is pregnant.)	■ Retilt the head and attempt a ventilation. ■ Give 30 chest compressions. ■ Look inside the mouth and remove the object if seen. ■ Attempt ventilations.
Infant	■ 5 back blows ■ 5 chest trusts	(Same steps as adult.)
Continue the cycle of care until:	■ The object is forced out. ■ The victim begins to cough forcefully or breathe. ■ The victim becomes unconscious.	■ The object is forced out. ■ The victim begins to cough forcefully or breathe. ■ Ventilation attempts are successful and effective.

When providing care:

■ Use less force on a child than you would on an adult when giving abdominal thrusts.

■ Use two or three fingers on the center of the chest just below the nipple line when giving chest trusts to an infant.

■ Keep one hand on the infant's forehead to maintain an open airway when giving chest thrusts to an infant.

blows and 5 abdominal thrusts, but with less force. Using too much force could cause internal injuries. For a conscious choking infant, perform a combination of 5 back blows and 5 chest thrusts. Use even less force when giving back blows and chest thrusts to an infant.

If you cannot reach far enough around the victim to give effective abdominal thrusts or if the victim is obviously pregnant or known to be pregnant, give back blows followed by chest thrusts (Figure 8-9).

For all victims, continue 5 back blows and 5 abdominal or chest thrusts until the object is dislodged and the victim can cough or breathe, or until the victim becomes unconscious.

Conscious Choking Victim Who Becomes Unconscious

If a conscious victim becomes unconscious, carefully lower the victim to the ground and provide care for an unconscious choking victim.

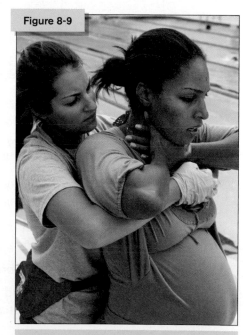

Figure 8-9

If a victim is obviously pregnant, use chest thrusts instead of abdominal thrusts to dislodge the object.

Unconscious Choking

Unlike the conscious victim suffering foreign body airway obstruction, consent is implied when a victim is unconscious. However, you must get consent from a parent or guardian, if present, before helping an unconscious choking child.

You should provide care to an unconscious adult, child or infant who is choking on a firm, flat surface. The objective is to clear the airway of the obstruction, allowing adequate ventilations. If an unconscious victim's chest does not clearly rise after giving a ventilation, assume the airway is blocked by a foreign object and position yourself to give chest compressions as you would when performing CPR chest compressions. (See Chapter 9, Cardiac Emergencies, for information on how to give chest compressions.) After compressions, look in the mouth for an object and, if you see one, remove it with a gloved finger. For an infant, use your little finger to remove the object. Reattempt 2 ventilations.

Repeat cycles of 30 chest compressions, foreign object check/removal and 2 ventilations until the chest clearly rises. If the chest clearly rises, quickly check for breathing and a pulse for *no more than 10 seconds.* Provide care based on the conditions found.

EMERGENCY OXYGEN

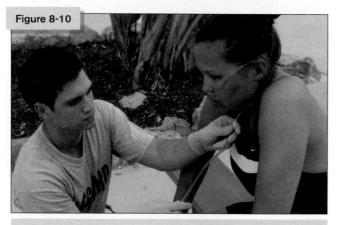

Figure 8-10

Administering emergency oxygen

When someone has a breathing or cardiac emergency, the supply of oxygen to the brain and heart, as well as the rest of the body, is reduced, resulting in hypoxia, in which an insufficient amount of oxygen reaches the cells. If breathing stops (respiratory arrest), the brain and heart will soon be starved of oxygen, resulting in cardiac arrest and ultimately death if not managed quickly and appropriately.

The air a person normally breathes is about 21 percent oxygen. When giving ventilations or performing CPR, the air exhaled into the victim is about 16 percent oxygen. This may not be enough oxygen to save the victim's life. By administering emergency oxygen, you can deliver a higher percentage of oxygen, thus increasing the victim's chance of survival (Figure 8-10).

Emergency oxygen can be given for many breathing and cardiac emergencies. Consider administering emergency oxygen for:

- An adult breathing fewer than 12 or more than 20 breaths per minute.
- A child breathing fewer than 15 or more than 30 breaths per minute.
- An infant breathing fewer than 25 or more than 50 breaths per minute.

Oxygen should be delivered using equipment that is properly sized for the victim and flow rates that are appropriate for the delivery device.

Emergency oxygen units are available without prescription for first aid use, provided that they contain at least a 15-minute supply of oxygen and are designed to deliver a pre-set flow rate of at least 6 liters per minute (LPM). Oxygen cylinders are labeled "U.S.P." and marked with a yellow diamond containing the word "Oxygen" (Figure 8-11). The U.S.P. stands for United States Pharmacopeia and indicates that the oxygen is medical grade.

Oxygen cylinders come in different sizes and various pressure capacities. In the United States, oxygen cylinders typically have green markings. However, the color scheme is not regulated, so different manufacturers and countries other than the United States may use differently colored markings. Oxygen cylinders are under high pressure and should be handled carefully.

Variable-Flow-Rate Oxygen

Many EMS systems use variable-flow-rate oxygen, which allows the rescuer to vary the flow of oxygen. These systems are practical because they are able to deliver a large amount of oxygen.

To administer emergency oxygen using a variable-flow-rate system, assemble the following pieces of equipment: an oxygen cylinder, a regulator with pressure gauge and flowmeter, and a delivery device.

The regulator lowers the pressure of the oxygen as it comes out of the cylinder so that the oxygen can be used safely. The regulator also has a pressure gauge that shows the pressure in the cylinder (Figure 8-12). The pressure gauge shows if the cylinder is full (2000 pounds per square inch [psi]), nearly empty or in between). The regulator must be carefully attached to the oxygen cylinder. An "O-ring" gasket makes the seal tight (Figure 8-13). The flowmeter controls how rapidly the oxygen flows from the cylinder to the victim. The flow can be set from 1 to 25 LPM.

Fixed-Flow-Rate Oxygen

Some emergency oxygen systems have the regulator set at a fixed-flow rate. Most fixed-flow rate tanks are set at 15 LPM; however, you may come across tanks set at 6 LPM, 12 LPM or another rate. Some fixed-flow-rate systems have a dual (high/low) flow setting. Fixed-flow-rate oxygen systems typically come with the delivery device, regulator and cylinder already assembled (Figure 8-14), which makes it quick and simple to administer emergency oxygen.

A drawback to fixed-flow-rate oxygen systems is that the flow rate cannot be adjusted, which limits how it can be used as well as the concentration of oxygen

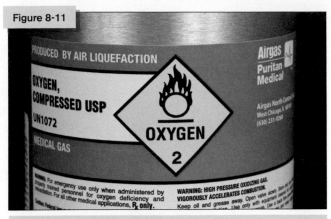

Figure 8-11

Oxygen cylinders are marked with a yellow diamond that says "Oxygen" and, in the United States, typically have green markings.

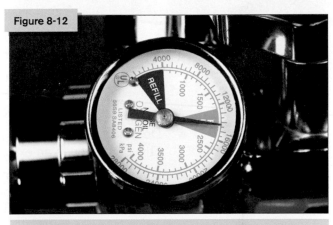

Figure 8-12

A pressure regulator is attached to an oxygen cylinder to reduce the pressure of oxygen to a safe level.

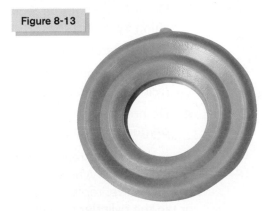

Figure 8-13

An O-ring gasket

Figure 8-14

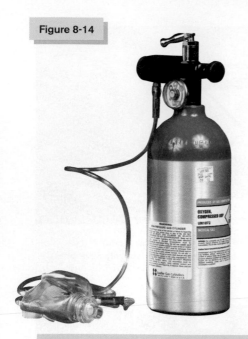

A fixed-flow-rate oxygen system

that can be delivered. For example, a fixed-flow-rate unit with a preset flow of 6 LPM can be used only with a nasal cannula or resuscitation mask, whereas a preset flow rate of 12 LPM allows the use of only a resuscitation mask or non-rebreather mask.

To operate this type of device, simply turn it on according to the manufacturer's instructions, check that oxygen is flowing and place the delivery device on the victim.

Oxygen Safety Precautions

When preparing and administering emergency oxygen, safety is a major concern. Use emergency oxygen equipment according to the manufacturer's instructions and in a manner consistent with federal and local regulations.

Also, follow these recommended guidelines:

- Be sure that oxygen is flowing before putting the delivery device over the victim's face.
- Do not use oxygen around flames or sparks, including smoking materials, such as cigarettes, cigars and pipes. Oxygen causes fire to burn more rapidly and intensely.
- Do not use grease, oil or petroleum products to lubricate or clean the regulator. This could cause an explosion.
- Do not stand oxygen cylinders upright unless they are well secured. If the cylinder falls, the regulator or valve could become damaged or cause injury due to the intense pressure in the tank.
- Do not drag or roll cylinders.
- Do not carry a cylinder by the valve or regulator.
- Do not hold onto protective valve caps or guards when moving or lifting cylinders.
- Do not deface, alter or remove any labeling or markings on the oxygen cylinder.
- Do not attempt to mix gases in an oxygen cylinder or transfer oxygen from one cylinder to another.
- Do not use a defibrillator when around flammable materials, such as free-flowing oxygen or gasoline.

Never attempt to refill an oxygen cylinder; only an appropriately licensed professional should do this. When high-pressure oxygen cylinders have been emptied, close the cylinder valve, replace the valve protection cap or outlet plug if provided, and mark or tag the cylinder as empty. Promptly return the cylinder to be refilled according to state and local regulations.

Pay specific attention to the following areas concerning oxygen cylinders:

- Check for cylinder leaks, abnormal bulging, defective or inoperative valves or safety devices.
- Check for the physical presence of rust or corrosion on a cylinder or cylinder neck, and any foreign substances or residues, such as adhesive tape, around the cylinder neck, oxygen valve or regulator assembly. These substances can hamper oxygen delivery and in some cases have the potential to cause a fire or explosion.

OXYGEN DELIVERY DEVICES

An oxygen delivery device is the equipment used by a victim for breathing emergency oxygen. Tubing carries the oxygen from the regulator to the delivery device, which is placed on the victim's face. When administering emergency oxygen, make sure that the tubing does not get tangled or kinked, which could stop the flow of oxygen to the mask. Oxygen delivery devices include nasal cannulas, resuscitation masks, non-rebreather masks and BVMs (Table 8-3). Various sizes of these devices are available for adults, children and infants. Appropriate sizing is important to ensure adequate airway management.

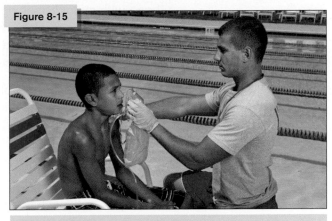

Figure 8-15

Use the blow-by technique for children and infants who are frightened by having oxygen masks on their faces.

If young children or infants are frightened by a mask being placed on their face, use the "blow-by" technique. To perform this technique, you or a parent or guardian holds the mask about 2 inches from the child's or infant's face, waving it slowly from side to side, allowing the oxygen to pass over the face and be inhaled (Figure 8-15).

Table 8-3: Oxygen Delivery Devices

Delivery Device	Common Flow Rate	Oxygen Concentration	Suitable Victims
Nasal Cannula	1–6 LPM	24–44%	■ Victims with breathing difficulty ■ Victims unable to tolerate mask
Resuscitation Mask	6–15 LPM	35–55%	■ Victims with breathing difficulty ■ Victims who are nonbreathing
Non-Rebreather Mask	10–15 LPM	Up to 90%	Breathing victims only
BVM	15 LPM or higher	90% or higher	Breathing and nonbreathing victims

Nasal Cannulas

Nasal cannulas are used only on victims who are able to breathe, most commonly on those with minor breathing difficulty or a history of respiratory medical conditions. They are useful for a victim who can breathe but cannot tolerate a mask over the face. Nasal cannulas are held in place over a victim's ears, and oxygen is delivered through two small prongs inserted into the nostrils.

These devices are not used often in an emergency because they do not give as much oxygen as a resuscitation mask, non-rebreather mask or BVM. Victims experiencing a serious breathing emergency generally breathe through the mouth and need a device that can supply a greater concentration of oxygen. Nasal cannulas may not be effective for victims with a nasal airway obstruction, nasal injury or severe cold.

With a nasal cannula, you should set the flow rate at 1 to 6 LPM. Avoid using rates above 6 LPM with this device since they tend to quickly dry out mucous membranes, which causes nose bleeds and headaches.

MONITORING OXYGEN SATURATION

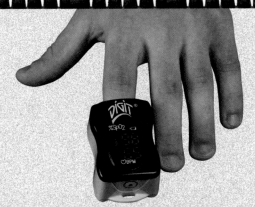

Pulse oximetry is used to measure the percentage of oxygen saturation in the blood. The reading is taken by a pulse oximeter and appears as a percentage of hemoglobin saturated with oxygen. Pulse oximetry readings are recorded using the percentage and then Sp02 (e.g., 95 to 99% Sp02).

Pulse oximetry should be used as an added tool for victim care, as it is possible for victims to show a normal reading but have trouble breathing, or have a low reading but appear to be breathing normally. When treating the victim, all symptoms should be assessed, along with the data provided by the device. The pulse oximeter reading never should be used to withhold oxygen from a victim who appears to be in respiratory distress or when it is the standard of care to apply oxygen despite good pulse oximetry readings, such as in a victim with chest pain.

To use a pulse oximeter, apply the probe to the victim's finger or any other measuring site, such as the ear lobe or foot, according to manufacturer's recommendation. If the victim is wearing nail polish, remove it using an acetone wipe. Let the machine register the oxygen saturation level and verify the victim's pulse rate on the oximeter with the actual pulse of the victim. Monitor the victim's saturation levels while administering emergency oxygen. If the oxygen level reaches 100 percent and local protocols allow, you may decrease the flow rate of oxygen and change to a lower flowing delivery device.

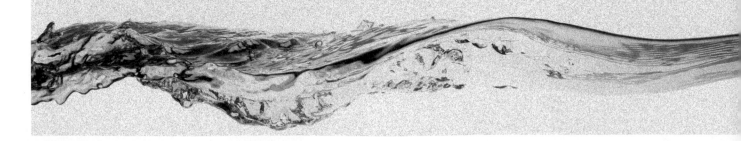

Resuscitation Masks

A resuscitation mask with oxygen inlet can be used to deliver emergency oxygen to a nonbreathing victim. It also can be used to deliver oxygen to someone who is breathing but still requires emergency oxygen. Some resuscitation masks come with elastic straps to place over the victim's head to keep the mask in place. If the mask does not have straps, you or the victim can hold the mask in place. With a resuscitation mask, set the oxygen flow rate at 6 to 15 LPM.

Non-Rebreather Masks

A non-rebreather mask is used to deliver high concentrations of oxygen to a victim who is breathing. It consists of a face mask with an attached oxygen reservoir bag and a one-way valve between the mask and bag, which prevents the victim's exhaled air from mixing with the oxygen in the reservoir bag.

Limitations

Some factors may reduce the reliability of the pulse oximetry reading, including:

- Hypoperfusion, poor perfusion (shock).
- Cardiac arrest (absent perfusion to fingers).
- Excessive motion of the patient during the reading.
- Carbon monoxide poisoning (carbon monoxide saturates hemoglobin).
- Fingernail polish.
- Hypothermia or other cold-related emergency.
- Sickle cell disease or anemia.
- Cigarette smokers (due to carbon monoxide).
- Edema (swelling).
- Time lag in detection of respiratory insufficiency. (The pulse oximeter could warn too late of a decrease in respiratory function based on the amount of oxygen in circulation.)

Range	Percent Value	Delivery Device
Normal	95 to 100	None
Mild hypoxia	91 to 94	Nasal cannula or resuscitation mask
Moderate hypoxia	86 to 90	Non-rebreather mask or BVM
Severe hypoxia	< 85	Non-rebreather mask or BVM

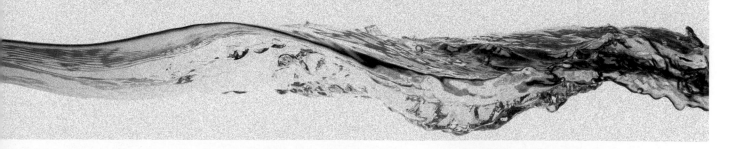

AIRWAY ADJUNCTS

The tongue is the most common cause of airway obstruction in an unconscious person. You can use a mechanical device, called an *airway adjunct*, to keep a victim's airway clear.

There are two types of airway adjuncts. One type, called an oropharyngeal airway (OPA), is inserted in the victim's mouth.

The other type, called a nasopharyngeal airway (NPA), is inserted in the victim's nose.

OPAs and NPAs come in a variety of sizes. The curved design fits the natural contour of the mouth and throat. Once you have positioned the device, use a resuscitation mask or BVM to ventilate a nonbreathing victim.

Oropharyngeal Airways

When properly positioned, an OPA keeps the tongue away from the back of the throat, helping to maintain an open airway. An improperly

placed airway device can compress the tongue into the back of the throat, further blocking the airway.

When preparing to insert an OPA, first be sure that the victim is unconscious. OPAs are used *only* on unconscious, unresponsive victims with

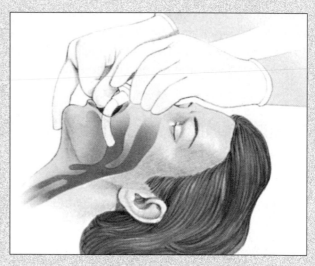

Insert an OPA with the curved tip along the roof of the mouth.

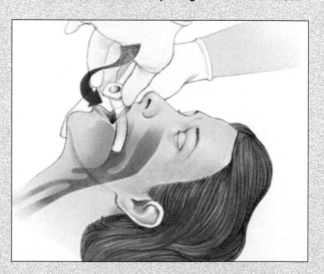

Rotate it to drop into the back of the throat.

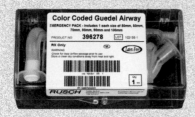

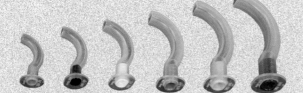

Oropharyngeal airways

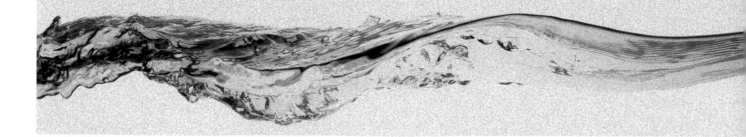

no gag reflex. If a victim begins to gag, remove the airway immediately. OPAs should not be used if the victim has suffered oral trauma, such as broken teeth, or has recently undergone oral surgery. To insert an OPA on an adult, select the appropriately sized OPA, point the tip upward toward the roof of the mouth and then rotate it 180 degrees into position. Follow local protocols for when, how and who can use OPAs.

Airways of children and infants are smaller than those of adults. The size of the airway also can vary according to the age of the child or infant, so it is important to use an appropriately sized OPA for pediatric victims. Also, the palate for children and infants is softer than for an adult. For a child or infant, insert the OPA sideways and then rotate it 90 degrees. Or, use a tongue depressor and insert with the tip of the device pointing toward the back of the tongue and throat in the position in which the device will rest after insertion. If an OPA is inserted with the tip pointing upward toward the roof of the mouth and rotated 180 degrees in a child or infant, it can cause injury to the child's or infant's palate.

Nasopharyngeal Airways

When properly positioned, an NPA keeps the tongue out of the back of the throat, keeping the airway open. An NPA may be used on a conscious, responsive victim or an unconscious victim. Unlike an OPA, the NPA does not cause the victim to gag. NPAs should not be used on victims with suspected head trauma or skull fracture. Follow local protocols for when, how and who can use NPAs.

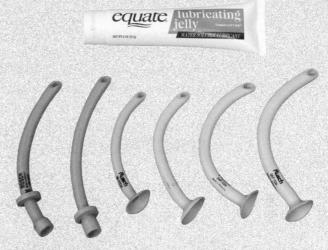

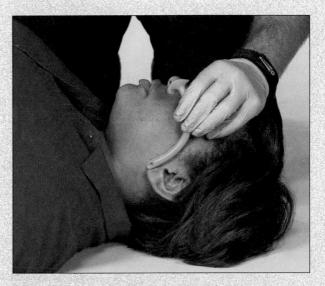

Nasopharyngeal airways

A properly positioned NPA keeps the tongue out of the back of the throat.

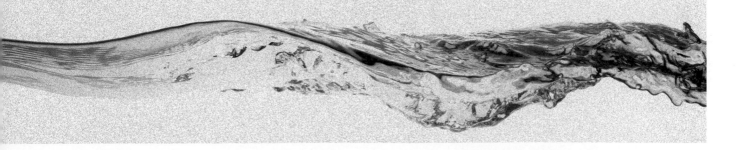

The victim inhales oxygen from the bag, and exhaled air escapes through flutter valves on the side of the mask. The flow rate should be set at 10 to 15 LPM. When using a non-rebreather mask with a high-flow rate of oxygen, you can deliver up to 90 percent oxygen concentration to the victim.

Bag-Valve-Mask Resuscitators

A BVM can be used on a breathing or nonbreathing victim. A conscious, breathing victim can hold the BVM to inhale the oxygen, or you can squeeze the bag as the victim inhales to deliver more oxygen. Set the oxygen flow rate at 15 LPM or higher when using a BVM. The BVM with an oxygen reservoir bag is capable of supplying 90 percent or more oxygen concentration when used at 15 LPM or higher.

SUCTIONING

Sometimes injury or sudden illness can cause mucus, fluids or blood to collect in a victim's airway. A finger sweep can be used to clear the airway on an unconscious victim when the blockage is visible, but a more effective method is to suction the airway clear. *Suctioning* is the process of removing foreign matter from the upper airway using a manual or mechanical device.

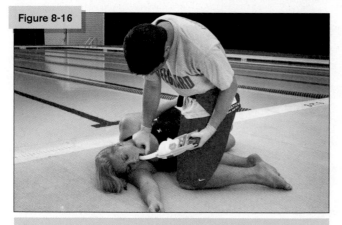

Figure 8-16

Suctioning devices are used to clear a victim's airway.

It is important to suction when fluids or foreign matter are present or suspected, because the airway must be open and clear in order for the victim to breathe. Manual suction units are operated by hand (Figure 8-16). They are lightweight, compact and relatively inexpensive. Because they do not require an energy source, they avoid some of the problems associated with mechanical units and are more suited to the aquatic environment.

If suctioning is part of facility protocols, there should be several sizes of sterile suction catheters on hand to use on victims of various sizes.

WRAP-UP

Breathing emergencies are extremely serious. As a lifeguard, you must know how to recognize the signs and symptoms of respiratory distress, hypoxia and respiratory arrest, and react immediately to provide care for victims. This includes knowing how to give ventilations and care for choking victims. If facility protocols allow, it also includes knowing how to administer emergency oxygen.

GIVING VENTILATIONS

Note: *Always follow standard precautions when providing care. Activate the EAP, size-up the scene for safety and then perform a primary assessment. Always select the right sized mask for the victim.*

If the victim is not breathing but has a pulse:

1 Position and seal the resuscitation mask.

2 Open the airway and blow into the mask.

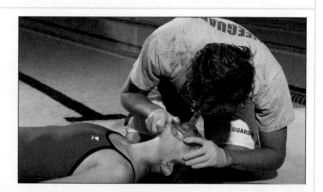

- For an adult, give **1** ventilation about every **5** seconds.
- For a child or infant, give **1** ventilation about every **3** seconds.
- Each ventilation should last about **1** second and make the chest clearly rise.
- The chest should fall before you give the next breath.
- Give ventilations for about **2** minutes.

Note: *For a child, tilt the head slightly past a neutral position. Do not tilt the head as far back as for an adult. For a victim with a suspected head, neck or spinal injury, use the jaw-thrust (without head extension) maneuver to open the airway to give ventilations.*

3 Recheck for breathing and pulse about every 2 minutes.

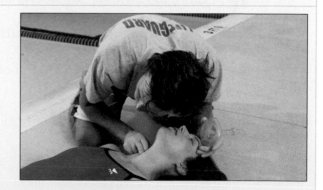

- Remove the mask and look, listen and feel for breathing and a pulse for *no more than **10** seconds.*

What to Do Next

If unconscious but breathing:

- Place in a recovery position.

If unconscious and no breathing but there is a pulse:

- Continue giving ventilations.

Continued on Next Page

GIVING VENTILATIONS *continued*

If unconscious and no breathing or pulse:

- Begin CPR.

If at any time the chest does *not* rise:

- The airway could be blocked—provide care for an unconscious choking victim:
  - o Retilt the head and try to give another ventilation.
  - o If the chest still does not clearly rise, give **30** chest compressions.
  - o Open the mouth to look for and remove a foreign object with a finger if seen.
  - o Give **2** ventilations.
  - o As long as the chest does not clearly rise, continue cycles of giving **30** chest compressions, looking for a foreign object and giving ventilations.

 # GIVING VENTILATIONS USING A BAG-VALVE-MASK RESUSCITATOR—**TWO RESCUERS**

Note: *Always follow standard precautions when providing care. Activate the EAP, size-up the scene for safety and then perform a primary assessment. Always select the right sized mask for the victim. Prepare the BVM for use during the primary assessment.*

If the victim is not breathing but has a pulse:

1 Rescuer 1 kneels behind the victim's head and positions the mask over the victim's mouth and nose.

2 To seal the mask and open the airway using the jaw-thrust (with head extension) maneuver:

- Using the elbows for support, place your thumbs and index fingers along each side of the resuscitation mask to create a "C."
- Slide your 3rd, 4th and 5th fingers into position to create an "E" on both sides of the victim's jawbone.
- Hold the mask in place while you tilt the head back and lift the jaw into the mask.

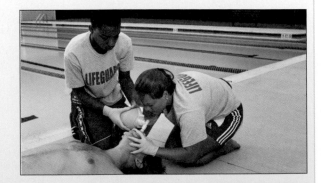

Note: *For a child, tilt the head back slightly past a neutral position. Do not tilt the head as far back as for an adult. For an infant, position the head in a neutral position.*

3 | Rescuer 2 gives ventilations.

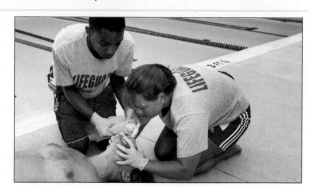

- Squeeze the bag slowly with both hands.

- For an adult, give **1** ventilation about every **5** seconds.

- For a child or infant, give **1** ventilation about every **3** seconds.

- Each ventilation should last about **1** second and make the chest clearly rise. The chest should fall before the next breath is given.

4 | Rescuer 2 rechecks for breathing and a pulse about every **2** minutes.

- Remove the mask and look, listen and feel for breathing and a pulse for *no more than 10 seconds*.

What to Do Next

If unconscious but breathing:

- Place in a recovery position.

If unconscious and not breathing but there is a pulse:

- Continue giving ventilations.

If unconscious and no breathing or pulse:

- Begin CPR.

If at any time the chest does *not* rise:

- The airway could be blocked—provide care for an unconscious choking victim:
  - Retilt the head and try to give another ventilation.
  - If the chest still does not clearly rise, give **30** chest compressions.
  - Open the mouth to look for a foreign object and remove with a finger if seen.
  - Give **2** ventilations.
  - As long as the chest does not clearly rise, continue cycles of giving **30** chest compressions, looking for a foreign object and giving ventilations.

CONSCIOUS CHOKING—**ADULT AND CHILD**

Notes:

- *Activate the EAP; size-up the scene for safety, which includes using appropriate PPE; and obtain consent.*
- *For a child, stand or kneel behind the child, depending on the child's size. Use less force on a child than you would on an adult.*

If the victim cannot cough, speak or breathe:

1   Give **5** back blows.

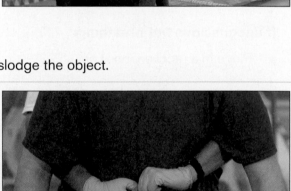

- Position yourself slightly behind the victim.
- Place one arm diagonally across the victim's chest and bend the victim forward at the waist. The victim's upper airway should be at least parallel to the ground.
- Firmly strike the victim between the shoulder blades with the heel of your hand.
- Each thrust should be a distinct attempt to dislodge the object.

2   Give **5** abdominal thrusts.

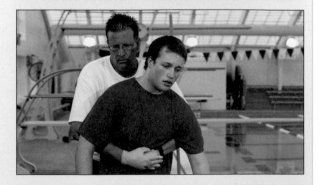

- Stand behind the victim.
- For a child, stand or kneel behind the child, depending on the child's size. Use less force on a child than you would on an adult.
- Place the thumb side of your fist against the middle of the abdomen, just above the navel.
- Grab your fist and give quick, upward thrusts.
- Each thrust should be a distinct attempt to dislodge the object.

What to Do Next

Continue giving 5 back blows and 5 abdominal thrusts until:

■ The object is forced out.

■ The victim begins to cough forcefully or breathe.

■ The victim becomes unconscious.

If the victim becomes unconscious:

■ Carefully lower the victim to the ground, open the mouth and look for an object.

■ Continue to provide care for an unconscious choking victim.

Use chest thrusts if:

■ You cannot reach far enough around the victim to give abdominal thrusts.

■ The victim is obviously pregnant or known to be pregnant.

To perform chest thrusts:

1 Stand behind the victim and place the thumb side of your fist against the center of the victim's chest, or slightly higher on the victim's chest if she is pregnant.

2 Grab your fist and give quick, inward thrusts. Look over the victim's shoulder so that his or her head does not hit your face when you perform the chest thrusts.

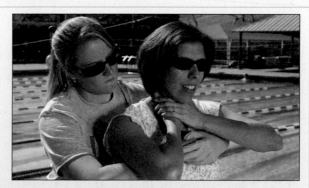

3 Repeat until the object is forced out, the victim begins to cough forcefully or breathe, or until the victim becomes unconscious.

CONSCIOUS CHOKING—**INFANT**

Note: *Activate the EAP; size-up the scene for safety, which includes using appropriate PPE; and obtain consent.*

If the infant cannot cough, cry or breathe:

1 Carefully position the infant face-down along your forearm.

- Support the infant's head and neck with your hand.
- Lower the infant onto your thigh, keeping the infant's head lower than his or her chest.

2 Give **5** back blows.

- Give back blows with the heel of your hand between the infant's shoulder blades.
- Each back blow should be a distinct attempt to dislodge the object.

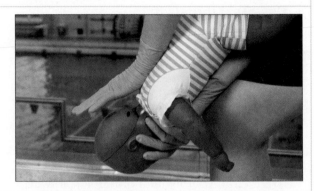

3 Position the infant face-up along your forearm.

- Position the infant between both of your forearms, supporting the infant's head and neck.
- Turn the infant face-up.
- Lower the infant onto your thigh with the infant's head lower than his or her chest.

4 Give **5** chest thrusts.

- Put two or three fingers on the center of the chest just below the nipple line and compress the chest about 1½ inches.
- Each chest thrust should be a distinct attempt to dislodge the object.

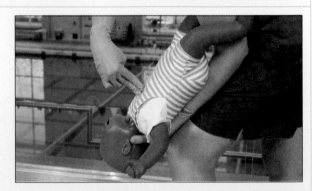

What to Do Next

Continue giving 5 back blows and 5 chest thrusts until:

- The object is forced out.
- The infant begins to cough forcefully or breathe.
- The infant becomes unconscious.

If the infant becomes unconscious:

- Carefully lower the infant to the ground, open the mouth and look for an object.
- Continue to provide care for an unconscious choking infant.

UNCONSCIOUS CHOKING

Notes:

- *Activate the EAP, size-up the scene for safety then perform a primary assessment.*
- *Ensure that the victim is on a firm, flat surface, such as the floor or a table.*

If at any time the chest does *not* clearly rise:

1 Retilt the head and give another ventilation.

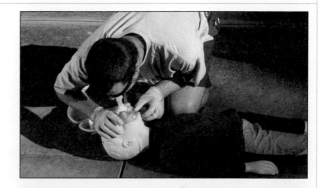

2 If the chest still does not clearly rise, give **30** chest compressions.

- Place the heel of one hand on the center of the chest.
- Place the other hand on top of the first hand and compress the chest **30** times.
- For an adult, compress the chest at least **2** inches.
- For a child, compress the chest about **2** inches.
- Compress at a rate of about **100** compressions per minute.

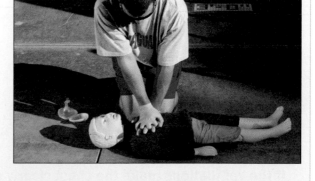

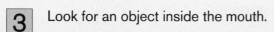

3 Look for an object inside the mouth.

- Grasp the tongue and lower jaw between your thumb and fingers, and lift the jaw.

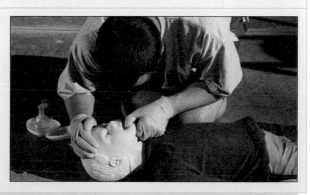

Continued on Next Page ▶

UNCONSCIOUS CHOKING *continued*

4 If you see an object, remove it.

- Slide your finger along the inside of the victim's cheek, using a hooking motion to sweep out the object.

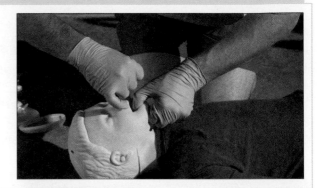

5 Give **2** ventilations.

- Replace the resuscitation mask and give **2** ventilations.

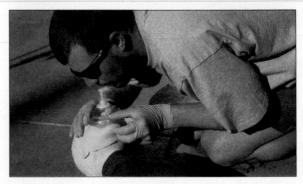

What to Do Next

If at any time the chest does *not* rise:

- Repeat Steps 2–5.

If the ventilations make the chest clearly rise:

- Remove the mask, check for breathing and a pulse for no more than **10** seconds.

If unconscious but breathing, place in a recovery position:

- Leave the victim face-up and continue to monitor the victim's condition.

If unconscious and no breathing but there is a pulse:

- Give ventilations.

If unconscious and no breathing or pulse:

- Begin CPR.

Notes:

- *Keep your fingers off the chest when giving chest compressions.*
- *Use your body weight, not your arms, to compress the chest.*
- *Position your shoulders over your hands with your arms as straight as possible.*

ASSEMBLING THE OXYGEN SYSTEM

Note: *Always follow standard precautions when providing care.*

1 Check the cylinder.

- Make sure that the oxygen cylinder is labeled "U.S.P." (United States Pharmacopeia) and is marked with a yellow diamond containing the word "Oxygen."

2 Clear the valve.

- Remove the protective covering.
- Remove and save the O-ring gasket, if necessary.
- Turn the cylinder away from you and others before opening for 1 second to clear the valve of any debris.

3 Attach the regulator.

- Put the O-ring gasket into the valve on top of the cylinder, if necessary.
- Make sure that it is marked "Oxygen Regulator" and that the O-ring gasket is in place.
- Check to see that the pin index corresponds to an oxygen cylinder.
- Secure the regulator on the cylinder by placing the two metal prongs into the valve.
- Hand-tighten the screw until the regulator is snug.

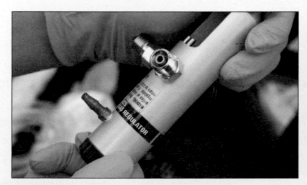 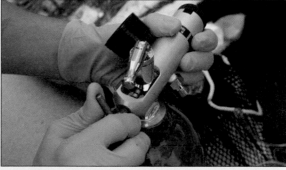

4 Open the cylinder counterclockwise one full turn.

- Check the pressure gauge.
- Determine that the cylinder has enough pressure (more than 200 psi). If the pressure is lower than 200 psi, DO NOT use.

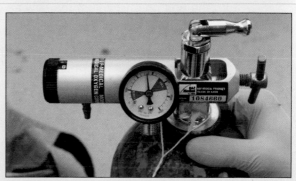

Continued on Next Page ➤

ASSEMBLING THE OXYGEN SYSTEM *continued*

5 Attach the delivery device.

- Attach the plastic tubing between the flowmeter and the delivery device.

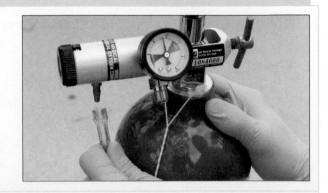

Note: *When breaking down the oxygen equipment, be sure to bleed the pressure regulator by turning on the flowmeter after the cylinder has been turned off.*

 # ADMINISTERING EMERGENCY OXYGEN

Notes:

- *Always follow standard precautions when providing care. Follow local protocols for using emergency oxygen.*
- *Check the cylinder to make sure the oxygen cylinder is labeled "U.S.P." and is marked with a yellow diamond containing the word "Oxygen."*
- *Determine that the cylinder has enough pressure (more than 200 psi). If the pressure is lower than 200 psi, DO NOT use. Assemble the cylinder, regulator and delivery device prior to delivery.*

1 Turn the unit on and adjust the flow as necessary.

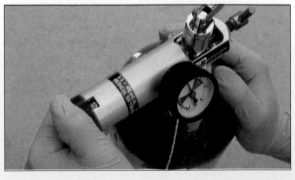

- For a variable-flow-rate oxygen system, turn the flowmeter to the desired flow rate.
  - Nasal cannula: 1–6 LPM
  - Resuscitation mask: 6–15 LPM
  - Non-rebreather mask: 10–15 LPM
    - Inflate the oxygen reservoir bag to two-thirds full by placing your thumb over the one-way valve until the bag is sufficiently inflated.
  - BVM: 15 LPM or higher

2 Verify the oxygen flow.

- Listen for a hissing sound and feel for oxygen flow through the delivery device.

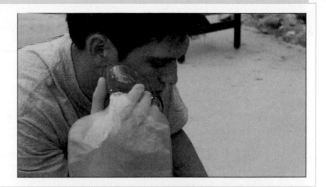

3 Place the delivery device on the victim and continue care until EMS personnel take over.

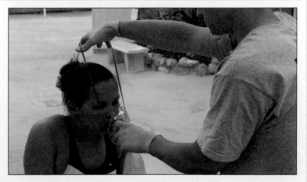

Note: *When monitoring a conscious victim's oxygen saturation levels using a pulse oximeter, you may reduce the flow of oxygen and change to a lower flowing delivery device if the blood oxygen level of the victim reaches 100 percent.*

 # USING A MANUAL SUCTIONING DEVICE

Note: *Follow standard precautions and then perform a primary assessment. If needed, assemble the device according to manufacturer's instructions.*

1 Position the victim.

- Roll the body as a unit onto one side.
- Open the mouth.

2 Remove any visible large debris from the mouth with a gloved finger.

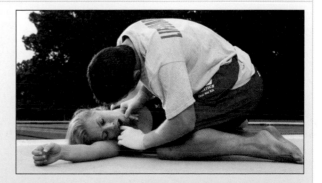

Continued on Next Page

USING A MANUAL SUCTIONING DEVICE *continued*

 3 Measure and check the suction tip.

- Measure from the victim's earlobe to the corner of the mouth.
- Note the distance to prevent inserting the suction tip too deeply.
- Check that the suction is working by placing your finger over the end of the suction tip as you squeeze the handle of the device.

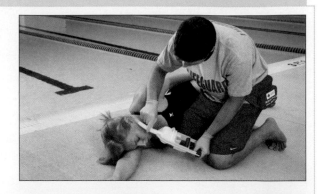

 4 Suction the mouth.

- Insert the suction tip into the back of the mouth.
- Squeeze the handle of the suction device repeatedly to provide suction.
- Apply suction as you withdraw the tip using a sweeping motion, if possible.
- Suction for *no more than 15 seconds at a time for an adult*, *10 seconds for a child* or *5 seconds for an infant*.

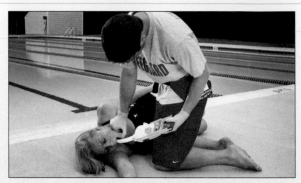

Cardiac Emergencies

A cardiac emergency is life threatening. It can happen at any time to a victim of any age, on land or in the water. You may be called on to care for a victim of a cardiac emergency. This care includes performing CPR and using an automated external defibrillator (AED)—two of the links in the Cardiac Chain of Survival. By following the Cardiac Chain of Survival, you can greatly increase a victim's chance of survival.

Chapter 7 describes how to identify and give initial care for life-threatening conditions by performing a primary assessment. Chapter 8 covers how to recognize and care for breathing emergencies. This chapter covers how to provide care for cardiac emergencies, such as heart attack and cardiac arrest. ∎

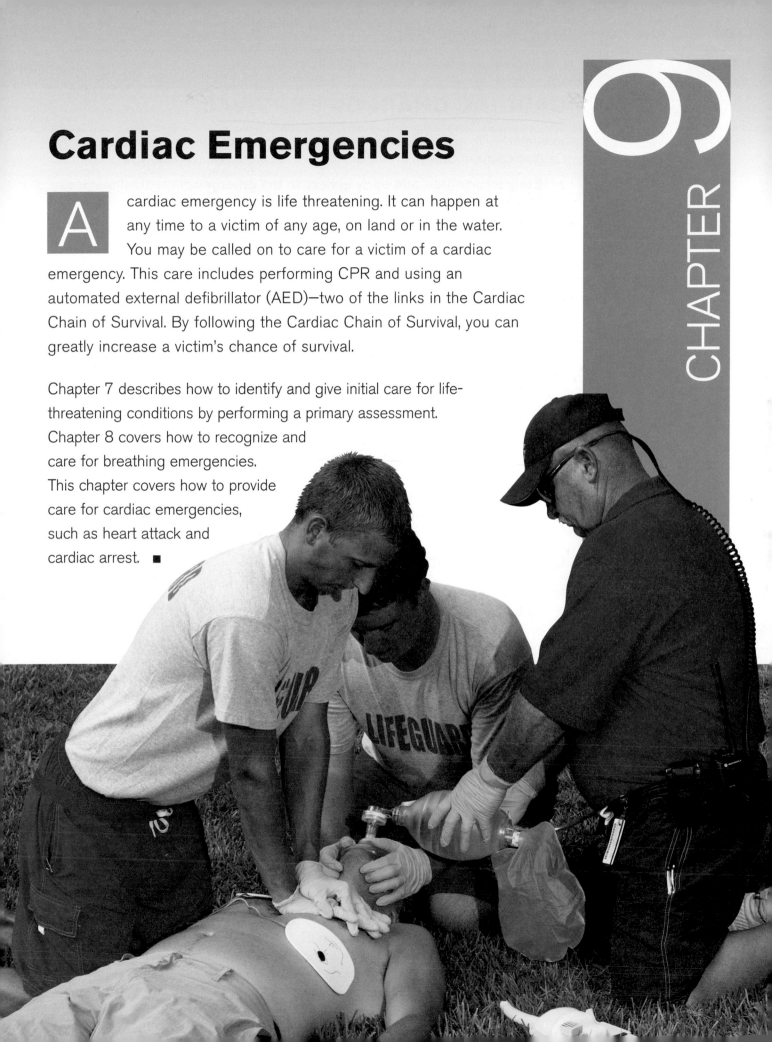

CARDIAC CHAIN OF SURVIVAL

To effectively respond to cardiac emergencies, it is important to understand the Cardiac Chain of Survival. The four links in the Cardiac Chain of Survival are:

- **Early recognition and early access to the emergency medical services (EMS) system.** The sooner someone calls 9-1-1 or the local emergency number, the sooner EMS personnel will arrive and take over.
- **Early CPR.** CPR helps supply oxygen to the brain and other vital organs. This helps keep the victim alive until an AED is used or more advanced medical care is provided.
- **Early defibrillation.** An electrical shock, called defibrillation, may help restore an effective heart rhythm. Defibrillation is delivered using an AED.
- **Early advanced medical care.** EMS personnel provide more advanced medical care and transport the victim to a hospital.

For each minute CPR and defibrillation are delayed, the victim's chance for survival is reduced by about 10 percent.

HEART ATTACK

When the muscle of the heart suffers a loss of oxygenated blood, the result is a *myocardial infarction* (MI), or heart attack.

Causes of a Heart Attack

Heart attacks usually result from cardiovascular disease. Other common causes of heart attack include respiratory distress, electrocution and traumatic injury. The most common conditions caused by cardiovascular disease include coronary heart disease (also known as coronary artery disease) and stroke.

Recognizing a Heart Attack

The sooner you recognize the signs and symptoms of a heart attack and act, the better the victim's chance of survival. Heart attack pain can be confused with the pain of indigestion, muscle spasms or other conditions, often causing people to delay getting medical care. Brief, stabbing pain or pain that gets worse when bending or breathing deeply usually is not caused by a heart problem.

Summon EMS personnel and provide prompt care if the victim shows or reports any of the signs and symptoms listed below. Ask open-ended questions, such as "How are you feeling?" to hear the symptoms described in the victim's own words.

- Chest discomfort or pain that is severe, lasts longer than 3 to 5 minutes, goes away and comes back, or persists even during rest
- Discomfort, pressure or pain that is persistent and ranges from discomfort to an unbearable crushing sensation in the center of the chest, possibly spreading to the shoulder, arm, neck, jaw, stomach or back, and usually not relieved by resting, changing position or taking medication
- Pain that comes and goes (such as angina pectoris)

- Difficulty breathing, such as at a faster rate than normal or noisy breathing
- Pale or ashen skin, especially around the face
- Sweating, especially on the face
- Dizziness or light-headedness
- Nausea or vomiting
- Fatigue, lightheadedness or loss of consciousness

Some individuals may show no signs at all. Women may experience different signs. The chest pain or discomfort experienced by women may be sudden, sharp, but short-lived pain and outside the breastbone. Women are somewhat more likely to experience some of the other warning signs, such as shortness of breath, nausea or vomiting, back or jaw pain and unexplained fatigue or malaise.

Caring for a Heart Attack

If you think someone is having a heart attack:

- Take immediate action and summon EMS personnel.
- Have the victim stop any activity and rest in a comfortable position.
- Loosen tight or uncomfortable clothing.
- Closely monitor the victim until EMS personnel take over. Note any changes in the victim's appearance or behavior.
- Comfort the victim.
- Assist the victim with prescribed medication, such as nitroglycerin or aspirin, and administer emergency oxygen, if is available and you are trained to do so.
- Be prepared to perform CPR and use an AED.

You should also ask questions to get information that relates to the victim's condition, such as what happened, whether the victim has any medical conditions or is taking any medications, or when was the last time the victim had anything to eat or drink.

Administering Aspirin for a Heart Attack

You may be able to help a conscious victim who is showing early signs of a heart attack by offering an appropriate dose of aspirin when the signs first begin, if local protocols allow or medical direction permits. Aspirin never should replace advanced medical care.

If the victim is conscious and able to take medicine by mouth, ask:

- Are you allergic to aspirin?
- Do you have a stomach ulcer or stomach disease?
- Are you taking any blood thinners, such as Coumadin® (warfarin)?
- Have you been told by a doctor not to take aspirin?

If the victim answers "no" to all of these questions and if local protocols allow, consider administering two chewable (162-mg) baby aspirins or up to one 5-grain (325-mg) adult aspirin tablet with a small amount of water. You also may offer these doses of aspirin if you have cared for the victim and he or she has regained consciousness and is able to take the aspirin by mouth.

Be sure that you give *only* aspirin and not acetaminophen (e.g., Tylenol®) or other nonsteroidal anti-inflammatory drugs (NSAIDs), such as ibuprofen (e.g., Motrin® or Advil®) or naproxen (e.g., Aleve®). Likewise, do not offer coated aspirin products since they take too long to dissolve, or products meant for multiple symptoms, such as cold, fever and headache.

CARDIAC ARREST

Cardiac arrest is a life-threatening emergency that may be caused by a heart attack, drowning, electrocution, respiratory arrest or other conditions. Cardiac arrest occurs when the heart stops beating, or beats too irregularly or weakly to circulate blood effectively. Cardiac arrest can occur suddenly and without warning. In many cases, the victim already may be experiencing the signs and symptoms of a heart attack.

The signs of a cardiac arrest include sudden collapse, unconsciousness, no breathing and no pulse.

CPR

A victim who is unconscious, not breathing and has no pulse is in cardiac arrest and needs CPR (Figure 9-1). The objective of CPR is to perform a combination of effective chest compressions and ventilations to circulate blood that contains oxygen to the victim's brain and other vital organs. In most cases, CPR is performed in cycles of 30 chest compressions followed by 2 ventilations.

Summoning EMS personnel immediately is critical for the victim's survival. If an AED is available, it should be used in combination with CPR and according to local protocols until EMS personnel take over.

To most effectively perform compressions, place your hands in the center of the chest. Avoid pressing directly on the *xiphoid process*, the lowest point of the breastbone. Compressing the chest straight down provides the best blood flow and is also less tiring for you. Kneel at the victim's side, opposite the chest, with your hands in the correct position. Keep your arms as straight as possible, with your shoulders directly over your hands.

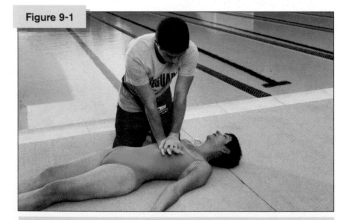

Figure 9-1

CPR is delivered in cycles of chest compressions and ventilations.

The effectiveness of compressions can be increased if:

■ The victim is on a firm, flat surface

■ Compressions are the proper depth.

■ Compression rate is appropriate.

■ The chest fully recoils after each compression (letting the chest come all the way back up).

■ CPR is performed without interruption.

Remember that when giving ventilations to a victim, you should:

■ Maintain an open airway by keeping the head tilted back in the proper position.

■ Seal the mask over the victim's mouth and nose.

■ Blow into the one-way valve, ensuring that you can see the chest clearly rise and fall. Each ventilation should last about 1 second, with a brief pause between breaths to let the chest fall.

After ventilations, quickly reposition your hands on the center of the chest and start another cycle of compressions and ventilations.

Table 9-1: **Summary of Techniques for CPR–Adult, Child and Infant**			
	Adult	**Child**	**Infant**
Hand position	Heel of one hand in center of chest (on lower half of sternum) with the other hand on top		Two or three fingers on the center of the chest (just below the nipple line)
Compression depth	At least **2** inches	About **2** inches	About **1½** inches
Ventilations	Until chest clearly rises (about **1** second per ventilation)		
Cycles (one rescuer)	**30** chest compressions and **2** ventilations		
Cycles (two rescuers)	**30** chest compressions and **2** ventilations	**15** chest compressions and **2** ventilations	
Rate	At least 100 compressions per minute		

Once you begin CPR, do not stop. Continue CPR until:

■ You see an obvious sign of life, such as breathing.

■ An AED is available and ready to use.

■ Another trained rescuer takes over, such as a member of your safety team.

■ EMS personnel take over.

■ You are too exhausted to continue.

■ The scene becomes unsafe.

When performing CPR, it is not unusual for the victim's ribs to break or cartilage to separate. The victim may vomit, there may be frothing at the nose and mouth, and the scene may be chaotic. The victim also may produce agonal gasps. Remember that agonal gasps are not breathing–this victim needs CPR.

Understand that, despite your best efforts, not all victims of cardiac arrest survive.

Two-Rescuer CPR

When an additional rescuer is available, you should provide two-rescuer CPR. One rescuer gives ventilations and the other gives chest compressions. Rescuers should change positions (alternate giving compressions and ventilations) about every 2 minutes to reduce the possibility of rescuer fatigue. Changing positions should take less than 5 seconds.

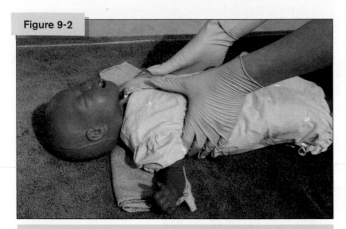

Figure 9-2

The two-thumb-encircling-hands chest compression technique with thoracic squeeze is used on an infant in two-person CPR.

When CPR is in progress by one rescuer and a second rescuer arrives, the second rescuer should confirm whether EMS personnel have been summoned. If EMS personnel have not been summoned, the second rescuer should do so before getting the AED or assisting with care. If EMS personnel have been summoned, the second rescuer should get the AED, or if an AED is not available, help perform two-rescuer CPR.

When performing two-rescuer CPR on a child or infant, rescuers should change the compression-to-ventilation ratio from 30:2 to 15:2. This provides more frequent respirations for children and infants. When providing two-rescuer CPR to an infant, rescuers should perform a different technique, called the *two-thumb-encircling-hands chest compression technique with thoracic squeeze* (Figure 9-2).

AEDS

AEDs are portable electronic devices that analyze the heart's rhythm and provide an electrical shock (Figure 9-3). Defibrillation is the delivery of an electrical shock that may help re-establish an effective rhythm. CPR can help by supplying blood that contains oxygen to the brain and other vital organs. However, the sooner an AED is used, the greater the likelihood of survival. You must assess victims quickly and be prepared to use an AED in cases of cardiac arrest.

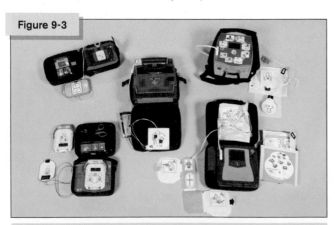

Figure 9-3

AEDs

When the Heart Stops

Any damage to the heart from disease or injury can disrupt the heart's electrical system, which normally triggers the contraction—or pumping action—of the heart muscle. This disruption can result in an abnormal heart rhythm, possibly stopping circulation. The two most common treatable abnormal rhythms that cause sudden cardiac arrest are *ventricular fibrillation* (V-fib) and *ventricular tachycardia* (V-tach). In V-fib, the ventricles quiver, or fibrillate, without any organized rhythm, and the electrical impulses fire at random, creating chaos and preventing the heart from pumping and circulating blood. There is no pulse. In V-tach, an abnormal electrical impulse controls the heart. This abnormal impulse fires so fast that the heart's chambers do not have time to fill, and the heart is unable to pump blood effectively. With little or no blood circulating, there may be either a pulse or no pulse.

In many cases, V-fib and V-tach can be corrected by early defibrillation. If V-fib or V-tach is not corrected, all electrical activity will eventually cease, a condition called *asystole*. Asystole cannot be corrected by defibrillation. You cannot tell what, if any, rhythm the heart has by feeling for a pulse. An AED will analyze the heart's rhythm and determine if there is a treatable rhythm.

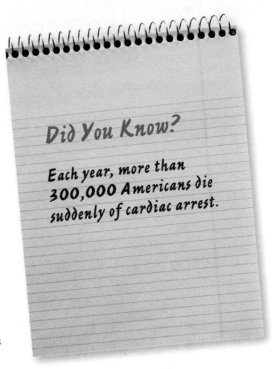

Did You Know?

Each year, more than 300,000 Americans die suddenly of cardiac arrest.

Using an AED on Adults

When cardiac arrest occurs, use an AED as soon as it is ready to use. First, apply the AED pads and allow the AED to analyze the heart rhythm. Then, follow the prompts of the AED. If CPR is in progress, do not interrupt chest compressions until the AED is turned on, the AED pads are applied and the AED is ready to analyze the heart rhythm.

After a shock is delivered, or if no shock is advised, perform about 2 minutes of CPR before the AED analyzes the heart rhythm again. If at any time you notice an obvious sign of life, such as breathing, stop CPR and monitor the victim's condition. Administer emergency oxygen if available and you are trained to do so.

Using an AED on Children and Infants

While the incidence of cardiac arrest in children and infants is relatively low compared with that of adults, cardiac arrest does happen to young children. Causes of cardiac arrests in children include:

- Airway and breathing problems.
- Traumatic injuries or accidents (e.g., drowning, motor-vehicle collision, electrocution and poisoning).
- A hard blow to the chest.
- Congenital heart disease.
- Sudden infant death syndrome (SIDS).

AEDs equipped with pediatric AED pads are capable of delivering the lower levels of energy considered appropriate for infants and children up to 8 years old or weighing less than 55 pounds. Use pediatric AED pads and/or equipment for a pediatric victim, if available. If pediatric-specific equipment is not available, an AED designed for adults can be used on children and infants.

Always follow local protocols, medical direction and the manufacturer's instructions. For a child or infant in cardiac arrest, follow the same general steps and precautions as when using an AED on an adult. If the pads risk touching each other because of the victim's smaller chest size, place one pad on the child or infant's chest and the other on the back.

AED Precautions

When operating an AED, follow these general precautions:

- Do *not* use alcohol to wipe the victim's chest dry; alcohol is flammable.
- Do *not* touch the victim while the AED is analyzing. Touching or moving the victim could affect the analysis.
- Before shocking a victim with an AED, make sure that *no one* is touching or is in contact with the victim or the resuscitation equipment.
- Do *not* touch the victim while the device is defibrillating. You or someone else could be shocked.
- Do *not* defibrillate a victim when around flammable or combustible materials, such as gasoline or free-flowing oxygen.
- Do *not* use an AED in a moving vehicle. Movement could affect the analysis.
- Do *not* use an AED on a victim wearing a nitroglycerin patch or other patch on the chest. With a gloved hand, remove any patches from the chest before attaching the device.
- Do *not* use a mobile phone or radio within 6 feet of the AED. Electromagnetic and infrared interference generated by radio signals can disrupt analysis.

Special AED Situations

Some situations require special precautions when using an AED. These include using AEDs around water, on victims with implantable devices or transdermal patches, on victims of trauma or hypothermia, or when confronted with AED protocols that differ from those discussed here. Be familiar with these situations and know how to respond appropriately. Always follow manufacturer's recommendations.

AEDs Around Water

A shock delivered *in* water could harm rescuers or bystanders; however, AEDs are safe to use on victims who have been removed from the water. If the victim is in water:

- Remove the victim from the water before defibrillation. A shock delivered in water could harm rescuers or bystanders.
- Be sure that there are no puddles of water around you, the victim or the AED (Figure 9-4).
- Remove the victim's wet clothing to place the AED pads properly, if necessary.
- Dry the victim's chest and attach the AED pads.

If it is raining, take steps to make sure that the victim is as dry as possible and sheltered from the rain. Ensure that the victim's chest is wiped dry. Do not delay defibrillation when taking steps to create a dry environment. AEDs are safe, even in rain and snow, when all precautions and manufacturer's operating instructions are followed. Avoid getting the AED or AED pads wet.

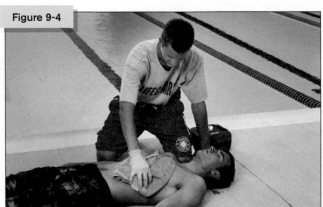

Figure 9-4

Before using an AED, be sure the victim is not lying in any puddles of water. Dry the victim's chest, then attach the AED pads.

Pacemakers and Implantable Cardioverter-Defibrillators

Pacemakers are small implantable devices sometimes located in the area below the right collarbone. There may be a small lump that can be felt under the skin (Figure 9-5). An implantable cardioverter-defibrillator (ICD) is a miniature version of an AED that automatically recognizes and restores abnormal heart rhythms. Sometimes, a victim's heart beats irregularly, even if the victim has a pacemaker or an ICD.

Figure 9-5

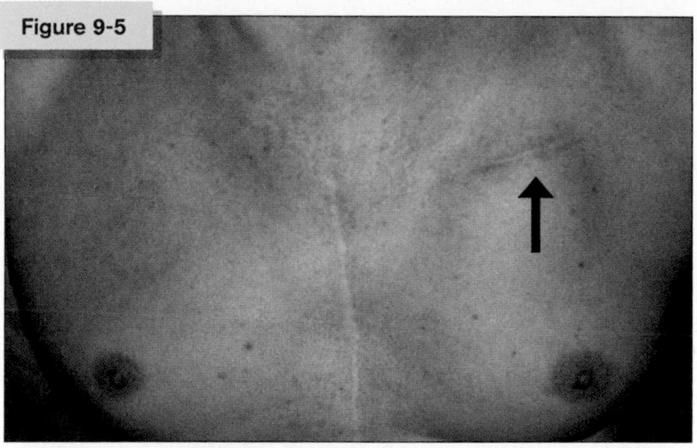

Scars or a small lump may indicate that the patient has had some sort of device implanted.

■ If the implanted device is visible, or you know that the victim has one, do not place the AED pad directly over the device. This may interfere with the delivery of the shock. Adjust AED pad placement if necessary and continue to follow the AED instructions.

■ If you are not sure whether the victim has an implanted device, use the AED as needed. It will not harm the victim or rescuer.

■ Follow any special precautions associated with ICDs, but do not delay CPR or defibrillation.

It is possible to receive a mild shock if an implantable ICD delivers a shock to the victim while CPR is performed. This risk of injury to rescuers is minimal and the amount of electrical energy involved is low.

Transdermal Medication Patches

A transdermal medication patch automatically delivers medication through the skin. The most common of these patches is the nitroglycerin patch, used by those with a history of cardiac problems. Since you might absorb nitroglycerin or other medications, remove the patch from the victim's chest with a gloved hand before defibrillation. Nicotine patches used to stop smoking look similar

Figure 9-6

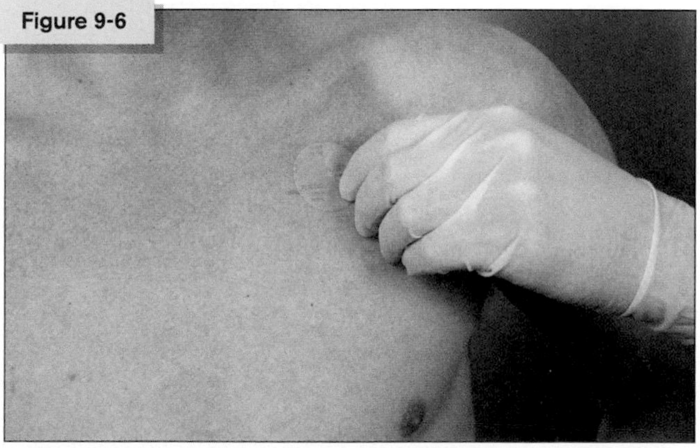

Remove any type of transdermal medication patch from the victim's chest with a gloved hand before defibrillation.

to nitroglycerin patches. To avoid wasting time trying to identify patches, remove any patch on the victim's chest with a gloved hand (Figure 9-6). *Never* place AED electrode pads directly on top of medication patches.

Hypothermia

Hypothermia is a life-threatening condition in which the entire body cools because its ability to keep warm fails. Some people who have experienced hypothermia have been resuscitated successfully even after prolonged exposure to the cold. During your primary assessment, you may have to check for breathing and a pulse for up to 30 to 45 seconds.

If the victim is not breathing and does not have a pulse begin CPR until an AED becomes available. Follow local protocols regarding whether you should use an AED in this situation.

If the victim is wet:

- Remove wet clothing, dry the victim's chest and protect the victim from further heat loss.
- Attach the AED pads.
- If a shock is indicated, deliver it, following the instructions of the AED.
- Follow local protocols regarding whether additional shocks should be delivered.
- Do not withhold CPR or defibrillation to re-warm the victim.
- Be careful not to unnecessarily shake a victim who has experienced hypothermia as this could result in an irregular heart rhythm.

Chest Hair

Some men have excessive chest hair that may cause difficulty with pad-to-skin contact. Since the time it takes to deliver the first shock is critical, and chest hair *rarely* interferes with pad adhesion, attach the pads and analyze the heart's rhythm as soon as possible.

- Press firmly on the pads to attach them to the victim's chest. If you get a "Check pads" or similar message from the AED, remove the pads and replace with new ones. The pad adhesive may pull out some of the chest hair, which may solve the problem.
- If you continue to get the "Check pads" message, remove the pads, carefully shave the victim's chest and attach new pads to the victim's chest.

Trauma

If a victim is in cardiac arrest resulting from traumatic injuries, you may still use an AED. Administer defibrillation according to local protocols.

Metal Surfaces

It is safe to deliver a shock to a victim in cardiac arrest on a metal surface, such as bleachers, as long as appropriate safety precautions are taken. Care should be taken that AED pads do not contact the conductive (metal) surface and that no one is touching the victim when the shock button is pressed.

Jewelry and Body Piercings

You do not need to remove jewelry and body piercings when using an AED. Leaving them on the victim will do no harm. However, do *not* place the AED pad directly over metallic jewelry or body piercings. Adjust pad placement if necessary and continue to follow established protocols.

Pregnancy

Defibrillation shocks transfer no significant electrical current to the fetus. Follow local protocols and medical direction.

AED Maintenance

For defibrillators to perform optimally, they must be maintained. AEDs require minimal maintenance. These devices have various self-testing features. Familiarize yourself with any visual or audible prompts the AED may have to warn of malfunction or a low battery. Read the operator's manual thoroughly and check with the manufacturer to obtain all necessary information regarding maintenance.

In most instances, if the machine detects any malfunction, you should inform management, who will contact the manufacturer. The device may need to be returned to the manufacturer for service. While AEDs require minimal maintenance, it is important to remember the following:

- Follow the manufacturer's specific recommendations for periodic equipment checks.
- Make sure that the batteries have enough energy for one complete rescue. (A fully charged backup battery should be readily available.)
- Make sure that the correct defibrillator pads are in the package and are properly sealed.
- Check any expiration dates on AED pads and batteries, and replace as necessary.
- After use, make sure that all accessories are replaced and that the machine is in proper working order before placing the unit back in service.
- If at any time the machine fails to work properly, or you recognize any warning indicators, discontinue use, place the unit out of service and contact the manufacturer immediately.

MULTIPLE-RESCUER RESPONSE

In the aquatic environment, more than two rescuers often respond to an emergency. In many cases, three or more rescuers provide care for an unconscious victim. When an unconscious victim has been removed from the water and needs CPR, care might begin with one rescuer until other rescuers arrive on the scene with additional equipment and begin assisting in providing care.

Roles for multiple-rescuer response for an unconscious victim may include (Figure 9-7):

- **Airway.** The rescuer is positioned behind the victim's head to maintain an open airway and ensure the mask is positioned and sealed to provide effective ventilations.
- **Breathing.** The rescuer provides ventilations by using a bag-valve-mask resuscitator (BVM). Emergency oxygen may be attached to the BVM if rescuers are trained to administer emergency oxygen. If there is froth or the victim vomits during CPR, the rescuer clears the obstructed airway from the victim's mouth by using a finger sweep or a manual suction device.

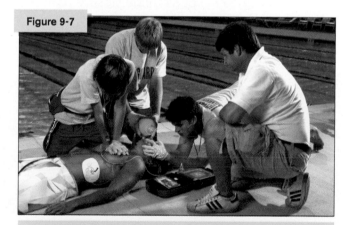

Figure 9-7

In a multi-rescuer response for an unconscious victim, lifeguards and other staff work together to provide care.

- **Circulation.** The rescuer provides compressions and also may operate the AED. If an additional rescuer is available, he or she should place the pads and operate the AED.

Practice multiple-rescuer response drills regularly with your team. Each member of the team should be able to arrive on the scene and be able to perform any of the roles necessary in providing the appropriate care. See the flowchart on the next page for an example of how multiple-rescuer response operates.

Example of a Multiple-Rescuer Response

This is an example of how multiple rescuers come on to the scene and help care for the victim. Follow the protocols for the EAP for your facility. A victim may not exhibit all of the symptoms or exhibit the symptoms in this order (e.g., obstructed airway). Always provide the appropriate care for the conditions found.

You should use an AED as soon as it is available and ready to use. Using an AED has priority over using a BVM or administering emergency oxygen. If a rescuer is needed to get or prepare the AED, stop using the BVM and perform two-person CPR until the AED is ready to analyze.

This example assumes that the EAP has been activated, EMS personnel have been called and a primary assessment has been done. The victim is not breathing and has no pulse. Additional rescuers are coming in to support the efforts of the initial rescuers and are bringing equipment.

The initial rescuers begin two-rescuer CPR.

- Rescuers 1 and 2 perform two-rescuer CPR.
- Rescuer 1 gives ventilations while Rescuer 2 gives chest compressions.

An additional rescuer arrives with the AED. CPR continues until the AED pads are placed on the victim and it is ready to begin analyzing.

Rescuer 3:

- Turns on the AED and follows the prompts.
  - Attaches the pads to the victim's bare chest.
  - Plugs in the connector, if necessary.
  - Says "Everyone, stand clear!"
  - Pushes the "Analyze" button, if necessary.
  - If a shock is advised, delivers the shock by pressing the "Shock" button, if necessary.

After the shock or if no shock is advised:

- Rescuers 1, 2 and 3 perform about **2** minutes of CPR.

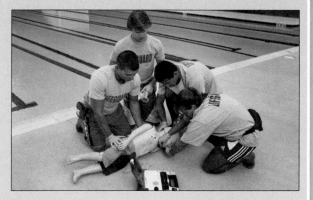

■ Rescuer 4 assembles the BVM, if necessary. Administer emergency oxygen if trained to do so.

■ Rescuer 1 places and seals the mask of the BVM and maintains an open airway.

■ Rescuer 4 provides ventilations by squeezing the bag.

■ Rescuer 2 performs compressions.

  ○ **If the victim vomits:**

    ● Rescuers quickly roll the victim onto the side.

    ● After vomiting stops, a rescuer on the side of the victim clears the victim's mouth out using a finger sweep and suction if necessary.

    ● Turn the victim onto the back and continue providing care.

  ○ **If ventilations do not make the chest clearly rise:**

    ● Rescuer 1 retilts the head.

    ● Rescuer 3 attempts **1** ventilation.

  ○ **If ventilation attempt still does not make the chest clearly rise:**

    ● Rescuer 2 gives **30** chest compressions.

    ● Rescuer 3 looks inside the mouth and removes any visible large debris from the mouth using a finger sweep and suction if necessary.

    ● Rescuer 4 replaces the mask.

    ● Rescuer 1 opens the airway and seals the mask.

    ● Rescuer 4 provides ventilations.

    ● Rescuer 2 performs compressions.

Notes:

■ *If at any time you notice breathing or a pulse, stop CPR and monitor the victim's condition.*

■ *Rescuers should change positions (alternate performing compressions and giving ventilations) about every **2** minutes to reduce the possibility of rescuer fatigue. Changing positions should take less than **5** seconds.*

WRAP-UP

As a professional lifeguard, you should be able to recognize and respond to cardiac emergencies, including heart attacks and cardiac arrest. To do this, you must understand the importance of the four links of the Cardiac Chain of Survival: early recognition of the emergency and early access to EMS, early CPR, early defibrillation and early advanced medical care.

When using an AED, always follow local protocols. AEDs are relatively easy to operate, and generally require minimal training and retraining. Remember that AEDs are safe to use on victims who have been removed from the water, but you must first make sure you, the victim and the AED are not in or near puddles.

ONE-RESCUER CPR

Notes:

- *Activate the EAP, size-up the scene for safety and then perform a primary assessment.*
- *Always follow standard precautions when providing care.*
- *Ensure the victim is on a firm, flat surface, such as the floor or a table.*

If the victim is not breathing and has no pulse:

1 Give **30** chest compressions.

- Push hard, push fast.
  - Compress the chest at least **2** inches for an adult, about **2** inches for a child and about **1½** inches for an infant at a rate of at least **100** per minute.
  - Let the chest rise completely before pushing down again.
- For an adult or a child:
  - Place the heel of one hand on the center of the chest with the other hand on top.
  - Keep your arms as straight as possible and shoulders directly over your hands.
- For an infant:
  - Place one hand on the infant's forehead.
  - Place two or three fingers on the center of the chest just below the nipple line (toward the infant's feet).

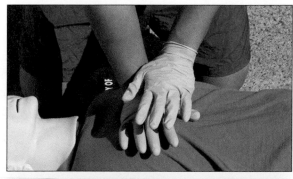

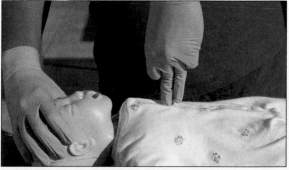

2 Give **2** ventilations.

3 Perform cycles of **30** compressions and **2** ventilations.

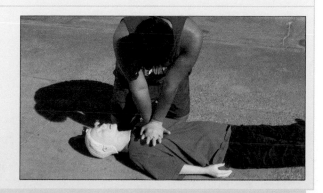

Continued on Next Page

ONE-RESCUER CPR *continued*

Do not stop CPR except in one of the following situations:

- You see an obvious sign of life, such as breathing.
- An AED is ready to use.
- Another trained responder takes over.
- More advanced medical personnel take over.
- You are too exhausted to continue.
- The scene becomes unsafe.

Notes:

- *Keep your fingers off the chest when performing compressions on an adult or child.*
- *Use your body weight, not your arms, to compress the chest.*
- *Count out loud or to yourself to help keep an even pace.*

 # TWO-RESCUER CPR—**ADULT AND CHILD**

Notes:

- *Activate the EAP, size-up the scene for safety and then perform a primary assessment.*
- *Always follow standard precautions when providing care.*
- *Ensure the victim is on a firm, flat surface, such as the floor or a table.*

If the victim is not breathing and has no pulse:

 Rescuer 2 finds the correct hand position to give chest compressions.

- Place two hands on the center of the chest.

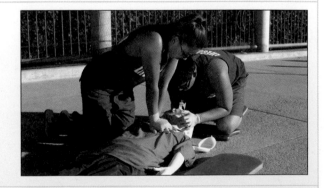

 Rescuer 2 gives chest compressions.

- Push hard, push fast.
  - Compress the chest at least **2** inches for an adult and about **2** inches for a child at a rate of at least **100** per minute.

3 Rescuer 1 gives **2** ventilations.

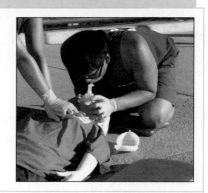

4 Perform about **2** minutes of compressions and ventilations.

- Adult: Perform cycles of **30** compressions and **2** ventilations.
- Child: Perform cycles of **15** compressions and **2** ventilations.

5 Rescuers change positions about every **2** minutes.

- Rescuer 2 calls for a position change by using the word "change" at the end of the last compression cycle:
  - For an adult, use the word "change" in place of the word "30."
  - For a child, use the word "change" in place of the word "15."
- Rescuer 1 gives **2** ventilations.
- Rescuer 2 quickly moves to the victim's head with his or her own mask.
- Rescuer 1 quickly moves into position at the victim's chest and locates correct hand position on the chest.
- Changing positions should take less than **5** seconds.

6 Rescuer 1 begins chest compressions.

- Continue cycles of compressions and ventilations.

Continue CPR until:

- You see an obvious sign of life, such as breathing.
- An AED is ready to use.
- Another trained responder takes over.
- EMS personnel take over.
- You are too exhausted to continue.
- The scene becomes unsafe.

Notes:

- *Keep your fingers off the chest when performing compressions for an adult or child.*
- *Use your body weight, not your arms, to compress the chest.*
- *Count out loud or to yourself to help keep an even pace.*

TWO-RESCUER CPR—**INFANT**

Notes:

- *Activate the EAP, size-up the scene for safety and then perform a primary assessment.*
- *Always follow standard precautions when providing care.*
- *Ensure the victim is on a firm, flat surface, such as the floor or a table.*

If the victim is not breathing and has no pulse:

1 Rescuer 2 finds the correct hand position to give chest compressions.

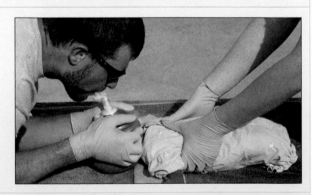

- Use the two-thumbs-encircling technique on the infant's chest.
  - Place thumbs next to each other on the center of the chest just below the nipple line.
  - Place both hands underneath the infant's back and support the infant's back with your fingers.
  - Ensure that your hands do not compress or squeeze the side of the ribs.
- If available, a towel or padding can be placed underneath the infant's shoulders to help maintain the head in the neutral position.

2 Rescuer 2 gives chest compressions.

- Push hard, push fast.
  - Compress the chest about **1½** inches for an infant at a rate of at least **100** per minute.

3 Rescuer 1 gives **2** ventilations.

4 Perform about **2** minutes of compressions and ventilations.

- Perform cycles of **15** compressions and **2** ventilations.

5 Rescuers change positions about every **2** minutes.

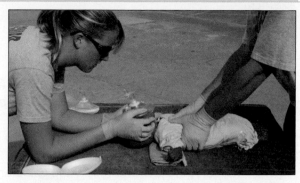

- Rescuer 2 calls for a position change by using the word "change" in place of saying "15" at the end of the last compression cycle.

- Rescuer 1 gives **2** ventilations.

- Rescuer 2 quickly moves to the victim's head with his or her own mask.

- Rescuer 1 quickly moves into position at the victim's chest and locates correct hand position on the chest.

- Changing positions should take less than **5** seconds.

6 Rescuer 1 begins chest compressions.

- Continue cycles of compressions and ventilations.

Continue CPR until:

- You see an obvious sign of life, such as breathing.
- An AED is ready to use.
- Another trained responder takes over.
- EMS personnel take over.
- You are too exhausted to continue.
- The scene becomes unsafe.

Note:

- *Count out loud or to yourself to help keep an even pace.*

USING AN AED

Note: *Activate the EAP, size-up the scene for safety and then perform a primary assessment. Always follow standard precautions when providing care.*

If the victim is not breathing and has no pulse:

1 Turn on the AED and follow the voice and/or visual prompts.

2 Wipe the victim's bare chest dry.

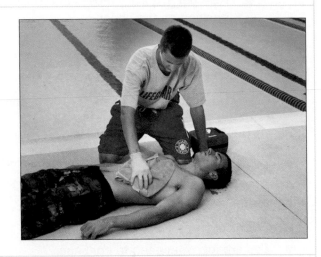

Tip: *Remove any medication patches with a gloved hand.*

3 Attach the AED pads to the victim's bare, dry chest.

- Place one pad on the victim's upper right chest and the other pad on the left side of the chest.
  - For a child or an infant: Use pediatric AED pads, if available. If the pads risk touching each other, place one pad in the middle of the child's chest and the other pad on the child's back, between the shoulder blades.

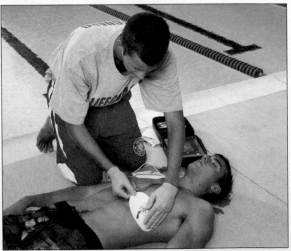

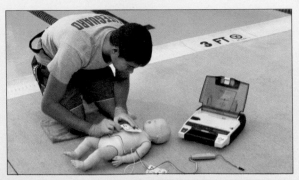

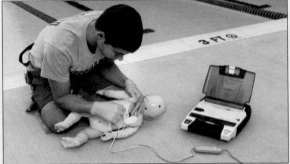

4 Plug in the connector, if necessary.

5 Stand clear.

- Make sure that *no one*, including you, is touching the victim.
- Say, "Everyone, stand clear!"

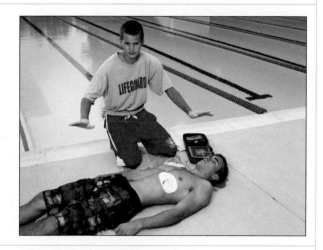

6 Analyze the heart rhythm.

- Push the "Analyze" button, if necessary. Let the AED analyze the heart rhythm.

7 Deliver a shock or perform CPR based on the AED recommendation.

- If a shock is advised:
  - Make sure *no one*, including you, is touching the victim.
  - Say, "Everyone, stand clear."
  - Deliver the shock by pushing the "Shock" button, if necessary.
  - After delivering the shock, perform about **2** minutes of CPR.
  - Continue to follow the prompts of the AED.
- If no shock is advised:
  - Perform about **2** minutes of CPR.
  - Continue to follow the prompts of the AED.

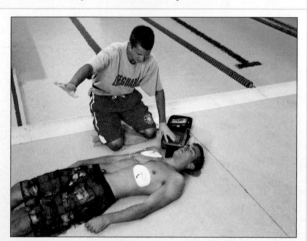

Notes:

- *If at any time you notice an obvious sign of life, such as breathing, stop CPR and monitor the victim's condition.*
- *The AED will not advise a shock for normal or absent heart rhythms.*
- *If two trained rescuers are present, one should perform CPR while the second rescuer operates the AED.*

First Aid

A s covered in Chapter 7, when you encounter an ill or injured victim, you must follow a series of general procedures designed to ensure a proper assessment and response. These include activating the emergency action plan (EAP), sizing up the scene, performing a primary assessment and summoning emergency medical services (EMS) personnel for any life-threatening emergencies. If you do not find a life-threatening situation, you should perform a secondary assessment and provide first aid as needed.

This chapter covers how to perform a secondary assessment, including how to check a conscious victim and how to take a brief history. It also describes how to recognize and provide first aid for some of the injuries, illnesses and medical conditions that you might encounter while on the job. ■

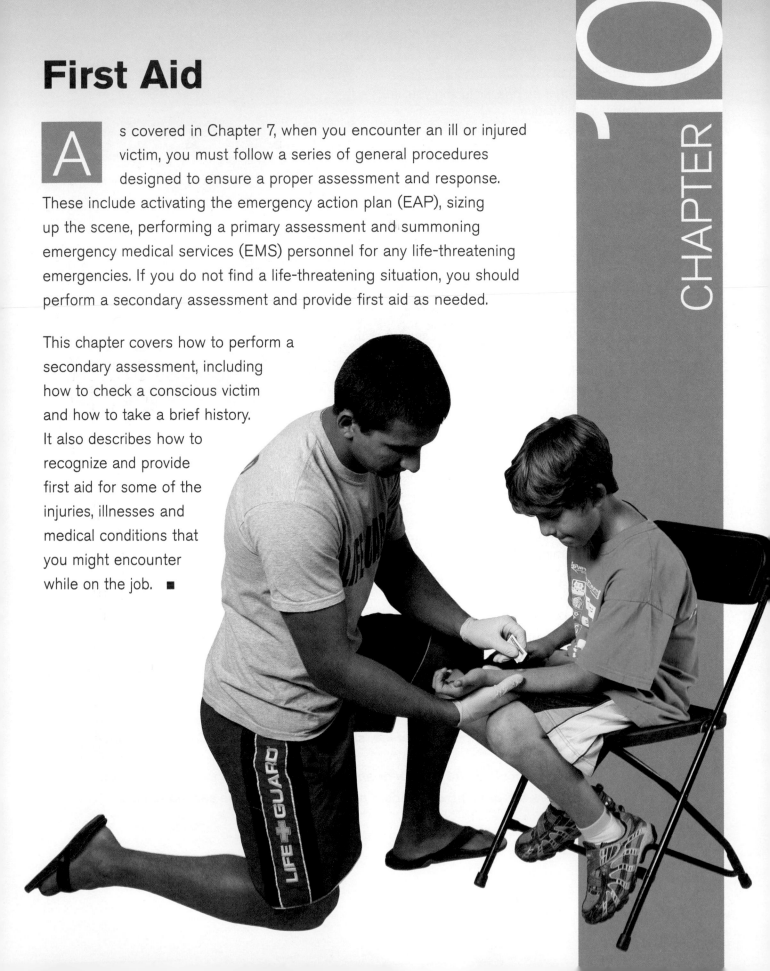

RESPONDING TO INJURIES AND ILLNESSES

Even when everyone works to prevent emergencies, injuries and illnesses do occur at aquatic facilities. With some injuries, such as a nosebleed, the problem will be obvious and easy to treat by following the first aid care steps described in this chapter. In other situations, such as a sudden illness, it may be harder to determine what is wrong.

In all cases, remember to follow the general procedures for injury or sudden illness on land and to use appropriate personal protective equipment, such as disposable gloves and CPR breathing barriers. It is a common practice to carry a few first aid supplies in your hip pack (Figure 10-1).

Also, be aware that every facility should have a first aid area where an injured or ill person can receive first aid and rest, and where first aid supplies are available (Figure 10-2). Some facilities staff the first aid area with highly trained personnel, such as emergency medical technicians (EMTs). You should know where your facility's first aid area is located, the type of equipment and supplies available, how to provide first aid correctly and whether staff with more advanced training are present.

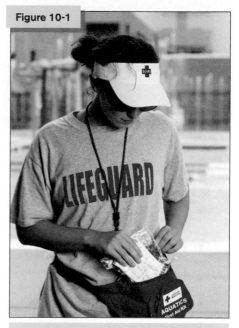

Figure 10-1

A few first aid supplies can be carried in your hip pack

Considerations for Responding to Injuries and Illnesses

Your job as a lifeguard requires you to juggle many responsibilities. Injuries happen suddenly, and in a first aid emergency you must decide how best to respond to the situation, including when to activate the EAP. The ability to recognize that an emergency has occurred is the first step toward taking appropriate action. Once you recognize that an emergency has occurred, you must decide to act. To help make decisions in an emergency situation, consider the following:

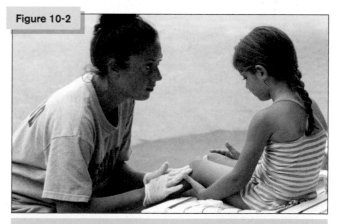

Figure 10-2

Every facility should have first aid supplies that are available from a first aid area.

- Should I provide care where the victim was found, or move him or her to the first aid room?
- Is the safety of the victim or others compromised?
- Is there a risk of further injury to the victim?
- Is there a risk of exposing the victim or others to pathogens (e.g., by leaving a trail of blood or body fluids)?
- Should I summon EMS personnel?
- When should I recommend that the victim see a health care provider to seek further medical treatment?

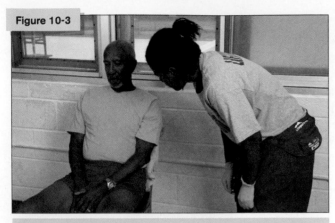

Figure 10-3

When conducting a secondary assessment on a conscious victim, perform a head-to-toe physical exam.

SECONDARY ASSESSMENT

During the secondary assessment, you should take a brief history and perform a quick head-to-toe physical exam (Figure 10-3). If any life-threatening conditions develop during your secondary assessment, stop the assessment and provide appropriate care immediately.

Using SAMPLE to Take a Brief History

Use the SAMPLE mnemonic as an easy way to remember what you should ask about when you are taking the brief history:

S = Signs and symptoms

- These include bleeding, skin that is cool and moist, pain, nausea, headache and difficulty breathing.

A = Allergies

- Determine if the victim is allergic to any medications, food, or environmental elements, such as pollen or bees.

M = Medications

- Find out if the victim is using any prescription or nonprescription medications.

P = Pertinent past medical history

- Determine if the victim is under the care of a health care provider for any medical condition, has had medical problems in the past or recently has been hospitalized.

L = Last oral intake

- Find out what the victim most recently took in by mouth as well as the volume or dose consumed. This includes food, drinks and medication.

E = Events leading up to the incident

- Determine what the victim was doing before and at the time of the incident.

When talking to a child, get down at eye level with the child, speak slowly and in a friendly manner, use simple words and ask questions that the child can easily understand.

Checking a Conscious Person

Check the victim by performing a head-to-toe exam. Before beginning the exam, tell the person what you are going to do. Visually inspect the person's body, looking carefully for any bleeding, cuts, bruises and obvious deformities. Look for a medical identification (ID) tag, necklace or bracelet on the person's wrist, neck or ankle (Figure 10-4). These will provide medical information about the person, explain how to care for the conditions identified and list whom to call for help. Do not ask the person to move any areas in which he or she has discomfort or pain or if a head, neck or spinal injury is suspected.

When checking a child or infant for non-life-threatening conditions, observe the child or infant before touching him or her. Look for signs and symptoms that indicate changes in the level of consciousness (LOC), trouble breathing and any apparent injuries or conditions. If a child or an infant becomes extremely upset, conduct the check from toe to head. This will allow the child or infant to become familiar with the process and see what is happening. Check for the same things on a child or an infant that you would look for with an adult.

See the Checking a Conscious Person skill sheet at the end of this chapter for steps to follow when performing a head-to-toe exam.

If the person is unable to move a body part or is experiencing dizziness or pain on movement:

- Help the person rest in a comfortable position.
- Keep the person from getting chilled or overheated.
- Reassure the person.
- Determine whether to summon EMS personnel.
- Continue to watch for changes in LOC and breathing.

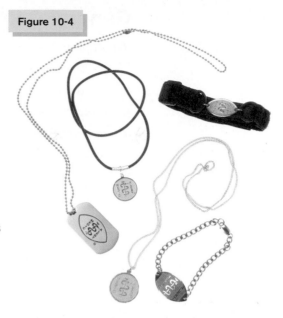

Figure 10-4

Medical ID tags, necklaces and bracelets can provide important information about an injured or ill person.

SUDDEN ILLNESS

Sudden illness can happen to anyone, anywhere. You may not be able to identify the illness, but you still can provide care. Victims of sudden illness usually look and feel ill. If you suspect something is wrong, check the victim and look for a medical ID tag, necklace or bracelet on the person's wrist, neck or ankle. The victim may try to say nothing is seriously wrong, but the victim's condition can worsen rapidly. Do not be afraid to ask the victim questions.

There are many types of sudden illness, including diabetic emergencies, fainting, seizures and stroke.

Signs and Symptoms of Sudden Illness

Many sudden illnesses have similar signs and symptoms. These include:

- Changes in LOC, such as feeling light-headed, dizzy or becoming unconscious.
- Nausea or vomiting.
- Difficulty speaking or slurred speech.
- Numbness or weakness.
- Loss of vision or blurred vision.
- Changes in breathing; the person may have trouble breathing or may not be breathing normally.

- Changes in skin color (pale, ashen or flushed skin).
- Sweating.
- Persistent pressure or pain.
- Diarrhea.
- Seizures.
- Paralysis or an inability to move.
- Severe headache.

General Care Steps for Sudden Illness

When providing care for sudden illness, follow the general procedures for injury or sudden illness on land:

- Care for any life-threatening conditions first.
- Monitor the victim's condition and watch for changes in LOC.
- Keep the victim comfortable, reassure him or her and keep the victim from getting chilled or overheated.
- Do not give the victim anything to eat or drink unless the victim is fully conscious and is not in shock.
- Care for any other problems that develop, such as vomiting.

Diabetic Emergencies

People who are diabetic sometimes become ill because there is too much or too little sugar in their blood. Many people who are diabetic use diet, exercise or medication to control their diabetes. The person may disclose that he or she is diabetic or you may learn this from the information on a medical ID tag or from a bystander. Often, people who have diabetes know what is wrong and will ask for something with sugar if they are experiencing symptoms of low blood sugar (*hypoglycemia*). They may carry some form of sugar with them.

If the person is conscious and can safely swallow fluids or food, give him or her sugar. If it is available, give glucose paste or tablets to the victim. If not available, sugar in liquid form is preferred. Most fruit juices (e.g., about 12 ounces of orange juice), milk and non-diet soft drinks have enough sugar to be effective (Figure 10-5). You also can give table sugar dissolved in a glass of water. If the person has hypoglycemia, sugar will help quickly. If the problem is high blood sugar (*hyperglycemia*), giving the sugar will not cause any further harm. Give something by mouth only if the victim is fully conscious.

Always summon EMS personnel for any of the following circumstances:

- The person is unconscious or about to lose consciousness.
- The person is conscious and unable to swallow.
- The person does not feel better within about 5 minutes after taking sugar.
- A form of sugar cannot be found immediately. Do not spend time looking for it.

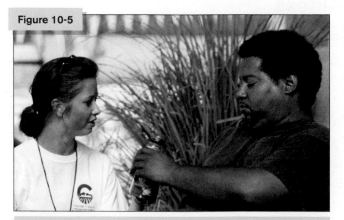

Figure 10-5

Give a victim experiencing a diabetic emergency fruit juice, milk or a non-diet soft drink.

Fainting

When a person suddenly loses consciousness and then reawakens, he or she may simply have fainted. Fainting is not usually harmful, and the person will usually quickly recover. Lower the person to the ground or other flat surface and position the person on his or her back. Loosen any tight clothing, such as a tie or collar. Make sure the victim is breathing. Do not give the victim anything to eat or drink. If the victim vomits, position the victim on his or her side.

Seizures

There are many different types of seizures. Generalized seizures usually last 1 to 3 minutes and can produce a wide range of signs and symptoms. When this type of seizure occurs, the person loses consciousness and can fall, causing injury. The person may become rigid and then experience sudden, uncontrollable muscular convulsions, lasting several minutes. Breathing may become irregular and even stop temporarily.

Seeing someone have a seizure may be intimidating, but you can provide care for the person. The person cannot control any muscular convulsions that may occur, and it is important to allow the seizure to run its course because attempting to restrain the person can cause further injury. To provide care to a person having a seizure:

- Protect the person from injury by moving nearby objects away from the person.
- Position the person on his or her side, if possible, after the seizure passes so that fluids (saliva, blood, vomit) can drain from the mouth.

When the seizure is over, the person usually begins to breathe normally. He or she may be drowsy and disoriented or unresponsive for a period of time. Check to see if the person was injured during the seizure. Be reassuring and comforting. If the seizure occurred in public, the person may be embarrassed and self-conscious. Ask bystanders not to crowd around the person. He or she will be tired and want to rest. Stay with the person until he or she is fully conscious and aware of his or her surroundings.

If the person is known to have periodic seizures, there is no need to summon EMS personnel. He or she usually will recover from a seizure in a few minutes. However, summon EMS personnel if:

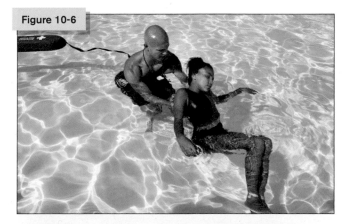

Figure 10-6

- The seizure occurs in the water.
- The seizure lasts more than 5 minutes.
- The person has repeated seizures with no sign of slowing down.
- The person appears to be injured.
- The cause of the seizure is unknown.
- The person is pregnant.
- The person is known to have diabetes.
- The person fails to regain consciousness after the seizure.
- The person is elderly and may have suffered a stroke.
- This is the person's first seizure.

Seizures in the Water

If a person has a seizure in the water:

1. Summon EMS personnel.
2. Support the person with his or her head above water until the seizure ends (Figures 10-6 and 10-7).

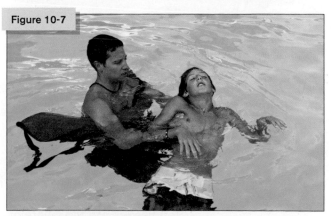

Figure 10-7

If someone experiences a seizure while in the water, support the victim's head above the water until the seizure ends.

3. Remove the person from the water as soon as possible after the seizure (since he or she may have inhaled or swallowed water).

4. Once on land, position the person on his or her back and perform a primary assessment. Give ventilations or CPR if needed. If the person vomits, turn the victim on his or her side to drain fluids from the mouth. Sweep out the mouth (or suction out the mouth if you are trained to do so).

Stroke

As with other sudden illnesses, the signs and symptoms of a stroke or mini-stroke are a sudden change in how the body is working or feeling. This may include sudden weakness or numbness of the face, an arm or a leg. Usually, weakness or numbness occurs only on one side of the body. Other signs and symptoms include difficulty with speech (trouble speaking and being understood, and difficulty understanding others); blurred or dimmed vision; sudden, severe headache; dizziness or confusion; loss of balance or coordination; trouble walking; and ringing in the ears.

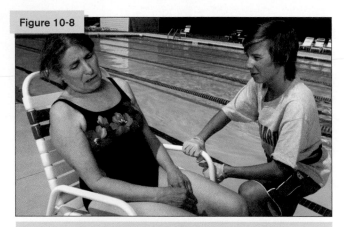

Figure 10-8

Signals of a stroke include facial drooping.

If the person shows any signs or symptoms of stroke, time is critical. The objective is to recognize a possible stroke and summon EMS personnel immediately. To identify and care for a victim of stroke, think FAST:

- Face—Weakness on one side of the face (Figure 10-8)
  - Ask the person to smile. This will show if there is drooping or weakness in the muscles on one side of the face. Does one side of the face droop?

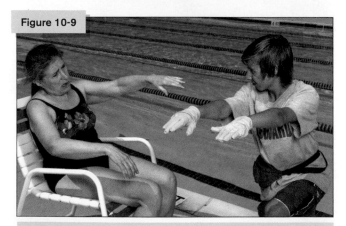

Figure 10-9

Weakness on one side of the body is another signal of a stroke.

- Arm—Weakness or numbness in one arm (Figure 10-9)
  - Ask the person to raise both arms to find out if there is weakness in the limbs. Does one arm drift downward?

- Speech—Slurred speech or trouble speaking
  - Ask the person to speak a simple sentence to listen for slurred or distorted speech. Example: "The sky is blue." Can the victim repeat the sentence correctly?

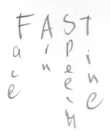

- Time—Time to summon EMS personnel if any of these signs or symptoms are seen
  - Note the time of onset of signs and symptoms, and summon EMS personnel immediately.

SKIN AND SOFT TISSUE INJURIES

Soft tissues are the layers of skin and the fat and muscle beneath the skin's outer layer. A physical injury to the body's soft tissue is called a *wound*. Any time the soft tissues are damaged or torn, the body is threatened. Injuries may damage the soft tissues at or near the skin's surface or deep in the body. Germs can enter the body through a scrape, cut, puncture or burn and cause infection. Severe bleeding can occur at or under the skin's surface, where it is harder to detect.

Burns are a special kind of soft tissue injury. Like other types of soft tissue injury, burns can damage the top layer of skin or the skin and the layers of fat, muscle and bone beneath.

Soft tissue injuries typically are classified as either closed or open wounds.

Closed Wounds

Closed wounds occur beneath the surface of the skin. The simplest closed wound is a bruise or *contusion*. Bruises result when the body is subjected to blunt force, such as when you bump your leg on a table or chair. Such a blow usually results in damage to soft tissue layers and blood vessels beneath the skin, causing internal bleeding. Most closed wounds do not require special medical care. However, a significant violent force can cause injuries involving larger blood vessels and the deeper layers of muscle tissue. These injuries can result in severe bleeding beneath the skin. In these cases, medical care is needed quickly.

Caring for Internal Bleeding

Summon EMS personnel immediately if:

- The victim complains of severe pain or cannot move a body part without pain.
- The force that caused the injury was great enough to cause serious damage.
- An injured arm or leg is blue or extremely pale.
- The victim has excessive thirst, becomes confused, faint, drowsy or unconscious.
- The victim is vomiting blood or coughing up blood.
- The victim has skin that feels cool or moist, or looks pale or bluish.
- The victim has a rapid, weak pulse.
- The victim has tender, swollen, bruised or hard areas of the body, such as the abdomen.

While waiting for EMS personnel to arrive, the objectives are to:

- Care for any life-threatening conditions first.
- Help the victim rest in a comfortable position and reassure him or her.
- Monitor the victim's condition and watch for any changes in LOC.
- Keep the victim from getting chilled or overheated (care for shock).
- Care for other problems that develop, such as vomiting.

If the closed wound is not serious:

1. Apply direct pressure on the area to decrease bleeding under the skin.
2. Elevate the injured part to reduce swelling if you do not suspect a muscle, bone or joint injury and if doing so does not cause more pain.
3. Apply ice or a cold pack on the area to help control swelling and pain.
    o When applying ice or a chemical cold pack, place a gauze pad, towel or other cloth between the source of cold and the victim's skin.

○ If an ice pack is not available, fill a plastic bag with ice and water or wrap ice with a damp cloth.

○ Apply the ice or cold pack for no more than 20 minutes. If continued icing is needed, remove the pack for 20 minutes and re-chill it, then replace it.

Open Wounds

In an open wound, the break in the skin can be as minor as a scrape of the surface layers (*abrasion*) or as severe as a deep penetration. The amount of external bleeding depends on the location and severity of the injury. Most external bleeding injuries that you encounter will be minor, such as a small cut that can be cared for by cleaning the wound and applying an adhesive bandage. Minor bleeding, such as results from a small cut, usually stops by itself within 10 minutes when the blood clots.

However, some cuts are too large or the blood is under too much pressure for effective clotting to occur. In these cases, you need to recognize the situation and provide care quickly. Remember to always wear non-latex disposable gloves and follow all other standard precautions when giving care.

The following are the four main types of open wounds:

■ Abrasion (Figure 10-10)
  ○ Skin has been rubbed or scraped away (e.g., scrape, road rash, rug burn). The area usually is painful.
  ○ Dirt and other matter may have entered the wound. Cleaning the wound is important to prevent infection.
■ Laceration (Figure 10-11)
  ○ Cuts bleed freely, and deep cuts can bleed severely.
  ○ Deep cuts can damage nerves, large blood vessels and other soft tissues.
■ Avulsion (Figure 10-12)
  ○ An avulsion is a cut in which a piece of soft tissue or even part of the body, such as a finger, is torn loose or is torn off entirely (e.g., amputation).
  ○ Often, deeper tissues are damaged, causing significant bleeding.
■ Puncture (Figure 10-13)
  ○ Puncture wounds often do not bleed profusely and can easily become infected.
  ○ Bleeding can be severe, with damage to major blood vessels or internal organs.
  ○ An object embedded in the wound should be removed only by EMS personnel.

Figure 10-10

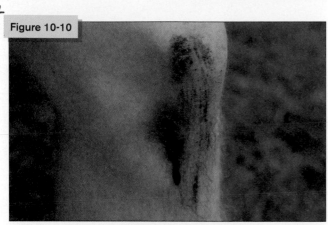

Abrasion

Figure 10-11

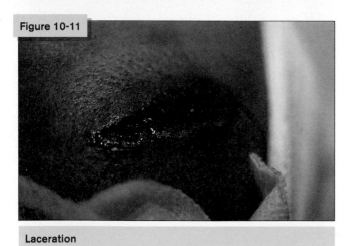

Laceration

Figure 10-12

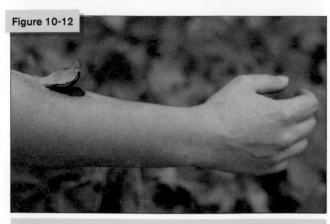

Avulsion

Caring for External Bleeding

To care for a minor wound, such as an abrasion, follow these general guidelines:

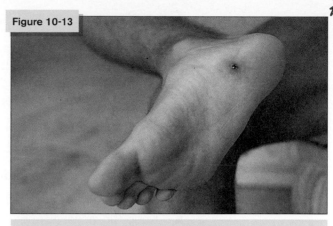

Figure 10-13

Puncture

■ Control any bleeding.
  ○ Place a sterile dressing over the wound.
  ○ Apply direct pressure until bleeding stops (Figure 10-14, A).

■ Clean the wound thoroughly with soap (if available) and water. If possible, irrigate an abrasion with clean, warm running tap water for about 5 minutes to remove any dirt and debris.

■ If bleeding continues, use a new sterile dressing and apply more pressure.

■ After bleeding stops, remove the dressing and apply antibiotic ointment, if one is available, the victim has no known allergies or sensitivities to the medication and local protocols allow you to do so.

■ Cover the wound with a sterile dressing and bandage (or with an adhesive bandage) to keep the wound moist and prevent drying. (Figure 10-14, B).

■ Wash your hands immediately after providing care.

To care for a major wound:

■ Activate the EAP, summon EMS personnel and follow the general procedures for injury or sudden illness on land.

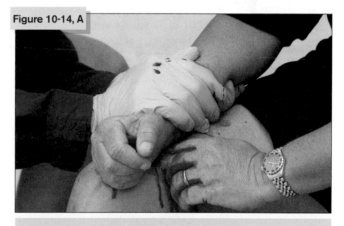

Figure 10-14, A

Apply direct pressure firmly against a wound for a few minutes to control any bleeding.

■ Cover the wound with a sterile gauze dressing and apply direct pressure using the flat part of your fingers. A large wound may require more pressure; use pressure from your full hand with gauze dressings to try to stop the bleeding. For an open fracture, do not apply direct pressure over the broken bones, but instead pack sterile gauze around the area to control bleeding and prevent infection.

■ If the dressing becomes saturated with blood while you are applying pressure, do not remove it. Instead, place additional dressings over the soaked bandage and reapply direct pressure. Then cover the dressings with a bandage to hold them in place.

■ Keep the victim warm and position the victim on his or her back.

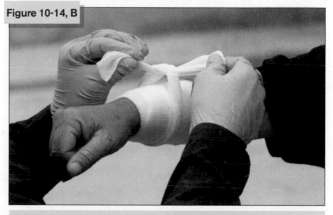

Figure 10-14, B

Use a sterile dressing and bandage to cover the wound.

■ Care for other conditions, including shock.

■ Wash your hands immediately after providing care.

If conscious and able, the victim may use his or her hand to apply pressure while you put your gloves on and prepare the necessary supplies.

Shock

Any serious injury or illness can result in a condition known as shock. Shock is a natural reaction by the body. It usually means the victim's condition is serious. Signs and symptoms of shock include restlessness or irritability; altered LOC; pale or ashen, cool, moist skin; nausea or vomiting; rapid breathing and pulse; and excessive thirst.

To minimize the effects of shock:

- Make sure that EMS personnel have been summoned.
- Monitor the victim's condition and watch for changes in LOC.
- Control any external bleeding.
- Keep the victim from getting chilled or overheated.
- Have the victim lie flat on his or her back.
- Cover the victim with a blanket to prevent loss of body heat. Do not overheat the victim—your goal is to maintain a normal body temperature.
- Comfort and reassure the victim until EMS personnel take over.
- Administer emergency oxygen, if available and trained to do so.

Note: *Do not give food or drink to a victim of shock, even if the victim asks for them.*

Care for Wounds–Specific Situations

Patrons at aquatic facilities can suffer a variety of wounds, from a minor nosebleed to a severed body part. No matter how seriously the victim is wounded, you must remain calm and follow the general procedures for injury or sudden illness on land. This section covers how to care for some of the specific wounds that you might encounter on the job.

Nosebleeds

To care for a nosebleed:

- Have the victim sit leaning slightly forward to prevent swallowing or choking on the blood (Figure 10-15).

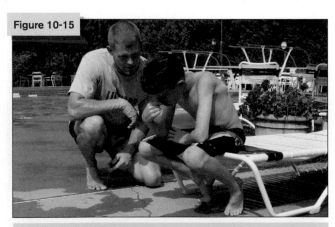

Figure 10-15

Control a nosebleed by having the victim sit with the head slightly forward, pinching the nostrils together.

- Pinch the nostrils together for about 5 to 10 minutes or until the bleeding stops.
  - Other methods of controlling bleeding include applying an ice pack to the bridge of the nose or putting pressure on the upper lip just beneath the nose.
  - Do not pack the victim's nose to stop the bleeding.
- After the bleeding stops, have the victim avoid rubbing, blowing or picking the nose, which could restart the bleeding.
- Medical attention is needed if the bleeding persists or recurs, or if the victim says the nosebleed was a result of high blood pressure.
- If the victim loses consciousness, place the victim on his or her side to allow blood to drain from the nose. Summon EMS personnel immediately.

Eye Injuries

Care for open or closed wounds around the eyeball as you would for any soft tissue injury. Never put direct pressure on the eyeball. For embedded objects in the eye:

■ Summon EMS personnel.

■ Help the victim into a comfortable position.

■ Do not try to remove any object from the eye.

■ Bandage loosely and do not put pressure on the injured eyeball.

■ Stabilize the object as best as possible. Depending on the size of the object, you may be able to stabilize it by encircling the eye with a gauze dressing or soft sterile cloth, being careful *not* to apply any pressure to the area. Position bulky dressings, such as roller gauze, around the impaled object and then cover it with a shield such as a paper cup (Figure 10-16). The shield should *not* touch the object. Bandage the shield and dressing in place with a self-adhering bandage and roller bandage covering the patient's injured eye, to keep the object stable and minimize movement.

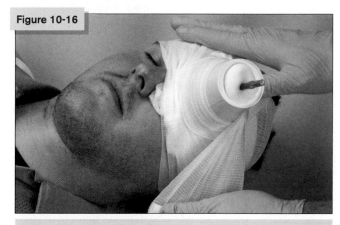

Figure 10-16

To care for an impaled object in the eye, stabilize the object with a shield, such as a paper cup, and bandage the cup in place.

For small foreign bodies in the eye, such as sand:

■ Tell the victim to blink several times to try to remove the object.

■ Gently flush the eye with water.

■ Seek medical attention if the object remains.

For chemicals in the eye, flush the eye continuously with water for 10 minutes or until EMS personnel take over. Always flush away from the uninjured eye.

Injuries to the Mouth and Teeth

If a head, neck or spinal injury is *not* suspected:

■ Rinse out the victim's mouth with cold tap water, if available.

■ Have the victim lean slightly forward or place the victim on his or her side.

■ Try to prevent the victim from swallowing the blood, which could cause nausea or vomiting.

■ Apply a dressing.

   o For injuries inside the cheek, place folded sterile dressings inside the mouth against the wound.

   o For injuries outside the cheek, apply direct pressure using a sterile dressing (Figure 10-17).

   o For injuries to the tongue or lips, apply direct pressure using a sterile dressing. Apply cold to reduce swelling and ease pain.

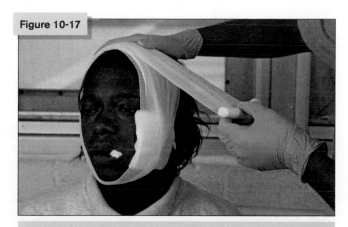

Figure 10-17

Apply direct pressure using a sterile dressing to injuries outside the cheek.

- If a tooth is knocked out:
  - ○ Rinse out the victim's mouth with cold tap water, if available.
  - ○ Have the victim bite down on a rolled sterile dressing in the space left by the tooth (or teeth).
  - ○ Save any displaced teeth.
    - Carefully pick up the tooth by the crown (white part), not the root.
    - Rinse off the root of the tooth in water if it is dirty. Do not scrub it or remove any attached tissue fragments.
    - Place the tooth in milk. If milk is not available, place the tooth in clean water and keep the tooth with the victim.
  - ○ Advise the victim to get to a dentist with the tooth as soon as possible.

Scalp Injuries

Scalp injuries often bleed heavily. Putting pressure on the area around the wound can control the bleeding.

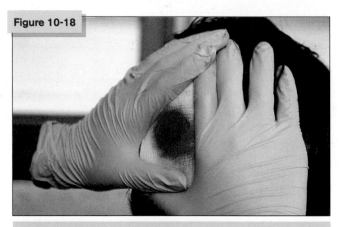

Figure 10-18

Control bleeding from a scalp injury by applying pressure around the wound. Avoid direct pressure.

- Apply gentle pressure at first because there may be a skull fracture (Figure 10-18). If you feel a depression, spongy areas or bone fragments, do not put direct pressure on the wound.
- Summon EMS personnel if you cannot determine the seriousness of the scalp injury.
- For an open wound with no sign of a fracture, control the bleeding with several dressings secured with a bandage.

If you suspect a head, neck or spinal injury, minimize movement of the head, neck and spine. See Chapter 11, Caring for Head, Neck and Spinal Injuries, on how to care for a head, neck or spinal injury.

Embedded Objects

An object that remains in an open wound is called an embedded object. Take the following steps to care for an embedded object:

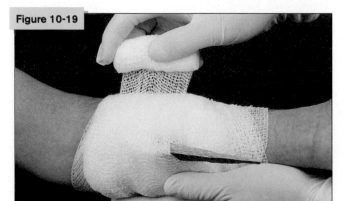

Figure 10-19

Place several dressing around an embedded objective to keep it from moving. Bandage the dressings in place around the object.

- Summon EMS personnel.
- Place several dressings around the object to keep it from moving. Avoid placing pressure on or moving the object.
- Bandage the dressings in place around the object (Figure 10-19). Do not remove the object.

Injuries to the Abdomen

Be aware that wounds through the abdomen can cause internal organs to push outside of the body. To care for an abdominal injury:

- Summon EMS personnel.

- Carefully remove clothing from around the wound.
- If organs are protruding:
  - Do not attempt to put them back into the abdomen.
  - Cover the organs with a moist, sterile dressing and cover the dressing with plastic wrap.
  - Place a folded towel or cloth over the dressing to keep the organs warm.
- Care for shock.

Animal and Human Bites

An animal or human bite may be serious because of the nature of the wound and risk of infection. A person who is bitten by an animal should be removed from the situation if possible, but only without endangering yourself or others. Do not try to restrain or capture the animal. Tetanus and rabies immunizations may be necessary, so it is vital to report bites from any wild or unknown domestic animal to the local health department or other agency according to local protocols. For animal or human bites:

- Summon EMS personnel if the wound bleeds severely or if the animal is suspected to have rabies.
- For severe bleeding, control the bleeding first. Do not clean the wound; it will be properly cleaned at the hospital.
- If the bleeding is minor, wash the wound with large amounts of clean water. Saline may be used, if available. Control the bleeding and cover with a sterile bandage.

Severed Body Parts

Caring for a victim with a severed body part can be disturbing. Remain calm and take the following steps:

- Summon EMS personnel.
- Control the bleeding, and wrap and bandage the wound to prevent infection.
- Wrap the severed body part(s) in sterile gauze (or clean material) (Figure 10-20).
- Place the severed body part(s) in a plastic bag and seal the bag. Put the plastic bag in a container of an ice and water slurry (not on ice alone).
- Care for shock.
- Be sure that the body part is taken to the hospital with the victim immediately.

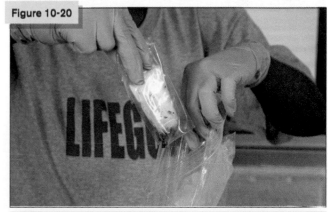

Figure 10-20

Wrap a severed body part in sterile gauze, put in a plastic bag and put the bag on ice.

Burns

Burns are a special kind of soft tissue injury. Like other types of soft tissue injury, burns can damage the top layer of skin or the skin and the layers of fat, muscle and bone beneath. There are four sources of burns: heat, radiation, chemicals and electricity.

Burns are classified by their depth. The deeper the burn, the more severe. Burns can be superficial (first degree), partial thickness (second degree) or full thickness

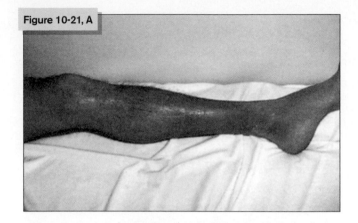

Figure 10-21, A

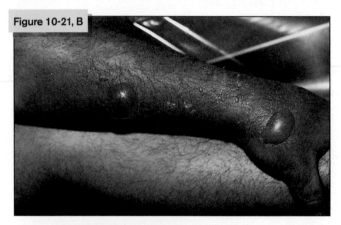

Figure 10-21, B

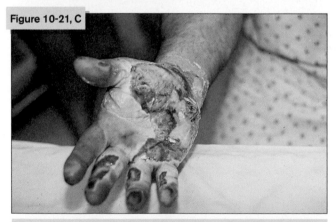

Figure 10-21, C

The three classifications of burns are: (A) superficial (first degree), (B) partial thickness (second degree) and (C) full thickness (third degree)

(third degree) (Figure 10-21, A–C). The severity of the burn depends on the temperature or strength of the heat or other source, length of exposure to the burn source, location of the burn, area and size of the burn and the victim's age and general medical condition.

Certain burns can lead to shock and need immediate medical attention. These include burns:

- That cause a victim to have difficulty breathing.
- That cover more than one body part or a large body surface area.
- To the head, neck, hands, feet or genitals.
- To the airway (burns to the mouth and nose may be a signal of this).
- To a child or an elderly person (other than very minor burns).
- From chemicals, explosions or electricity.

Caring for Burns

To care for burns, follow the general procedures for a land emergency. If the scene is safe, check the victim for life-threatening conditions. Summon EMS personnel if the condition is life threatening. The following general guidelines apply for all types of burns:

- Stop the burning by removing the victim from the source of the burn.
- Cool the burned area with large amounts of cold tap water at least until pain is relieved.
- Cover the burned area loosely with a sterile dressing.
- Take steps to minimize shock, such as by keeping the victim from getting chilled or overheated.
- Comfort and reassure the victim.

Table 10-1 outlines specific considerations and care steps for the different sources of burns.

BITES AND STINGS

Spider Bites and Scorpion Stings

Only two spiders in the United States are poisonous: the black widow and the brown recluse. A bite from one of these spiders can cause serious illness or fatality. Some scorpion stings also can be fatal. When patrons are bitten by spiders at aquatic facilities, it is usually when they are reaching or rummaging in dark places, such as lockers or storage areas. They are typically bitten on their hands or arms.

Table 10-1: Care Steps Based on Source of Burn

Electrical	Chemical	Radiation (Sun)
■ Summon EMS personnel. ■ Check the scene for safety and check for life-threatening injuries. If a power line is down, wait for the fire department or the power company to disconnect the power source. ■ Cool the burn with cold tap water until pain is relieved. ■ Cover the burn with a dry, sterile dressing. ■ Be aware that electrocutions can cause cardiac and breathing emergencies. Be prepared to perform CPR or defibrillation. Take steps to minimize shock.	■ Summon EMS personnel. ■ Brush off dry chemicals with a gloved hand, being careful not to get the chemical on yourself or to brush it into the victim's eyes. Flush the affected area continuously with large amounts of cool water. ■ Keep flushing the area for at least 20 minutes or until EMS personnel arrive. ■ If a chemical gets into an eye, flush the eye with cool, clean running water until EMS personnel arrive. Always flush the affected eye from the nose outward and downward to prevent washing the chemical into the other eye. ■ If possible, have the victim remove contaminated clothes to prevent further contamination while continuing to flush the area.	■ Cool the burned area and protect the area from further damage by keeping it out of the sun.

If someone has been bitten by a black widow or brown recluse spider or stung by a scorpion:

■ Summon EMS personnel.

■ Wash the wound thoroughly.

■ Bandage the wound. Apply a topical antibiotic ointment to the bite to prevent infection if the person has no known allergies or sensitivities to the medication.

■ Apply a cold pack to the site to reduce swelling and pain.

■ If it is available and local protocols allow, give the victim antivenin—a medication that blocks the effects of the black widow spider's poisonous venom.

■ Care for life-threatening conditions.

■ Monitor the victim's condition and watch for changes in LOC.

■ Keep the victim comfortable.

Snakebites

Snakebites kill few people in the United States. Whereas 7000 to 8000 venomous snakebites are reported each year in the United States, fewer than five victims die from the snakebite.

To provide care for a bite from a venomous snake:

- Summon EMS personnel.
- Keep the injured area still and lower than the heart. The victim should walk only if absolutely necessary.
- Wash the wound.
- Apply an elastic roller bandage. Use a narrow bandage to wrap a hand or wrist, a medium-width bandage to wrap an arm or ankle and a wide bandage to wrap a leg.
    - Check for feeling, warmth and color of the limb beyond where the bandage will be placed, and note changes in skin color and temperature.
    - Place the end of the bandage against the skin and use overlapping turns (Figure 10-22).
    - Gently stretch the bandage while wrapping. The wrap should cover a long body section, such as an arm or a calf, beginning at the point farthest from the heart. For a joint like a knee or ankle, use figure-eight turns to support the joint.
    - Always check the area above and below the injury site for warmth and color, especially fingers and toes, after applying an elastic roller bandage. By checking before and after bandaging, you will be able to determine if any tingling or numbness is a result of the bandaging or of the injury itself.
    - Check the snugness of the bandage—a finger should easily, but not loosely, pass under the bandage.

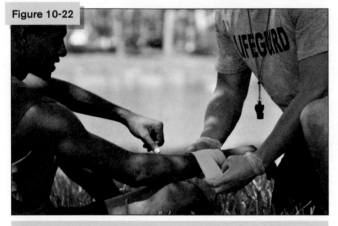

Figure 10-22

Apply an elastic roller bandage using overlapping turns to slow the spread of venom.

For *any* snakebite do not apply ice, cut the wound, apply suction or apply a tourniquet.

Insect Stings

Insect stings can be painful. They also can be fatal for people who have severe allergic reactions. Allergic reactions can result in a breathing emergency. If someone is having a breathing emergency, summon EMS personnel.

To care for an insect sting:

- Examine the sting site to see if the stinger is in the skin (if there is one). Remove the stinger if it is still present. Scrape it away with the edge of a plastic card, such as a credit card.
- Wash the wound with soap and water, cover the site with a dressing and keep the wound clean.
- Apply a cold pack to the site to reduce pain and swelling.

- Watch the victim for signals of an allergic reaction—shortness of breath; swelling of the face, neck or tongue; rash or hives; or a tight feeling in the chest and throat.
- Care for life-threatening conditions.
- Monitor the victim's condition, look for changes in LOC and keep the victim comfortable.

Marine Life

The stings of some forms of marine life not only are painful, but they can make the victim feel sick, and in some parts of the world, can be fatal (Figure 10-23, A–D). The side effects of a sting from an aquatic creature can include allergic reactions that can cause breathing and heart problems, as well as paralysis and death. If the sting occurs in water, the victim should be moved to dry land as soon as possible. Emergency care is necessary if the victim has been stung by a lethal jellyfish, does not know what caused the sting, has a history of allergic reactions to stings from aquatic life, has been stung on the face or neck, or starts to have difficulty breathing.

Basic care steps for jellyfish stings are to remove the victim from the water, prevent further injection of poisonous material by deactivating or removing nematocysts (stingers) and control pain.

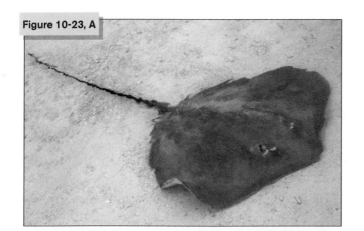
Figure 10-23, A

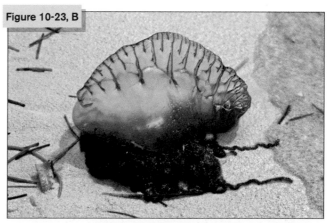
Figure 10-23, B

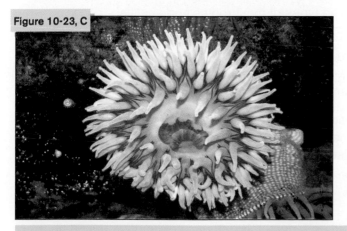
Figure 10-23, C

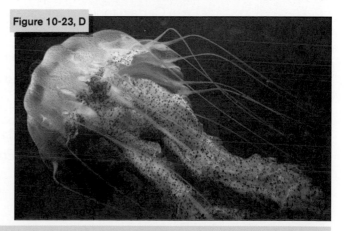
Figure 10-23, D

(A) Stingray, iStockphoto.com/Dia Karanouh; (B) Bluebottle jellyfish/Portuguese man-of-war, iStockphoto/Mark Kostich; (C) Sea anemone, iStockphoto/Omers; (D) Jellyfish, Shutterstock/Johan1900

There are some differences in specific care based on the region and the species of jellyfish. The supervisor of the aquatic facility should inform you of the types of jellyfish in the region, specific treatment recommendations and photographs of the jellyfish to aid in identification.

To deactivate the stingers/tentacles for most types of jellyfish in most waters in the United States, flush the injured part in vinegar as soon as possible for at least 30 seconds to offset the toxin. A baking soda slurry also may be used if vinegar is not available. For "bluebottle" jellyfish, also known as Portuguese man-of-war, which are found in tropical waters, flush with ocean water instead of vinegar. Vinegar triggers further injection of poisonous material. Do not rub the wound or apply fresh water, ammonia or rubbing alcohol, because these substances may increase pain.

Carefully remove any stingers/tentacles with gloved hands or a towel. When stingers are removed or deactivated, use hot-water immersion (as hot as can be tolerated) for at least 20 minutes or until pain is relieved. If hot water is not available, dry hot packs or, as a second choice, dry cold packs also may be helpful in decreasing pain. Do not apply a pressure immobilization bandage.

POISONING

A poison is any substance that can cause injury, illness or death when introduced into the body. Poisons can be in the form of solids, liquids, sprays or fumes (gases and vapors). If a person is showing signals of poisoning, call the Poison Control Center at 1-800-222-1222. If the person is unconscious or experiences a change in LOC, or if another life-threatening condition is present, summon EMS personnel.

In an aquatic facility, the Material Safety Data Sheet (MSDS) is required on site for every product/chemical in use. In the case of a known poisoning by a product or chemical, the MSDS should accompany the victim to the doctor or hospital.

Ingested Poison

Ingested poisons are poisons that are swallowed and include the following:

- Certain foods, such as specific types of mushrooms and shellfish
- Drugs, such as excessive amounts of alcohol
- Medications, such as too much aspirin
- Household items, such as cleaning products, pesticides and certain household plants

A person who has ingested poison generally looks ill and displays symptoms common to other sudden illnesses. If you have even a slight suspicion that a person has been poisoned, call the Poison Control Center.

Inhaled Poison

Poisoning by inhalation occurs when a person breathes in poisonous gases or fumes. Poisonous fumes can come from a variety of sources. They may or may not have an odor. Common inhaled poisons include:

- Carbon monoxide, which can come from car exhaust, fires or charcoal grills.

- Chlorine gas, which is highly toxic. You will need special training to recognize and treat this type of poisoning.
- Fire extinguisher gases.

If someone has inhaled poisonous fumes:

- Size-up the scene to be sure that it is safe to help the victim.
- Summon EMS personnel.
- Move the victim to fresh air.
- Care for life-threatening conditions.
- Monitor the victim's condition and watch for changes in the LOC.
- If conscious, keep the victim comfortable.

Absorbed Poison

An absorbed poison enters through the skin or mucous membranes in the eyes, nose and mouth. Absorbed poisons come from plants, as well as from chemicals and medications. Poison ivy, poison oak and poison sumac are the most common poisonous plants in the United States. Some people are allergic to these poisons and have life-threatening reactions after contact, whereas others may not even get a rash.

If someone has been exposed to a poisonous substance, remove exposed clothing and jewelry and immediately rinse the exposed area thoroughly with water for 20 minutes, using a shower or garden hose if possible. If a rash or wet blisters develop, advise the victim to see his or her health care provider. If the condition spreads to large areas of the body or face, have the victim seek medical attention.

HEAT-RELATED ILLNESSES AND COLD-RELATED EMERGENCIES

Exposure to extreme heat or cold can make a person ill. A person can develop a heat-related illness or a cold-related emergency even when temperatures are not extreme. Factors that may contribute to these emergencies include environmental conditions, such as wind speed, humidity level and general working or living conditions, as well as the victim's personal physical attributes, such as age and state of health and recent physical exertion.

Once the signs and symptoms of a cold-related emergency or heat-related illness appear, the victim's condition can quickly get worse and lead to death.

Heat-Related Illnesses

Heat-related illnesses are progressive conditions caused by overexposure to heat. If recognized in the early stages, heat-related emergencies usually can be reversed. If not recognized early, they may progress to heat stroke, a life-threatening condition. There are three types of heat-related illnesses:

- Heat cramps are painful muscle spasms that usually occur in the legs and abdomen. Heat cramps are the least severe of the heat-related illnesses.
- Heat exhaustion is an early indicator that the body's cooling system is becoming overwhelmed. Signs and symptoms of heat exhaustion include cool, moist,

pale, ashen or flushed skin; headache, nausea and dizziness; weakness and exhaustion; and heavy sweating.

- Heat stroke occurs when the body's systems are overwhelmed by heat and stop functioning. Heat stroke is a life-threatening condition. Signs and symptoms of heat stroke include red, hot, dry skin; changes in LOC; and vomiting.

Caring for Heat-Related Illnesses

Take the following steps to care for someone suffering from a heat-related illness:

- Move the victim to a cool place.
- Loosen tight clothing and remove perspiration-soaked clothing.
- Cool the victim by spraying with cool water or applying cool, wet towels to the skin.
- Fan the victim.
- Encourage the victim to drink small amounts of a commercial sports drink, milk or water if the victim is conscious and able to swallow.

If the victim refuses water, vomits or starts to lose consciousness:

- Send someone to summon EMS personnel.
- Place the victim on his or her side.
- Continue to cool the victim by using ice or cold packs on his or her wrists, ankles, groin and neck, and in the armpits. If possible, wrap the victim's entire body in ice-water-soaked towels.
- Continue to check for breathing and a pulse.

Cold-Related Emergencies

Temperatures do not have to be extremely cold for someone to suffer a cold-related emergency, especially if the victim is wet or if it is windy.

Hypothermia

Hypothermia occurs when a victim's entire body cools because its ability to keep warm fails. A victim with hypothermia will die if care is not provided. The signs and symptoms of hypothermia include shivering; numbness; glassy stare; apathy, weakness or impaired judgment; and loss of consciousness.

To care for hypothermia:

- Perform a primary assessment, including a pulse check for up to 30 to 45 seconds.
- Summon EMS personnel.
- Gently move the victim to a warm place. Sudden movements may cause a heart arrhythmia and possibly cardiac arrest.
- Remove any wet clothing.
- Warm the victim by wrapping all exposed body surfaces in blankets or by putting dry clothing on the victim. Be sure to cover the head since a significant amount of body heat is lost through the head.
  - Do not warm the victim too quickly, such as by immersing him or her in warm water.

- If the victim is alert, have him or her drink liquids that are warm, but not hot, and do not contain alcohol or caffeine.

- If you are using hot water bottles or chemical hot packs, first wrap them in a towel or blanket before applying.

- Monitor the victim's condition and watch for changes in LOC.

Frostbite

Frostbite occurs when body parts freeze from having been exposed to the cold. Severity depends on the air temperature, length of exposure and the wind speed. Frostbite can cause the loss of the nose, fingers, hands, arms, toes, feet and legs. The signs and symptoms of frostbite include a lack of feeling in an affected area, swelling and skin that appears waxy, is cold to the touch or discolored (flushed, white, yellow or blue).

To care for frostbite:

- Get the victim out of the cold.

- Do not attempt to warm the frostbitten area if there is a chance that it might refreeze or if you are close to a medical facility.

- Handle the area gently; never rub the affected area.

- Warm the affected area by soaking it in water not warmer than about 105° F until normal color returns and the area feels warm (for 20 to 30 minutes). If you do not have a thermometer, test the water temperature yourself. If the temperature is uncomfortable to your touch, it is too warm.

- Loosely bandage the area with dry, sterile dressings.

- If the victim's fingers or toes are frostbitten, separate them with dry, sterile gauze.

- Avoid breaking any blisters.

- Take precautions to prevent hypothermia.

- Monitor the person and care for shock.

- Summon EMS personnel to seek emergency medical care as soon as possible.

INJURIES TO MUSCLES, BONES AND JOINTS

Accidents, such as falls, are a common cause of injuries to muscles, bones and joints. There are four types of muscle, bone and joint injuries:

- Fracture—A complete break, a chip or a crack in a bone. Factures can be open or closed.
  - Closed fractures: The skin over the broken bone is intact.
  - Open fractures: There is an open wound in the skin over the fracture.
- Dislocation—Displacement of a bone away from its normal position at a joint. These usually are more obvious than fractures.
- Sprain—Tearing ligaments at a joint.
- Strain—Stretching and tearing muscles or tendons.

It is difficult to know whether a muscle, bone or joint injury is a closed fracture, dislocation, sprain or strain. However, you do not need to be able to identify the type of injury because the type of care provided is universal. The objective is to keep the injured area stable in the position found until EMS personnel take over.

R I C E
e m o l
s m e
t o v
b a
i t
l e
i
z
e

Caring for Muscle, Bone and Joint Injuries

When caring for muscle, bone and joint injuries, except for an open fracture, use the general procedures for a land emergency and:

- Summon EMS personnel if the victim cannot move or use the injured area.
- Support the injured area above and below the site of the injury.
- Check for circulation and sensation below the injured area.
- Immobilize and secure the injured area only if the victim must be moved and it does not cause further pain or injury. In many cases, it may be best to allow EMS personnel to immobilize the injury prior to transport.

RICE

The general care for all musculoskeletal injuries is similar: *rest, immobilize, cold* and *elevate* or "RICE."

Rest

Avoid any movements or activities that cause pain. Help the victim to find the most comfortable position. If you suspect head, neck or spinal injuries, leave the victim lying flat.

Immobilize

Stabilize the injured area in the position in which it was found. In most cases, applying a splint will *not* be necessary. For example, the ground can provide support to an injured leg, ankle or foot, or the victim may cradle an injured elbow or arm in a position of comfort.

Cold

Apply ice or a cold pack for periods of 20 minutes. If 20 minutes cannot be tolerated, apply ice for periods of 10 minutes. If continued icing is needed, remove the pack for 20 minutes, refreeze and then replace it.

Cold helps to reduce swelling, and eases pain and discomfort. Commercial cold packs can be stored in a kit until ready to use, or you can make an ice pack by placing ice (crushed or cubed) with water in a plastic bag and wrapping it with a towel or cloth. Place a thin layer of gauze or cloth between the source of cold and the skin to prevent injury to the skin. Do *not* apply an ice or cold pack directly over an open fracture because doing so would require you to put pressure on the open fracture site and could cause discomfort to the victim. Instead, place cold packs *around* the site. Do *not* apply heat as there is no evidence that applying heat helps.

Elevate

Elevating the injured area above the level of the heart helps slow the flow of blood, helping to reduce swelling. Elevation is particularly effective in controlling swelling in extremity injuries. However, *never* attempt to elevate a seriously injured area of a limb unless it has been adequately immobilized.

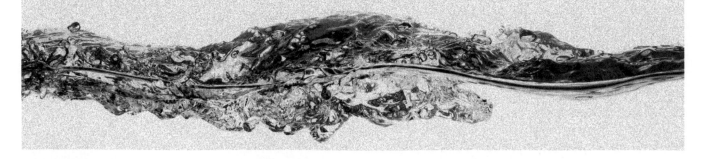

- Recheck for circulation and sensation below the injured area.

Caring for an open fracture is described in a later section.

Immobilizing Muscle, Bone and Joint Injuries

Immobilizing a muscle, bone or joint injury helps keep the injured body part from moving. This also may help to reduce any pain. Splinting is a method of immobilizing an injured extremity and should be used *only* if moving or transporting a person to seek medical attention and if splinting does not cause more pain.

If splinting is necessary, splint the injury in the position in which the injured area was found. Splint the injured area and the joints or bones above and below the injury site. Check for circulation and sensation before and after splinting.

A tool or device used to immobilize an injury is called a splint. Commercially manufactured splints are widely available, but if necessary you can improvise one from items available at the scene. The following can be used to immobilize common muscle, bone and joint injuries:

- **Anatomic splints.** The person's body is the splint. For example, an arm can be splinted to the chest, or an injured leg to the uninjured leg.
- **Soft splints.** Soft materials, such as a folded blanket, towel, pillow or folded triangular bandage, can be used to form a splint. A sling is a specific kind of soft splint that uses a triangular bandage tied to support an injured arm, wrist or hand.
- **Rigid splints.** Boards, folded magazines or newspapers, or metal strips that do not have sharp edges can serve as splints.

See the splinting skill sheets at the end of this chapter for specific steps to follow when caring for arm, leg and foot injuries.

Caring for Open Fractures

An open fracture occurs when a broken bone tears through the skin and surrounding soft tissue. To care for a victim with an open fracture, summon EMS personnel, place sterile dressings around the open fracture, bandage the dressings in place around the fracture, and do not move the exposed bone and limb. This may cause further harm and great pain.

EMERGENCY CHILDBIRTH

If a pregnant woman is about to give birth, summon EMS personnel. Important information to give to the dispatcher includes the pregnant woman's name, age and expected due date; the length of time that she has been having labor pains; and whether this is her first child.

You should also speak with the woman to help her remain calm; place layers of clean sheets, towels or blankets under the woman and over her abdomen; control the scene so that the woman will have privacy; and position the woman on her back with her knees bent, feet flat and legs spread apart.

Remember, the woman delivers the baby, so be patient and let it happen naturally. The baby will be slippery, so take care to avoid dropping the newborn. After delivery, ensure that you clear the newborn's nasal passages and mouth thoroughly, wrap the newborn in a clean, warm blanket or towel and place him or her next to the mother.

Notes:

■ *Do not let the woman get up or leave to find a restroom (most women at this moment feel a desire to use the restroom).*

■ *Be sure to allow the woman's knees to be spread apart to avoid causing complications or harm to the baby.*

■ *Do not place your fingers in the woman's vagina for any reason.*

■ *Do not pull on the baby.*

Continue to meet the needs of the newborn while caring for the mother. Help the mother to begin nursing the newborn, if possible. This will stimulate the uterus to contract and help to slow the bleeding. The placenta still will be in the uterus, attached to the newborn by the umbilical cord. Contractions of the uterus usually will expel the placenta within 30 minutes. Do not pull on the umbilical cord. Catch the placenta in a clean towel or container. It is not necessary to separate the placenta from the newborn. Follow local protocols and medical direction for guidance on cutting the cord.

WRAP-UP

As a professional lifeguard, you may need to care for patrons with a variety of injuries and illnesses. An important part of your job is to provide these victims with effective care. Remember to follow the general procedures for injury or sudden illness on land until EMS personnel arrive and take over. This includes performing a primary assessment and, if you do not find a life-threatening emergency, performing a secondary assessment. You must know how to check a conscious person from head to toe, take a brief SAMPLE history and provide the victim with whatever first aid is needed.

SECONDARY ASSESSMENT—USING SAMPLE TO TAKE A BRIEF HISTORY

Notes:

- *When talking to children, get to eye level with the child, talk slowly and in a friendly manner, use simple words and ask questions a child can easily answer.*

- *If the child's parents are nearby, ask for consent. If a parent or guardian is not available, consent is implied.*

Take a brief history using SAMPLE:

1 Signs and symptoms:

- What happened?
- Where do you feel any pain or discomfort?
- Do you have any numbness or loss of sensation? If so, where?

2 Allergies:

- Do you have any allergies to medications or food? If so, what type of reactions have you experienced when you were exposed?

3 Medications:

- Do you have any medical conditions or are you taking any medications? If so, what conditions do you have or what medications are you taking?
- Have you taken any medications in the past 12 hours?

4 Pertinent past medical history:

- Have you recently been ill?
- Do you have any medical conditions?
- Have you experienced any recent falls, accidents or blows to the head?
- Have you had surgery, been in a traumatic accident or had a medical emergency?

5 Last oral intake:

- When did you last eat or drink?
- What did you last eat or drink?

6 Events leading up to the incident:

- What were you doing before the incident occurred?
- What were you doing when the incident occurred?

CHECKING A CONSCIOUS PERSON

Notes:

■ *When checking an adult or child, explain what you are about to do.*

■ *If a child or an infant becomes extremely upset, conduct the check from toe to head.*

■ *Look for a medical ID tag, necklace or bracelet on the victim's wrist, neck or ankle.*

■ *Do not ask the victim to move any area of the body that causes discomfort or pain, or if you suspect a head, neck or spinal injury.*

1 Check the head.

■ Look at the scalp, face, ears, eyes, nose and mouth for cuts, bumps, bruises and depressions.

■ Note if the victim has any changes in LOC, such as dizziness, or feels light-headed.

2 Check skin appearance and temperature.

■ Feel the victim's forehead with the back of your hand and note if the skin is cold or hot.

■ Look at the color of the victim's face and lips.

■ Look at the victim's skin and note if it is moist or dry; or if it is red, pale, flushed or ashen.

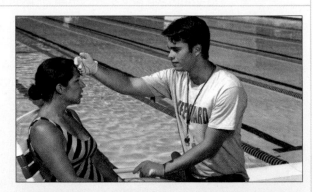

3 Check the neck.

■ Ask the victim to move his or her head from side to side if there is no discomfort and if an injury to the neck is not suspected.

■ Note pain, discomfort or inability to move.

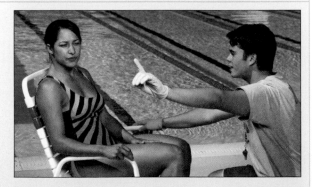

4 Check the shoulders.

■ Ask the victim to shrug his or her shoulders.

5 Check the chest and abdomen.

■ Ask the victim to take a deep breath and blow air out.

■ Listen for difficulty or changes in breathing.

■ Ask the victim if he or she is experiencing pain during breathing.

6 Check the arms.

- Check one arm at a time.
- Ask the victim to move his or her hand and fingers and to bend the arm.

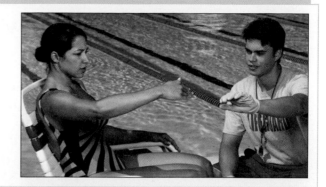

7 Check the legs.

- Check one leg at a time.
- Ask the victim to move his or her foot and toes and to bend the leg.

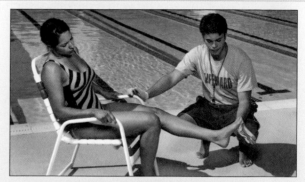

8 Provide care for any conditions found.

9 Have the victim rest in a comfortable position if he or she can move all body parts without pain or discomfort and has no other apparent signs or symptoms of injury or illness. Continue to watch for changes in consciousness and breathing.

CONTROLLING EXTERNAL BLEEDING

Note: *Always follow standard precautions when providing care. Activate the EAP and summon EMS personnel, if necessary. You can ask the victim to apply direct pressure with the dressing while you put on your gloves, if necessary.*

To control external bleeding:

1 Cover the wound with a dressing, such as a sterile gauze pad.

2 Apply direct pressure firmly against the wound until bleeding stops.

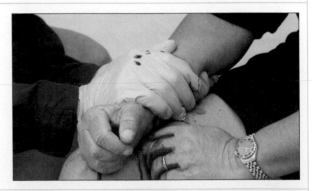

3 Cover the dressing with a roller bandage and secure it directly over the wound.

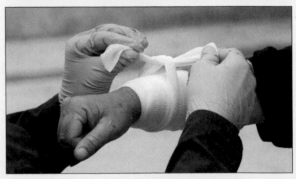

4 Check for circulation beyond the injury (check for pulse, skin temperature and feeling).

If the bleeding does not stop:

- Apply additional dressings and bandages on top of the first ones and continue to apply direct pressure.
- Take steps to minimize shock.
- Summon EMS personnel.
- Follow local protocols when considering other methods of bleeding control, such as applying a tourniquet.

SPLINTING

Note: *Splint only if necessary to move the victim before EMS personnel arrive.*

Arm Injuries

1 Leave the arm in the position in which it was found or in the position in which the victim is holding it.

2 Place a triangular bandage under the injured arm and over the uninjured shoulder to form a sling.

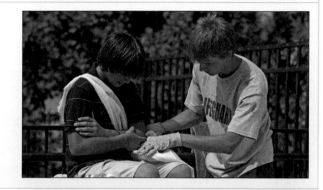

3 Tie the ends of the sling at the side of the neck. Place gauze pads under the knots to make it more comfortable for the victim.

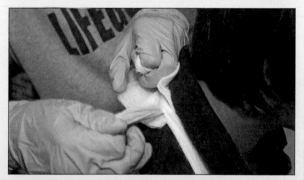

4 Secure the arm to the chest with a folded triangular bandage.

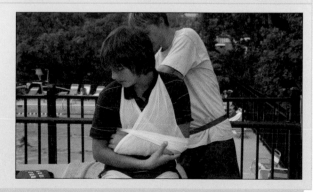

SPLINTING *continued*

Leg Injuries

1 Place several folded triangular bandages above and below the injured body area.

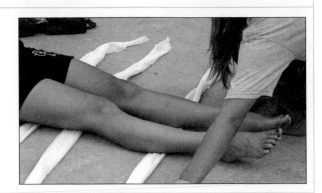

2 Place the uninjured leg next to the injured leg.

3 Tie triangular bandages securely with knots.

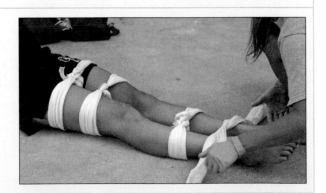

Foot Injuries

Note: *Do not remove the victim's shoes.*

1 Place several folded triangular bandages above and below the injured area.

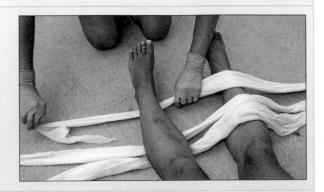

2 Gently wrap a soft object (pillow or folded blanket) around the injured area.

3 | Tie bandages securely with knots.

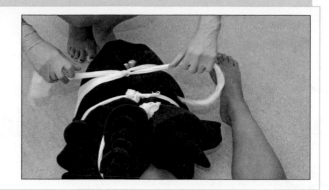

Rib and Breastbone Injuries

1 | Place a pillow or folded towel between the victim's injured ribs and arm.

2 | Bind the arm to the body to help support the injured area.

Hand and Finger Injuries

1 | For a hand injury, place a bulky dressing in the palm of the victim's hand and wrap with a roller bandage.

2 | For a possible fractured or dislocated finger, tape the injured finger to the finger next to it.

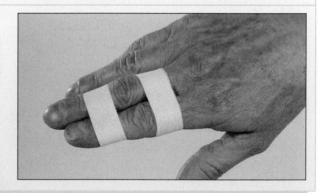

Caring for Head, Neck and Spinal Injuries

E very year, approximately 12,000 spinal cord injuries are reported in the United States. Nearly 8 percent of these injuries occur during sports and recreation, some from head-first entries into shallow water.

Although most head, neck and spinal injuries occur during unsupervised activities, they do sometimes happen while a lifeguard is on duty. These injuries are rare, but when they do occur, they can result in lifelong disability or even death. Prompt and effective care is required. As a professional lifeguard, you must be aware of the causes of head, neck and spinal injuries. You also must know how to recognize them and provide appropriate care. ■

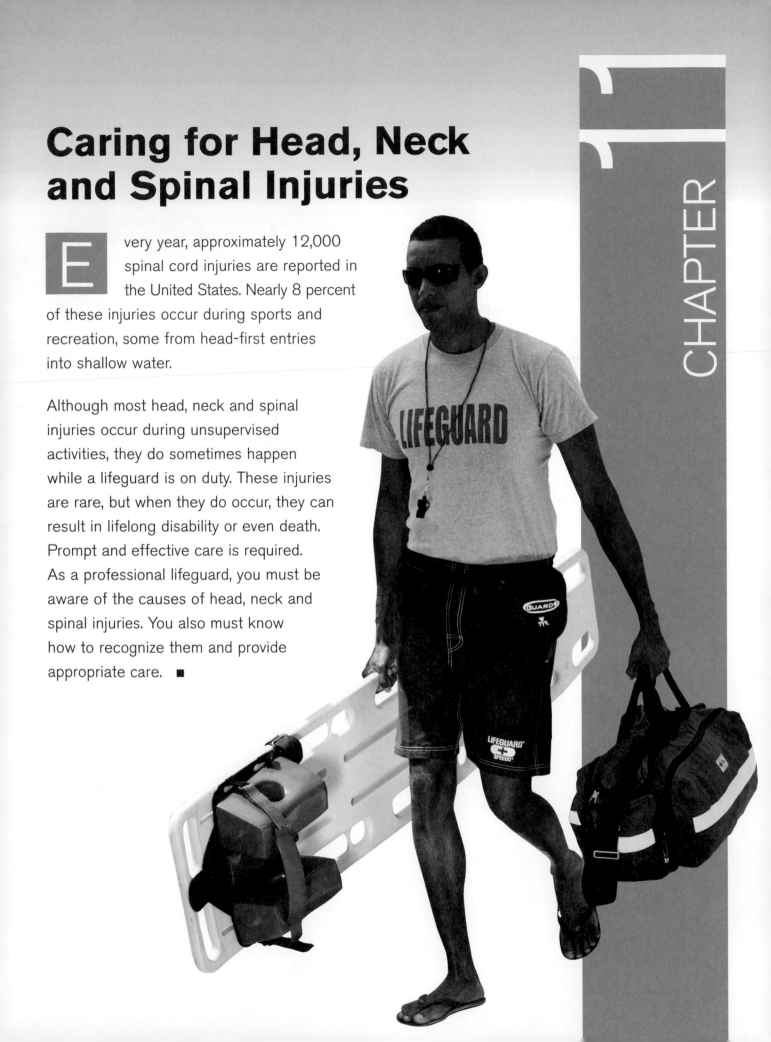

CAUSES OF HEAD, NECK AND SPINAL INJURIES

Head, neck and spinal injuries rarely happen during supervised diving into deep water. In pools, head, neck and spinal injuries most often occur at the shallow end, in a corner or where the bottom slopes from shallow to deep water. They also occur when someone strikes a floating object, like an inner tube or person, while diving. Head, neck or spinal injuries also happen out of the water, for example, when a person trips or falls on a pool deck or in a locker room.

At lakes, rivers and oceans, head, neck and spinal injuries usually occur in areas where depths change with the tide or current. At beaches, these injuries happen mainly when someone plunges head-first into shallow water or a breaking wave. These injuries also result from collisions with an underwater hazard, such as a rock, tree stump or sandbar.

Head, neck or spinal injuries often are caused by *high-impact/high-risk* activities. In aquatic environments, examples of these activities include:

- Entering head-first into shallow water.
- Falling from greater than a standing height.
- Entering the water from a height, such as a diving board, water slide, an embankment, cliff or tower.
- Striking a submerged or floating object.
- Receiving a blow to the head.
- Colliding with another swimmer.
- Striking the water with high impact, such as falling while water skiing or surfing.

Signs and Symptoms

You should suspect a possible head, neck or spinal injury only if the activity was high-impact or high-risk *and* signs or symptoms of injury are present.

The signs and symptoms of possible head, neck or spinal injury include:

- Unusual bumps, bruises or depressions on the head, neck or back.
- Heavy external bleeding of the head, neck or back.
- Bruising of the head, especially around the eyes and behind the ears.
- Blood or other fluids in the ears or nose.
- Seizures.
- Changes in level of consciousness.
- Impaired breathing or vision.
- Nausea or vomiting.
- Partial or complete loss of movement of any body area.
- Loss of balance.
- Victim holds his or her head, neck or back.
- Behavior resembling intoxication.
- Severe pain or pressure in the head, neck or back.
- Back pain, weakness, tingling or loss of sensation in the hands, fingers, feet or toes.
- Persistent headache.

CARING FOR HEAD, NECK AND SPINAL INJURIES

For a victim of a suspected head, neck or spinal injury, your objective is to minimize movement of the head, neck and spine. You must use specific rescue techniques to stabilize and restrict motion of the victim's head, neck and spine, regardless of whether the victim is on land or water. You must also be familiar with and train using your facility's equipment. Skill sheets that describe the steps to care for head, neck and spinal injuries are located at the end of the chapter.

If the victim is in the water and is breathing, you, along with at least one assisting lifeguard, will immobilize him or her using a backboard equipped with straps and a head-immobilizer device. If the victim is not breathing, immediately remove the victim from the water using a technique, such as the two-person-removal-from-the-water, and provide resuscitative care. Whether on land or in the water, higher priority is given to airway management, giving ventilations or performing CPR than to spinal immobilization.

The care that you provide to a victim with an injury to the head, neck or spine depends on:

- The victim's condition, including whether he or she is conscious and breathing.
- The location of the victim (shallow or deep water, at the surface of the water, submerged or not in the water).
- The availability of additional help, such as other lifeguards, bystanders, fire fighters, police or emergency medical services (EMS) personnel.
- The facility's specific procedures.
- The air and water temperature.

Caring for Head, Neck and Spinal Injuries in the Water

If you suspect a head, neck or spinal injury and the victim is in the water, follow these general rescue procedures:

1. Activate the facility's emergency action plan (EAP). Facilities may have a distinct signal to begin a suspected head, neck or spine injury rescue.
2. Safely enter the water. If the victim is near a pool wall or pier, minimize water movement by using a slide-in entry rather than a compact or stride jump. If you use a running entry, slow down before reaching the victim.
3. Perform a rescue providing in-line stabilization appropriate for the victim's location and whether the victim is face-up or face-down.
4. Move the victim to safety. If in deep water, move to shallow water if possible.
5. Check for consciousness and breathing (Figure 11-1).
   - If the victim is breathing, proceed with the spinal backboarding procedure (See page 250).
   - If the victim is not breathing, immediately remove the victim from the water using a technique, such as the two-person-removal-from-the-water, and provide resuscitative care.

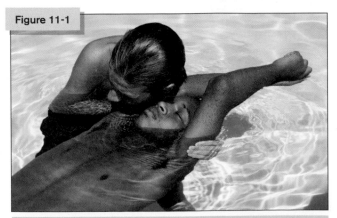

Figure 11-1

Check for consciousness and breathing while maintaining in-line stabilization.

    ○ Do not delay removal from the water by strapping the victim onto the board or using the head immobilizer device.

6. Backboard the victim using the spinal backboarding procedure.

7. Remove the victim from the water.

8. Re-assess the victim's condition and provide appropriate care. Additionally:

    ○ Minimize shock by keeping the victim from getting chilled or overheated.

    ○ If the victim vomits, tilt the backboard on one side to help clear the vomit from the victim's mouth.

Manual In-line Stabilization

The head splint technique is used for performing manual in-line stabilization for victims in the water (Figure 11-2). You can use this technique when the victim is face-up or face-down; in shallow or deep water; and at, near or below the surface. The technique is performed in subtly different ways, depending on the victim's location and position in the water. However, regardless of the variation used, your objective should remain the same—to get the victim into a face-up position while minimizing movement of the head, neck and spine.

Vary the technique in the following ways, based on the victim's position in the water:

- If the victim is face-up, approach from behind the victim's head.

- If the victim is face-down, approach from the victim's side.

- If the victim is in shallow water, you do not need to use the rescue tube to support yourself.

- If the victim is at the surface in deep water, you may need the rescue tube to support yourself and the victim.

- If the victim is submerged, do not use the rescue tube when you are submerging and bringing the victim to the surface. Once at the surface, another lifeguard can place a rescue tube under your armpits to help support you and the victim.

The head splint technique uses the victim's arms to help hold the victim's head in line with the body. Avoid lifting or twisting the victim when performing this skill. Do not move the victim any more than necessary. Minimize water movement by moving the victim away from crowded areas and toward the calmest water possible. Keep the victim's mouth and nose out of the water and minimize water splashing onto the victim's face.

As soon as the victim is stabilized in the head splint and is face-up in the water, immediately check the victim for consciousness and breathing.

Fortunately, injuries to the head, neck or spine rarely occur in deep water. Should this occur, the victim often can be moved to shallow water. Lane lines or safety lines

Head Injuries

Any significant force to the head can cause an injury, ranging from bleeding to a concussion. A *concussion* is a temporary impairment of brain function. In most cases, the victim may lose consciousness for only an instant. Be aware that a person in the water who receives a severe blow to the head could lose consciousness temporarily and submerge. Anyone suspected of having any head injury in or out of the water should be examined immediately by a health care provider.

Figure 11-2

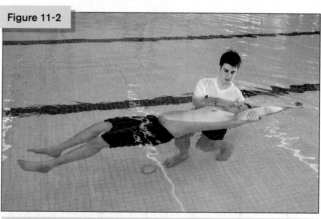

Use the head splint technique for performing manual in-line stabilization for victims in the water.

IMMOBILIZATION EQUIPMENT FOR VICTIMS OF HEAD, NECK OR SPINAL INJURIES

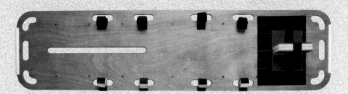

The backboard is the standard piece of rescue equipment used at aquatic facilities for immobilizing and removing a victim from the water. Backboards work best when they are equipped with:

- A minimum of three straps to secure the victim to the board.

- A head immobilizer device that can be attached to the top, or head-end, of the board.

Backboards vary in shape, size, buoyancy, number or style of body straps and style of head immobilizer device. Every aquatic facility develops its own backboarding procedures based on the facility type, equipment, number of rescuers available and local EMS protocols. Your facility should train you on using a backboard according to the facility's procedures.

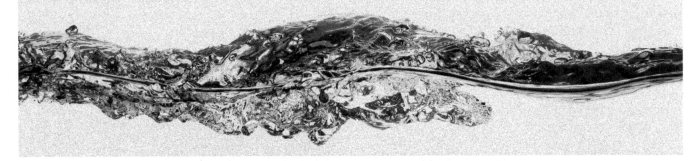

may need to be moved to clear a path to shallow water. If you cannot move the victim to shallow water, such as in a separate diving well, use the rescue tube under both armpits to help support yourself and the victim until the backboard arrives.

Spinal Backboarding Procedure

After stabilizing the victim's head, neck and spine, you and at least one other lifeguard should place and secure the victim on a backboard. Using a backboard helps to immobilize the victim during the process of removing him or her from the water. A minimum of two lifeguards is needed to place and secure a victim on a backboard, but additional lifeguards or bystanders should also help, if available.

To place a victim on a backboard, submerge the board, position it under the victim and carefully raise it up to the victim's body. You then secure the victim to the backboard with straps and a head immobilizer device. Throughout the spinal backboarding process, you or another lifeguard must maintain manual in-line stabilization of the victim's head and neck. To aid in floatation of the backboard, rescue tubes can be placed under the board (Figure 11-3). Additional lifeguards also can assist in keeping the board afloat.

Figure 11-3

Place rescue tubes under the backboard to help floatation of the board.

Communication between lifeguards is critical during the spinal backboarding procedure. Communication with the victim also is important. Let the victim know what you are doing and reassure him or her along the way. Tell the victim not to nod or shake his or her head, but instead to say "yes" or "no" in answer to your questions

Team Spinal Backboarding

Spinal backboarding and removal from the water can be a challenge in deep or shallow water. Having other lifeguards work with you is helpful and may be necessary to ensure your safety as well as that of the victim. Working together as a team, other lifeguards can help by:

- Submerging and positioning the backboard under the victim.
- Supporting the rescuer at the head of the backboard in deep water (Figure 11-4, A).
- Supporting the backboard while the straps and head immobilizer are secured.
- Securing the straps or the head immobilizer device (Figure 11-4, B–C).
- Communicating with and reassuring the victim.
- Guiding the backboard as it is being removed from the water (Figure 11-4, D).
- Removing the backboard from the water (Figure 11-4, E).

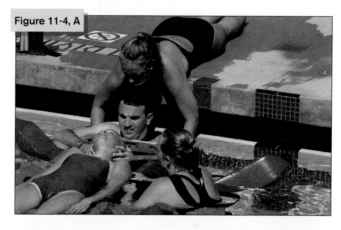
Figure 11-4, A

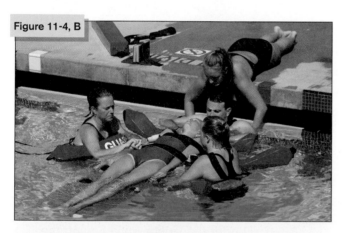
Figure 11-4, B

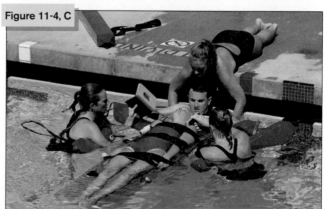
Figure 11-4, C

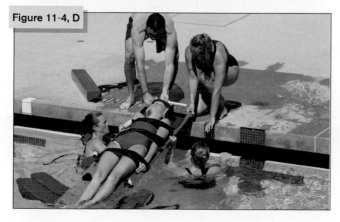
Figure 11-4, D

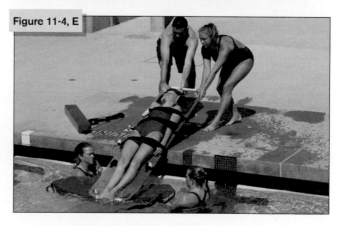
Figure 11-4, E

ALTERNATE METHOD FOR MANUAL IN-LINE STABILIZATION TECHNIQUE– HEAD AND CHIN SUPPORT

When caring for victims with head, neck or spinal injuries in the water, special situations may require a modification to the in-line stabilization technique used, such as when a victim has one arm or little flexibility in the shoulders. The head and chin support can be used for face-down or face-up victims who are at or near the surface in shallow water at least 3 feet deep or for a face-up victim. Be aware of the following situations:

■ Do not use the head and chin support for a face-down victim in water that is less than 3 feet deep. This technique requires you to submerge and roll under the victim while maintaining in-line stabilization. It is difficult to do this in water less than 3 feet deep without risking injury to yourself or the victim.

■ Do not use the rescue tube for support when performing the head and chin support on a face-down victim in deep water. This impedes your ability to turn the victim over. However, once the victim is turned face-up, another lifeguard can place a rescue tube under your armpits to help support you and the victim.

To perform the head and chin support for a face-up or face-down victim at or near the surface:

1. Approach the victim from the side

2. With your body about shoulder depth in the water, place one forearm along the length of the victim's breastbone and the other forearm along the victim's spine.

3. Use your hands to gently hold the victim's head and neck in line with the body. Place one hand on the victim's lower jaw and the

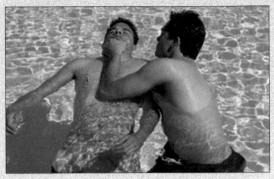

Place one hand on the victim's lower jaw and the other hand on the back of the lower head.

other hand on the back of the lower head. Be careful not to place pressure on the neck or touch the front or back of the neck.

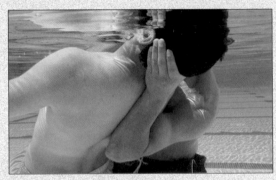

Be careful not to place pressure on the neck or touch the front or back of the neck.

4. Squeeze your forearms together, clamping the victim's chest and back. Continue to support the victim's head and neck.

   o If the victim is face-down, you must turn him or her face-up. Slowly move the victim forward to help lift the victim's legs. Turn the victim toward you while submerging.

   o Roll under the victim while turning the victim over. Avoid twisting the victim's body. The victim should be face-up as you surface on the other side.

   o Check for consciousness and breathing.

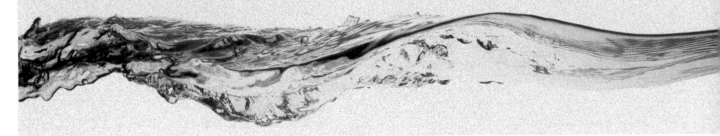

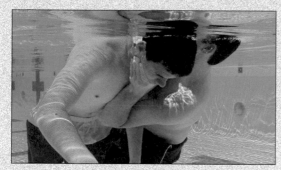

Turn the victim toward you while submerging.

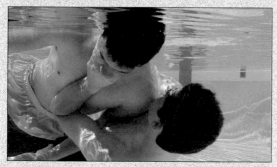

Roll under the victim while turning the victim over.

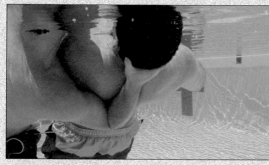

The victim should be face-up as you surface on the other side.

○ If the victim is not breathing, immediately remove the victim from the water using a technique, such as the two-person-removal-from-the-water. Do not delay removal from the water by strapping the victim onto the backboard or using the head immobilizer device.

○ If the victim is breathing, hold the victim face-up in the water and move toward safety until the backboard arrives. In deep water, move the victim to shallow water if possible.

Spinal Backboarding Procedure Using the Head and Chin Support

When using the head and chin support as the stabilization technique, modify the backboarding procedure in the following ways:

1. While an additional rescuer raises the backboard into place, the primary rescuer carefully removes his or her arm from beneath the victim and places it under the backboard while the other hand and arm remain on the victim's chin and chest.

2. The additional rescuer moves to the victim's head and places the rescue tube under the head of the backboard to aid in floatation of the board.

3. The additional rescuer then supports the backboard with his or her forearms and stabilizes the victim's head by placing his or her hands along side of the victim's head. The primary rescuer can now release.

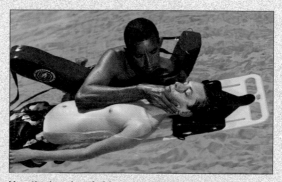

Use the head and chin support as a stabilization technique when performing spinal backboarding in deep water, but modify the backboarding procedure.

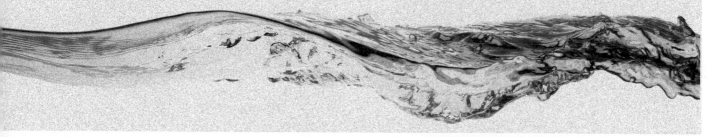

■ Providing care after the victim has been removed from the water.

Additional lifeguards should be able to arrive at the scene, identify what assistance is needed and begin helping.

Removal from the Water

Once the victim is secured onto the backboard, you should remove the victim from the water. Your technique will vary depending on the characteristics of your exit point (e.g., shallow or deep water, speed slide or sloping waterfront entry).

After the victim is out of the water, assess his or her condition and provide the appropriate care. Place a towel or blanket on the victim to keep him or her warm, if needed.

Use the following skills to secure a victim suspected of having a spinal injury to a backboard and remove him or her from the water:

■ **Spinal backboarding procedures–shallow water**
■ **Spinal backboarding procedures–deep water**
■ **Spinal injury removal from the water on a backboard**

Special Situations

In-line stabilization and backboarding can be more difficult to perform in facilities that have extremely shallow water, moving water or confined spaces. Caring for a victim of a head, neck or spinal injury in these situations requires modification of the techniques for in-line stabilization and removal from the water.

During orientation and in-service trainings, your facility's management should provide information and skills practice for in-line stabilization and backboarding procedures used at the facility for its specific attractions and environments. These trainings should include emergency shut-off procedures to stop water flow and movement.

Removal from Extremely Shallow Water

Many facilities have extremely shallow water, such as zero-depth pools, wave pools and sloping beaches. To remove a victim from a zero-depth or sloping entry, have sufficient lifeguards on each side of the backboard to support the victim's weight. After the victim is secured to the backboard:

■ Carefully lift up the backboard and victim using proper lifting techniques to prevent injuring yourself.
■ Remove the backboard and victim from the water by slowly walking out. Keep the board as level as possible during the removal.
■ Gently lower the backboard and the victim to the ground once out of the water using proper lifting techniques to prevent injuring yourself.

Moving Water

You may need to modify the way you care for a person with a head, neck or spinal injury if waves or currents are moving the water. In water with waves, move the victim to calmer water, if possible. At a waterfront, a pier or raft may break or block the waves. If there is no barrier from the waves, have other rescuers form a "wall" with their bodies to block the waves. At a wave pool, stop the waves by pushing the emergency stop button. Remember, even though the button has been pushed, residual wave action will continue for a short time.

Rivers, Streams and Winding River Attractions

A special problem in rivers, streams and winding rivers at waterparks is that the current can pull or move the victim. At waterparks, the facility's EAP may include signaling another lifeguard to stop the flow of water in a winding river by pushing the emergency stop button. In all cases:

- Ask other lifeguards or patrons for help in keeping objects and people from floating into the rescuer while he or she is supporting the victim.

- Do not let the current press sideways on the victim or force the victim into a wall. This would twist the victim's body. Keep the victim's head pointed upstream into the current (Figure 11-5). This position also reduces the splashing of water on the victim's face.

- Once the in-line stabilization technique is performed and the victim is turned face-up, slowly turn the victim so that the current pulls his or her legs around to point downstream.

- Place the victim on a backboard by following the facility's spinal backboarding procedures.

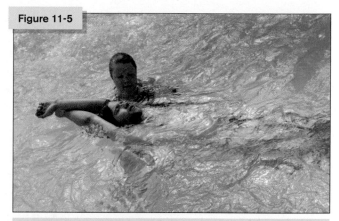

Figure 11-5

Position the victim's head so it is pointed upstream into the current.

Catch Pools

The water in a catch pool moves with more force than in a winding river and can make it difficult to hold a victim still.

- If a person is suspected of having a head, neck or spinal injury in a catch pool, immediately signal other lifeguards to stop sending riders.

- If possible, someone should stop the flow of water by pushing the emergency stop button.

- Once in-line stabilization is achieved and the victim is turned face-up, move the victim to the calmest water in the catch pool if water is still flowing (Figure 11-6). If there is only one slide, the calmest water is usually at the

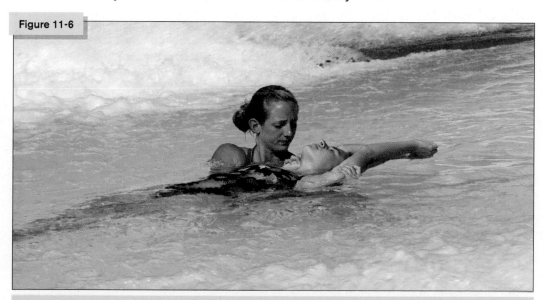

Figure 11-6

Move the victim to the calmest water in the catch pool once manual in-line stabilization is achieved.

Figure 11-7, A

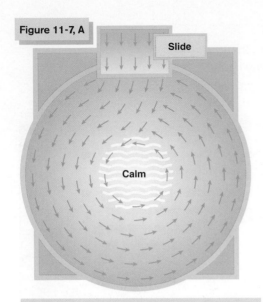

Slide

Calm

Catch pool with only one slide

Figure 11-7, B

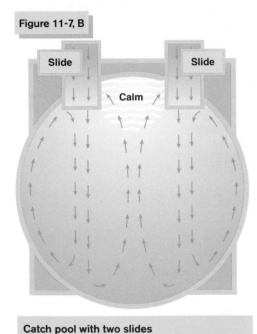

Slide   Slide

Calm

Catch pool with two slides

center of the catch pool. If several slides empty into the same catch pool, calmer water usually is between two slides (Figure 11-7, A–B).

■ Place the victim on a backboard following the facility's spinal backboarding procedures.

Speed Slides

A head, neck or spinal injury may happen on a speed slide if the patron twists or turns his or her body the wrong way, strikes his or her head on the side of the slide or sits up and tumbles down off the slide. The narrow space of a speed slide is problematic for rescuing a victim with a head, neck or spinal injury. Backboarding can be a challenge because the water in the slide is only 2 or 3 inches deep and does not help to support the victim.

Caring for Head, Neck and Spinal Injuries on Land

If you suspect that a victim on land has a head, neck or spinal injury, your goal is the same as for a victim in the water: minimize movement of the head, neck and spine. Activate the facility's EAP and follow the general procedures for injury or sudden illness on land:

■ Size-up the scene.

■ Perform a primary assessment.

■ Summon EMS personnel.

■ Perform a secondary assessment.

■ Provide the appropriate care.

Use appropriate personal protective equipment, such as disposable gloves and breathing barriers.

Approach the victim from the front so that he or she can see you without turning the head. Tell the victim not to nod or shake his or her head, but instead respond verbally to your questions, such as by saying "yes" or "no."

Caring for a Non-Standing Victim

If you suspect a victim on land has a head, neck or spinal injury, have the victim remain in the position in which he or she was found until EMS personnel assume control (Figure 11-8). Gently support the head in the position in which it was found. Do not attempt to align the head and neck, unless you cannot maintain an open airway. Gently position the victim's head in line with the body *only* if you cannot maintain an open airway.

Caring for a Standing Victim

If you encounter a patron who is standing but has a suspected head, neck or spinal injury, secure the victim to the backboard while he or she remains standing and slowly lower him or her to the ground (Figure 11-9). Follow the steps on the skill sheet, Caring for a Standing Victim Who Has a Suspected Head, Neck or Spinal Injury on Land.

If EMS personnel are available within a few minutes and the victim's safety is not compromised, you may maintain manual stabilization with the victim standing. Do not have the person sit or lie down. Minimize movement of the victim's head by placing your hands on both sides of the victim's head (Figure 11-10).

If the victim's condition becomes unstable (e.g., the victim complains of dizziness, has a potential life-threatening condition or begins to lose consciousness), slowly lower the victim to the ground with the assistance of other lifeguards. Try to maintain manual stabilization while the victim is being lowered.

WRAP-UP

Although they are rare, head, neck and spinal injuries do occur at aquatic facilities. They can cause life-long disability or even death. Prompt, effective care is needed. As a professional lifeguard, you must be able to recognize and care for victims with head, neck or spinal injuries. To decide whether an injury could be serious, consider both its cause and the signs and symptoms. If you suspect that a victim in the water has a head, neck or spinal injury, make sure to summon EMS personnel immediately. Minimize movement by using in-line stabilization. Secure the victim to a backboard to restrict motion of the head, neck and spine. When the victim is out of the water, provide the appropriate care until EMS personnel arrive and assume control of the victim's care.

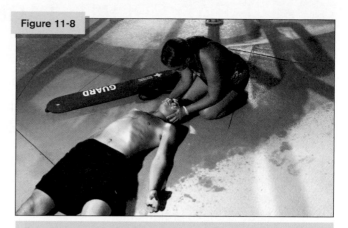

Figure 11-8

If a non-standing victim has a suspected head, neck or spinal injury, keep him in the position in which he was found until EMS personnel assume control.

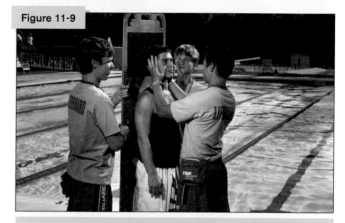

Figure 11-9

Secure a standing victim with a suspected head, neck or spinal injury to the backboard while he remains standing. Slowly lower him to the ground.

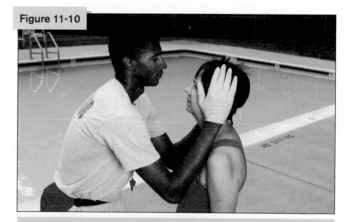

Figure 11-10

Maintain manual stabilization for a standing victim with a suspected head, neck or spinal injury by placing your hands on both sides of the person's head.

HEAD SPLINT—**FACE-UP VICTIM AT OR NEAR THE SURFACE**

1 Approach the victim's head from behind, or stand behind the victim's head.

- In shallow water, lower your body so that the water level is at your neck.
- In deep water, use the rescue tube under both of your arms for support.

2 Grasp the victim's arms midway between his or her shoulder and elbow. Grasp the victim's right arm with your right hand and the victim's left arm with your left hand. Gently move the victim's arms up alongside the head. Position yourself to the victim's side while trapping the victim's head with his or her arms.

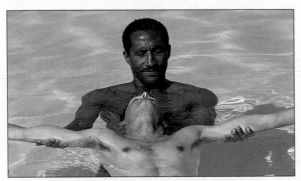 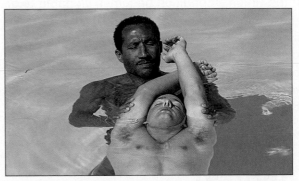

3 Slowly and carefully squeeze the victim's arms against his or her head to help hold the head in line with the body. Do not move the victim any more than necessary.

4 Position the victim's head close to the crook of your arm, with the head in line with the body.

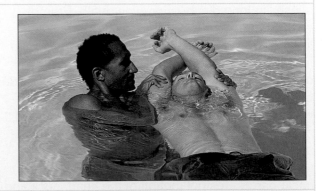

5 Check for consciousness and breathing.

- If the victim is not breathing, immediately remove the victim from the water using a technique, such as the two-person-removal-from-the-water, and provide resuscitative care. Do not delay removal from the water by strapping the victim in or using the head immobilizer device.
- If the victim is breathing, hold the victim with the head in line with the body and move toward safety until the backboard arrives. In deep water, move the victim to shallow water, if possible.

6 Continuously monitor for consciousness and breathing. If at any time the victim stops breathing, immediately remove the victim from the water then provide appropriate care.

HEAD SPLINT—**FACE-DOWN VICTIM AT OR NEAR THE SURFACE**

1 Approach the victim from the side.

- In deep water, use the rescue tube under both of your arms for support.

2 Grasp the victim's arms midway between the shoulder and elbow. Grasp the victim's right arm with your right hand and the victim's left arm with your left hand. Gently move the victim's arms up alongside the head.

3 Squeeze the victim's arms against his or her head to help hold the head in line with the body.

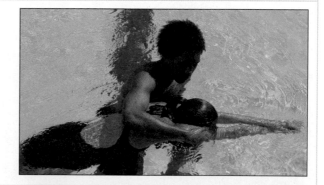

4 Glide the victim slowly forward.

- In shallow water, lower your body to shoulder depth before gliding the victim forward.

- Continue moving slowly and turn the victim until he or she is face-up. To do this, push the victim's arm that is closest to you under the water while pulling the victim's other arm across the surface toward you.

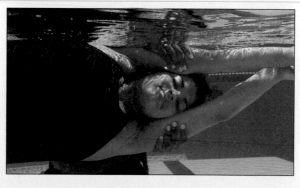

5 Position the victim's head in the crook of your arm, with the head in line with the body.

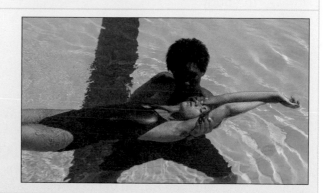

Continued on Next Page

HEAD SPLINT—**FACE-DOWN VICTIM AT OR NEAR THE SURFACE** *continued*

6 Check for consciousness and breathing.

- If the victim is not breathing, immediately remove the victim from the water using a technique, such as the two-person-removal-from-the-water, and provide resuscitative care. Do not delay removal from the water by strapping the victim in or using the head immobilizer device.

- If the victim is breathing, hold the victim with the head in line with the body and move toward safety until the backboard arrives. In deep water, move the victim to shallow water, if possible.

7 Continuously monitor for consciousness and breathing. If at any time the victim stops breathing, immediately remove the victim from the water then provide appropriate care.

HEAD SPLINT—**SUBMERGED VICTIM**

1 Approach the victim from the side. In deep water, release the rescue tube if the victim is more than an arm's reach beneath the surface.

2 Grasp the victim's arms midway between the shoulder and elbow. Grasp the victim's right arm with your right hand and the victim's left arm with your left hand. Gently move the victim's arms up alongside the head.

3 Squeeze the victim's arms against his or her head to help hold the head in line with the body.

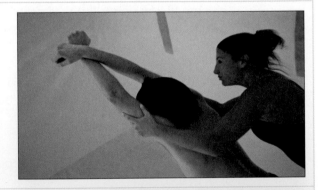

4 Turn the victim face-up while bringing the victim to the surface at an angle. To turn the victim face-up, push the victim's arm that is closest to you down and away from you while pulling the victim's other arm across the surface toward you. The victim should be face-up just before reaching the surface or at the surface.

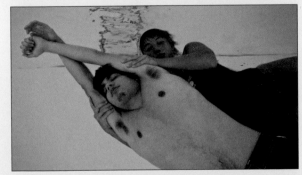

5 Position the victim's head close to the crook of your arm with the head in line with the body. Another lifeguard can place a rescue tube under your armpits to help support you and the victim.

6 Check for consciousness and breathing.

- If the victim is not breathing, immediately remove the victim from the water using a technique, such as the two-person-removal-from-the-water, and provide resuscitative care. Do not delay removal from the water by strapping the victim in or using the head immobilizer device.

- If the victim is breathing, hold the victim with the head in line with the body and move toward safety until the backboard arrives. In deep water, move the victim to shallow water, if possible.

7 Continuously monitor for consciousness and breathing. If at any time the victim stops breathing, immediately remove the victim from the water then provide appropriate care.

Note: *If the victim is submerged but face-up, approach the victim from behind and follow the same steps in the skill sheet, Head Splint—Face-Up Victim at or Near the Surface while you bring the victim to the surface.*

 HEAD SPLINT—**FACE-DOWN IN EXTREMELY SHALLOW WATER**

1 Approach the victim from the side. Grasp the victim's right arm with your right hand and the victim's left arm with your left hand, trapping the victim's head between his or her arms.

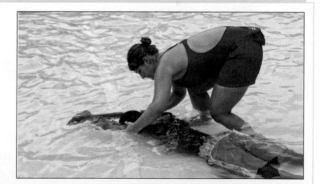

2 After the victim's head is trapped between his or her arms, begin to roll the victim toward you.

3 While rolling the victim, step from the victim's side toward the victim's head and begin to turn the victim face-up.

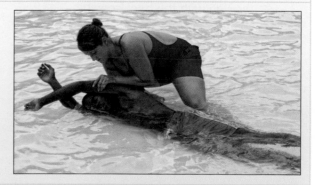

Continued on Next Page

HEAD SPLINT—**FACE-DOWN IN EXTREMELY SHALLOW WATER** *continued*

4 Lower your arm on the victim's side that is closest to you so that the victim's arms go over the top of your arm as you step toward the victim's head. Maintain arm pressure against the victim's head, since your hand rotates during this maneuver. You are now positioned above and behind the victim's head.

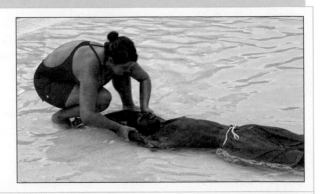

5 Check for consciousness and breathing.

- If the victim is not breathing, immediately remove the victim from the water and give the appropriate care.
- If the victim is breathing, hold the victim in this position. Place a towel or blanket on the victim to keep him or her from getting chilled.

6 Continuously monitor for consciousness and breathing. If at any time the victim stops breathing, immediately remove the victim from the water then provide appropriate care.

Note: *If you are unable to keep the victim from getting chilled and there are enough assisting lifeguards, follow the care steps for skill sheet, Spinal Backboarding Procedure and Removal from Water—Speed Slide.*

 # SPINAL BACKBOARDING PROCEDURE— **SHALLOW WATER**

Note: *If the victim is not breathing, immediately remove the victim from the water using the two-person-removal-from-the-water technique and provide resuscitative care. Do not delay removal from the water by strapping the victim in or using the head immobilizer device.*

1 The first lifeguard (primary rescuer) provides in-line stabilization until another lifeguard arrives with the backboard.

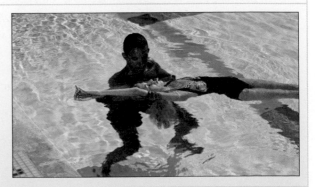

2 The assisting lifeguard removes the head-immobilizer device, enters the water, submerges the backboard and positions the board under the victim so that it extends slightly beyond the victim's head. The victim's head should be centered on the backboard's head space.

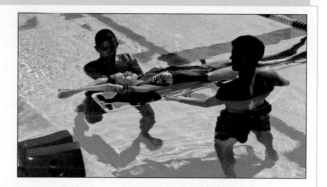

3 While an assisting lifeguard raises the backboard into place, the primary rescuer moves the elbow that is under the victim toward the top of the backboard while continuing to apply pressure on both of the victim's arms, using the victim's arms as a splint.

4 Once the backboard is in place, an assisting lifeguard then stabilizes the victim by placing one hand and arm on the victim's chin and chest, the other hand and arm under the backboard. The primary rescuer then releases his or her grip on the victim's arms.

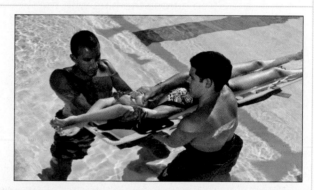

5 The primary rescuer lowers the victim's arms, moves behind the victim's head and places the rescue tube under the head of the backboard to aid in floatation of the board.

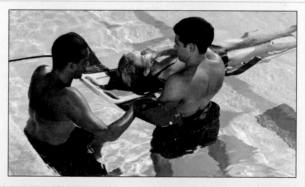

6 The primary rescuer balances the backboard on the rescue tube with his or her forearms and stabilizes the victim's head by placing his or her hands along each side of the victim's head.

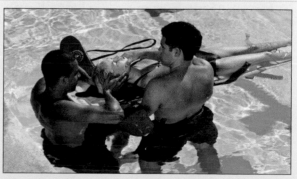

Continued on Next Page

SPINAL BACKBOARDING PROCEDURE—
SHALLOW WATER *continued*

7 An assisting lifeguard secures the victim on the backboard with a minimum of three straps: one each across the victim's chest, hips and thighs. Secure the straps in the following order:

- Strap high across the chest and under the victim's armpits. This helps prevent the victim from sliding on the backboard during the removal.

- Strap across the hips with the victim's arms and hands secured under the straps.

- Strap across the thighs.

- Recheck straps to be sure that they are secure.

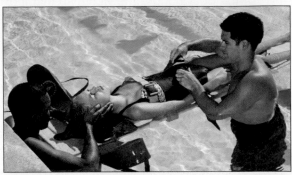

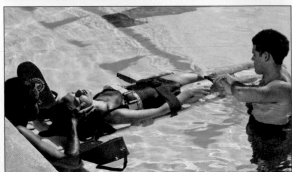

8 The rescuers secure the victim's head to the backboard using a head immobilizer and a strap across the victim's forehead.

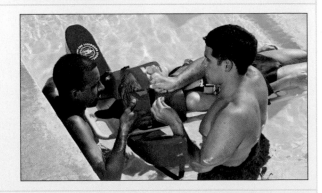

9 If not done already, bring the victim to the side.

SPINAL BACKBOARDING PROCEDURE—
DEEP WATER

Note: *If the victim is not breathing, immediately remove the victim from the water using the two-person removal-from-the-water technique and provide resuscitative care. Do not delay removal from the water by strapping the victim in or using the head immobilizer device.*

1 The first lifeguard (primary rescuer) provides in-line stabilization. If the victim is face-down, the primary rescuer turns the victim into a face-up position. If necessary, an assisting lifeguard retrieves the primary rescuer's rescue tube and inserts it under the primary rescuer's armpits.

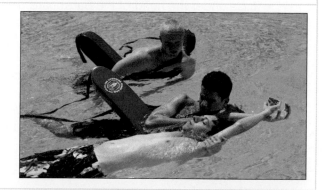

2 The primary rescuer moves the victim to the side, if possible, toward a corner. An assisting lifeguard places a rescue tube under the victim's knees to raise the legs. This makes placing the backboard under the victim easier.

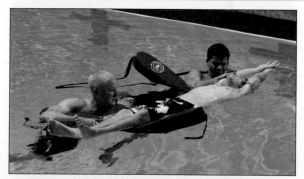

3 An assisting lifeguard places the backboard under the victim while the primary rescuer maintains stabilization.

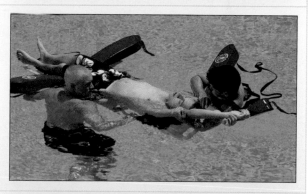

4 As an assisting lifeguard raises the backboard into place, the primary rescuer moves the elbow that is under the victim toward the top of the backboard while continuing to apply pressure on both of the victim's arms. An assisting lifeguard stabilizes the victim with one hand and arm on the victim's chin and chest, and the other hand and arm under the backboard.

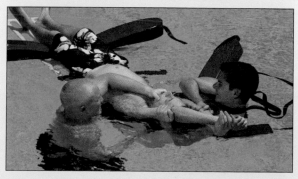

Continued on Next Page

SPINAL BACKBOARDING PROCEDURE—
DEEP WATER *continued*

5 Once the backboard is in place, the primary rescuer then lowers the victim's arms, moves behind the victim's head and places a rescue tube under the head of the backboard. The primary rescuer balances the board on the rescue tube with his or her forearms and stabilizes the victim's head by placing his or her hands along each side of the victim's head. The assisting rescuer moves to the foot of the board and removes the rescue tube under the victim's knees by sliding the rescue tube toward him or herself.

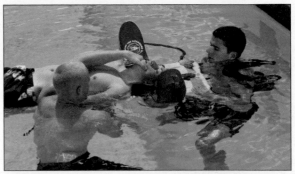

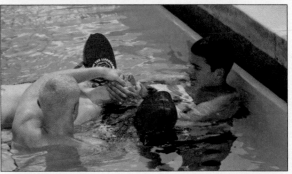

6 An assisting lifeguard secures the victim on the backboard by placing straps at least across the victim's chest, hips and thighs. After all the straps have been checked and properly secured, the rescuers secure the victim's head using a head immobilizer and a strap across the victim's forehead.

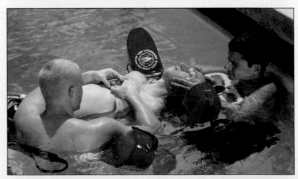

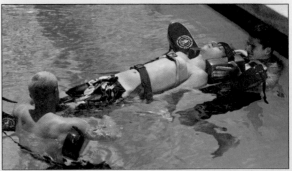

SPINAL INJURY–REMOVAL FROM THE WATER ON A BACKBOARD

1 Once the victim is properly secured to the backboard, position the backboard with the head-end by the side of the pool and the foot-end straight out into the water.

2 With one lifeguard at each side, lift the head of the backboard slightly and place it on the edge. Use one or two rescue tubes if needed to support the foot end of the board.

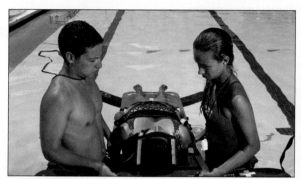
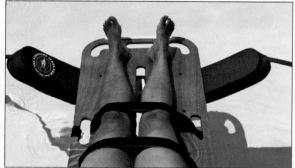

3 One lifeguard gets out of the pool while the other maintains control of the backboard. Once out of the water, the lifeguard on land grasps the head of the backboard while the other gets out of the water.

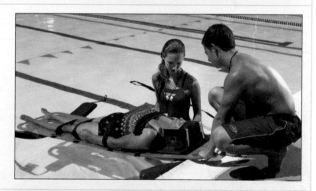

4 Together the lifeguards stand and step backward, pulling the backboard and sliding it up over the edge and out of and away from the water. If available, an assisting lifeguard remains in the water to help push the board.

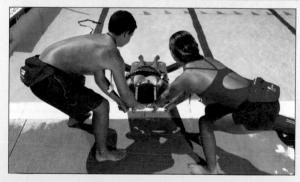

5 If available, additional lifeguards help guide and remove the backboard out of the water and onto land, then begin to assess the victim's condition and providing the appropriate care.

Continued on Next Page

SPINAL INJURY—**REMOVAL FROM THE WATER ON A BACKBOARD** *continued*

Notes:

- *Use proper lifting techniques to prevent injury to yourself:*
  - *Keep the back straight.*
  - *Bend at the knee.*
  - *Move in a controlled way without jerking or tugging.*
  - *Keep the board as level and low to the deck or pier as possible, consistent with proper lifting techniques.*
- *Additional lifeguards can assist by:*
  - *Supporting the primary rescuer at the head of the backboard.*
  - *Placing and securing the straps along the chest, hips and thighs.*
  - *Placing the head immobilizer and securing the strap across the forehead.*
  - *Removing the backboard from the water.*
  - *Begin assessing the victim's condition and providing the appropriate care.*

SPINAL BACKBOARDING PROCEDURE AND REMOVAL FROM WATER—**SPEED SLIDE**

| 1 | The primary rescuer performs in-line stabilization by placing his or her hands on both sides of the victim's head while the victim is on the slide. |

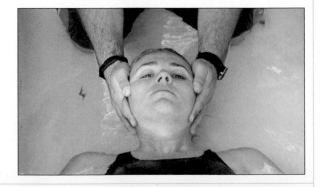

| 2 | Other lifeguards carefully lift the victim and slide the backboard into place from the feet to the head. |

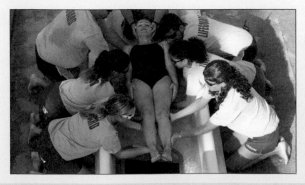
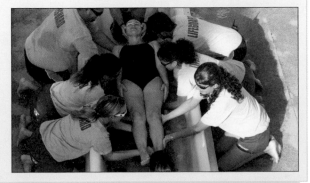

3	Lifeguards lower the victim onto the backboard.	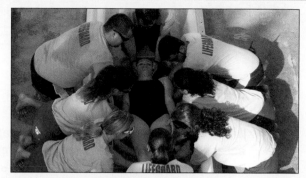

4	Lifeguards secure the victim to the backboard and immobilize the head.

5	Lifeguards lift the backboard and victim out of the slide.	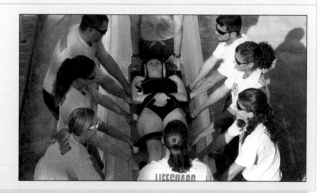

CARING FOR A STANDING VICTIM WHO HAS A SUSPECTED HEAD, NECK OR SPINAL INJURY ON LAND

Note: *Have another person call EMS personnel for a head, neck or spinal injury while you maintain in-line stabilization of the head, neck and spine.*

1	Lifeguard 1 approaches the victim from the front and performs manual stabilization of the victim's head and neck by placing one hand on each side of the head.

2	Lifeguard 2 retrieves a backboard and places it against the victim's back, being careful not to disturb stabilization of the victim's head. Lifeguard 3 helps to position the backboard so that it is centered behind the victim.	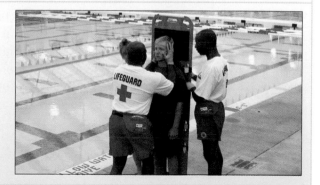

Continued on Next Page

CARING FOR A STANDING VICTIM WHO HAS A SUSPECTED HEAD, NECK OR SPINAL INJURY ON LAND *continued*

3 While Lifeguard 3 holds the backboard, Lifeguard 2 secures the victim to the backboard by placing and securing straps across the victim's chest, under the armpits, and across the hips and thighs. Lifeguard 2 rechecks the straps to be sure that they are secure, then secures the victim's head to the backboard using a head immobilizer and strap across the victim's forehead.

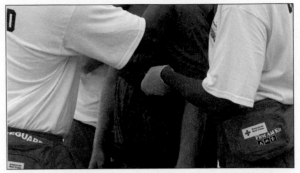

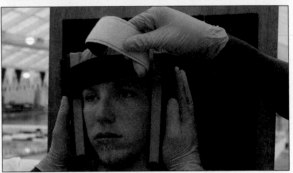

4 The lifeguards at the victim's side each place their inside hands underneath the victim's armpit, in between the victim's arm and torso, and grasp the backboard at a handhold at the victim's armpit level or higher.

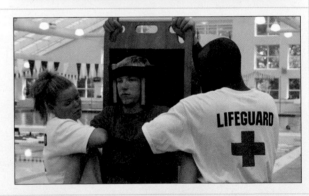

5 When the victim is secured to the board, the other lifeguard grasps the top. Lifeguard 1 informs the victim that they will lower him or her to the ground. When ready, signal to the other two lifeguards to begin. While lowering the victim, the lifeguards at the victim's sides should walk forward and bend at the knees to avoid back injury.

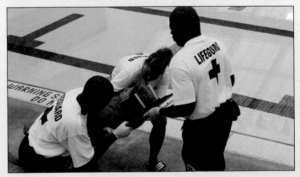

If the position of the head immobilizer cannot be adjusted to the height of a victim, consider one of the following options:

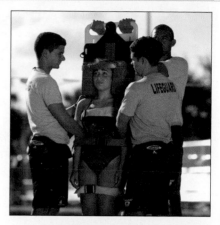

- Place the blocks on either side of the victim's head flush against the backboard. Place an additional strap across the victim's forehead.

  ○ If this not possible, have another lifeguard provide manual stabilization from the head of the board. At the beginning, this lifeguard stands behind the board and reaches around to provide stabilization. As the board is lowered, this lifeguard steps back, while maintaining stabilization, until the board is on the ground.

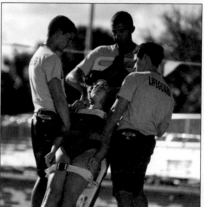

- If the victim is taller than the backboard, place an object such as a folded blanket or towel under the foot of the backboard so that the victim's head does not extend beyond the end of the board.

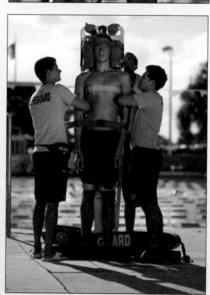

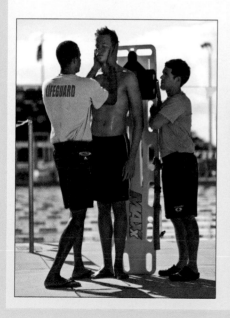

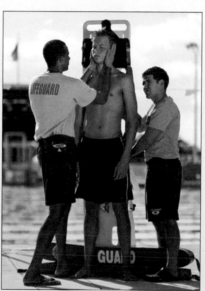

MANUAL STABILIZATION FOR A HEAD, NECK OR SPINAL INJURY ON LAND

Note: *Have someone call EMS personnel for a head, neck or spinal injury while you minimize movement of the head, neck and spine.*

1 Minimize movement by placing your hands on both sides of the victim's head.

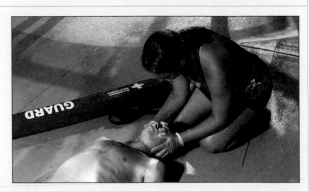

2 Support the head in the position found.

- Do not align the head and neck with the spine if the head is sharply turned to one side, there is pain on movement or if you feel any resistance when attempting to align the head and neck with the spine.

3 Maintain an open airway.

4 Keep the victim from getting chilled or overheated.

Note: *Gently position the victim's head in line with the body if you cannot maintain an open airway.*

GLOSSARY

Abandonment – Ending care of an ill or injured person without that person's consent or without ensuring that someone with equal or greater training will continue that care.

Abdomen – The middle part of the trunk (torso) containing the stomach, liver and other organs.

Abrasion – A wound in which skin is rubbed or scraped away.

Active drowning victim – A person exhibiting universal behavior that includes struggling at the surface in a vertical position and being unable to move forward or tread water.

Agonal gasps – Isolated or infrequent gasping in the absence of other breathing in an unconscious person.

AIDS – When an infected person has a significant drop in a certain type of white blood cells or shows signs of having certain infections or cancers caused by an HIV infection.

Airway adjunct – A mechanical device to keep a victim's airway clear.

Anaphylactic shock – A severe allergic reaction in which air passages may swell and restrict breathing; a form of shock. See also anaphylaxis.

Anaphylaxis – A severe allergic reaction; a form of shock. See also anaphylactic shock.

Anatomic splint – A part of the body used to immobilize an injured body part.

Anatomical airway obstruction – Complete or partial blockage of the airway by the tongue or swollen tissues of the mouth or throat.

Antihistamine – Drug used to treat the signals of allergic reactions.

Aquatic environment – An environment in which recreational water activities are played or performed.

Aquatic safety team – A network of people in the facility and emergency medical services system who can plan for, respond to and assist in an emergency at an aquatic facility.

Area of responsibility – The zone or area in which a lifeguard conducts surveillance.

Ashen – A grayish color; darker skin often looks ashen instead of pale.

Assess – To examine and evaluate a situation carefully.

Asthma – A condition that narrows the air passages and makes breathing difficult.

Asystole – A condition in which the heart has stopped generating electrical activity.

Atrioventricular node (AV) – The point along the heart's electrical pathway midway between the atria and ventricles that sends electrical impulses to the ventricles.

Automated external defibrillator (AED) – An automatic device used to recognize a heart rhythm that requires an electric shock and either delivers the shock or prompts the rescuer to deliver it.

Avulsion – A wound in which soft tissue is partially or completely torn away.

Backboard – A standard piece of rescue equipment at all aquatic facilities used to maintain in-line stabilization while securing and transporting a victim with a suspected head, neck or back injury.

Bag-valve-mask (BVM) resuscitator – A handheld breathing device used on a victim in respiratory distress or respiratory arrest. It consists of a self-inflating bag, a one-way valve and a mask; can be used with or without supplemental oxygen.

Bandage – Material used to wrap or cover an injured body part; often used to hold a dressing in place.

Blind spots – Areas within a lifeguard's area of responsibility that cannot be seen or are difficult to see.

Bloodborne pathogens – Bacteria and viruses present in blood and body fluids that can cause disease in humans.

Bloodborne pathogens standard – A federal regulation designed to protect employees from exposure to bodily fluids that might contain a disease-causing agent.

Body substance isolation (BSI) precautions – An approach to infection control that considers all body fluids and substances to be infectious.

Bone – A dense, hard tissue that forms the skeleton.

Buddy board – A board with identification tags used to keep track of swimmers and reinforce the importance of the buddy system.

Bulkhead – A moveable wall placed in a swimming pool to separate activities or water of different depths.

Buoy – A float in the water anchored to the bottom.

Buoyancy – The tendency of a body to float or to rise when submerged in a fluid.

Buoyant – Tending to float, capable of keeping an object afloat.

Bystanders – People at the scene of an emergency who do not have a duty to provide care.

Carbon dioxide – A colorless, odorless gas; a waste product of respiration.

Carbon monoxide – A clear, odorless, poisonous gas produced when carbon or other fuel is burned, as in gasoline engines.

Cardiac arrest – A condition in which the heart has stopped or beats too ineffectively to generate a pulse.

Cartilage – An elastic tissue in the body; in the joints, it acts as a shock absorber when a person is walking, running or jumping.

Catch pool – A small pool at the bottom of a slide where patrons enter water deep enough to cushion their landing.

Chain of command – The structure of employee and management positions in a facility or organization.

Chemical hazard – A harmful or potentially harmful substance in or around a facility.

Chest – The upper part of the trunk (torso), containing the heart, major blood vessels and lungs.

Chronic – Persistent over a long period of time.

Closed wound – An injury that does not break the skin and in which soft tissue damage occurs beneath the skin.

Cold-related emergencies – Emegencies, including hypothermia and frostbite, caused by overexposure to cold.

Concussion – A temporary impairment of brain function.

Confidentiality – Protecting a victim's privacy by not revealing any personal information learned about a victim except to law enforcement personnel or emergency medical services personnel caring for the victim.

Consent – Permission to provide care given by an ill or injured person to a rescuer.

Convulsions – Sudden, uncontrolled muscular contractions.

CPR – A technique that combines chest compressions and rescue breaths for a victim whose heart and breathing have stopped.

Critical incident – Any situation that causes a person to experience unusually strong emotional reactions that interfere with his or her ability to function during and after a highly stressful incident.

Critical incident stress – The stress a person experiences during or after a highly stressful emergency.

Cross bearing – A technique for determining the place where a submerged victim was last seen, performed by two persons some distance apart, each pointing to the place such that the position is where the lines of their pointing cross.

Current – Fast-moving water.

Cyanosis – A blue discoloration of the skin around the mouth and fingertips resulting from a lack of oxygen in the blood.

Daily log – A written journal kept by lifeguards, the head lifeguard and management containing a daily account of safety precautions taken and significant events.

Deep-water line search – An effective pattern for searching in water that is greater than chest deep.

Defibrillation – An electrical shock that disrupts the electrical activity of the heart long enough to allow the heart to spontaneously develop an effective rhythm on its own.

Diabetes – A condition in which the body does not produce enough insulin or does not use insulin effectively enough to regulate the amount of sugar (glucose) in the bloodstream.

Diabetic – A person with the condition called diabetes mellitus, which causes a body to produce insufficient amounts of the hormone insulin.

Diabetic emergency – A situation in which a person becomes ill because of an imbalance of sugar (glucose) and insulin in the bloodstream.

Direct contact transmission – Occurs when infected blood or body fluids from one person enter another person's body at a correct entry site.

Disability – The loss, absence or impairment of sensory, motor or mental function.

Dislocation – The movement of a bone away from its normal position at a joint.

Disoriented – Being in a state of confusion; not knowing place, identity or what happened.

Dispatch – The method for informing patrons when it is safe to proceed on a ride.

Distressed swimmer – A person capable of staying afloat, but likely to need assistance to get to safety. If not rescued, the person becomes an active drowning victim.

Dressing – A pad placed on a wound to control bleeding and prevent infection.

Drop-off slide – A slide that ends with a drop of several feet into a catch pool.

Droplet transmission – Transmission of disease through the inhalation of droplets from an infected person's cough or sneeze.

Drowning – Death by suffocation in water.

Drug – Any substance other than food intended to affect the functions of the body.

Duty to act – A legal responsibility of certain people to provide a reasonable standard of emergency care; may be required by case law, statute or job description.

Electrocardiogram (ECG) – A graphic record produced by a device that records the electrical activity of the heart from the chest.

Embedded object – An object that remains embedded in an open wound.

Emergency – A sudden, unexpected incident demanding immediate action.

Emergency action plan (EAP) – A written plan detailing how facility staff are to respond in a specific type of emergency.

Emergency back-up coverage – Coverage by lifeguards who remain out of the water during an emergency situation and supervise a larger area when another lifeguard must enter the water for a rescue.

Emergency medical services (EMS) personnel – Trained and equipped community-based personnel dispatched through a local emergency number to provide emergency care for injured or ill people.

Emergency medical technician (EMT) – A person who has successfully completed a state-approved emergency medical technician training program; paramedics are the highest level of EMTs.

Emergency stop button – A button or switch used to immediately turn off the waves or water flow in a wave pool, water slide or other water attraction in the event of an emergency.

Emphysema – A disease in which the lungs lose their ability to exchange carbon dioxide and oxygen effectively.

Engineering controls – Safeguards intended to isolate or remove a hazard from the workplace.

Epilepsy – A chronic condition characterized by seizures that vary in type and duration; can usually be controlled by medication.

Epinephrine – A form of adrenaline medication prescribed to treat the symptoms of severe allergic reactions.

Exhaustion – The state of being extremely tired or weak.

Facility surveillance – Checking the facility to help prevent injuries caused by avoidable hazards in the facility's environment.

Fainting – A temporary loss of consciousness.

Fibrillation – A quivering of the heart's ventricles.

Forearm – The upper extremity from the elbow to the wrist.

Fracture – A chip, crack or complete break in bone tissue.

Free-fall slide – A type of speed slide with a nearly vertical drop, giving riders the sensation of falling.

Frostbite – The freezing of body parts exposed to the cold.

Gasp reflex – A sudden involuntary attempt to "catch one's breath," which may cause the victim to inhale water into the lungs if the face is underwater.

Heat cramps – Painful spasms of skeletal muscles after exercise or work in warm or moderate temperatures; usually involve the calf and abdominal muscles.

Heat exhaustion – The early stage and most common form of heat-related illness; often results from strenuous work or exercise in a hot environment.

Heat stroke – A life-threatening condition that develops when the body's cooling mechanisms are overwhelmed and body systems begin to fail.

Heat-related illnesses – Illnesses, including heat exhaustion, heat cramps and heat stroke, caused by overexposure to heat.

Hemostatic agents – A substance that stops bleeding by shortening the amount of time it takes for blood to clot. They usually contain chemicals that remove moisture from the blood.

Hepatitis B – A liver infection caused by the hepatitis B virus; may be severe or even fatal and can be in the body up to 6 months before symptoms appear.

Hepatitis C – A liver disease caused by the hepatitis C virus; it is the most common chronic bloodborne infection in the United States.

HIV – A virus that destroys the body's ability to fight infection. A result of HIV infection is referred to as AIDS.

Hull – The main body of a boat.

Hydraulic – Strong force created by water flowing downward over an obstruction and then reversing its flow.

Hyperglycemia – Someone experiencing symptoms of high blood sugar.

Hyperventilation – A dangerous technique some swimmers use to stay under water longer by taking several deep breaths followed by forceful exhalations, then inhaling deeply before swimming under water.

Hypoglycemia – Someone experiencing symptoms of low blood sugar.

Hypothermia – A life-threatening condition in which cold or cool temperatures cause the body to lose heat faster than it can produce it.

Hypoxia – A condition in which insufficient oxygen reaches the cells, resulting in cyanosis and changes in consciousness and in breathing and heart rates.

Immobilize – To use a splint or other method to keep an injured body part from moving.

Implied consent – Legal concept that assumes a person would consent to receive emergency care if he or she were physically able to do so.

Incident – An occurrence or event that interrupts normal procedure or brings about a crisis.

Incident report – A report filed by a lifeguard or other facility staff who responded to an emergency or other incident.

Indirect contact transmission – Occurs when a person touches objects that have the blood or body fluid of an infected person, and that infected blood or body fluid enters the body through a correct entry site.

Inflatables – Plastic toys or equipment that are filled with air to function as recommended.

Inhaled poison – A poison that a person breathes into the lungs.

Injury – The physical harm from an external force on the body.

In-line stabilization – A technique used to minimize movement of a victim's head and neck while providing care.

In-service training – Regularly scheduled staff meetings and practice sessions that cover lifeguarding information and skills.

Instinctive drowning response – A universal set of behaviors exhibited by an active drowning victim that include struggling to keep the face above water, extending arms to the side and pressing down for support, not making any forward progress in the water and staying at the surface for only 20 to 60 seconds.

Intervals – A series of repeat swims of the same distance and time interval, each done at the same high level of effort.

Jaundice – Yellowing of the skin and eyes.

Joint – A structure where two or more bones are joined.

Laceration – A cut.

Laryngospasm – A spasm of the vocal cords that closes the airway.

Life jacket – A type of personal floatation device (PFD) approved by the United States Coast Guard for use during activities in, on or around water.

Lifeguard – A person trained in lifeguarding, CPR and first aid skills who ensures the safety of people at an aquatic facility by preventing and responding to emergencies.

Lifeguard competitions – Events and contests designed to evaluate the skills and knowledge of individual lifeguards and lifeguard teams.

Lifeguard team – A group of two or more lifeguards on duty at a facility at the same time.

Ligaments – A tough, fibrous connective tissue that holds bones together at a joint.

Line-and-reel – A heavy piece of rope or cord attached to rescue equipment that may be used to tow the lifeguard and the victim to safety.

Material Safety Data Sheet (MSDS) – A form that provides information about a hazardous substance.

Mechanical obstruction – Complete or partial blockage of the airway by a foreign object, such as a piece of food or a small toy, or by fluids, such as vomit or blood.

Muscle – Tissue in the body that lengthens and shortens to create movement.

Myocardial infarction – A heart attack.

Nasal cannula – A device used to deliver oxygen to a breathing person; used mostly for victims with minor breathing problems.

Negligence – The failure to follow the standard of care or to act, thereby causing injury or further harm to another.

Nonfatal drowning – To survive, at least temporarily, following submersion in water (drowning).

Non-rebreather mask – A mask used to deliver high concentrations of oxygen to breathing victims.

Occupational Safety and Health Administration (OSHA) – A government agency that helps protect the health and safety of employees in the workplace.

Open wound – An injury to soft tissue resulting in a break in the skin, such as a cut.

Opportunistic infections – Infections that strike people whose immune systems are weakened by HIV or other infections.

Oxygen – A tasteless, colorless, odorless gas necessary to sustain life.

Oxygen delivery device – Equipment used to supply oxygen to a victim of a breathing emergency.

Paralysis – A loss of muscle control; a permanent loss of feeling and movement.

Partial thickness burn – A burn that involves both layers of skin. Also called a second-degree burn.

Passive drowning victim – An unconscious victim face-down, submerged or near the surface.

Pathogen – A disease-causing agent. Also called a microorganism or germ.

Patron surveillance – Maintaining a close watch over the people using an aquatic facility.

Peripheral vision – What one sees at the edges of one's field of vision.

Personal floatation device (PFD) – Coast Guard-approved life jacket, buoyancy vest, wearable floatation aid, throwable device or other special-use floatation device.

Personal water craft – A motorized vehicle designed for one or two riders that skims over the surface of the water.

Pier – A wooden walkway or platform built over the water supported by pillars that is used for boats to dock, fishing or other water activities.

Poison – Any substance that causes injury, illness or death when introduced into the body.

Poison Control Center (PCC) – A specialized kind of health center that provides information in cases of poisoning or suspected poisoning emergencies.

Policies and procedures manual – A manual that provides detailed information about the daily and emergency operations of a facility.

Preventive lifeguarding – The methods that lifeguards use to prevent drowning and other injuries by identifying dangerous conditions or behaviors and then taking steps to minimize or eliminate them.

Primary responsibility – A lifeguard's main responsibility, which is to prevent drowning and other injuries from occurring at an aquatic facility.

Professional rescuers – Paid or volunteer personnel, including lifeguards, who have a legal duty to act in an emergency.

Public address system – An electronic amplification system, used at an aquatic facility so that announcements can be easily heard by patrons.

Puncture – An open wound created when the skin is pierced by a pointed object.

Rapids ride – A rough-water attraction that simulates white-water rafting.

Reaching assist – A method of helping someone out of the water by reaching to that person with your hand, leg or an object.

Reaching pole – An aluminum or fiberglass pole, usually 10- to 15-feet long, used for rescues.

Refusal of care – The declining of care by a victim; the victim has the right to refuse the care of anyone who responds to an emergency.

Rescue board – A plastic or fiberglass board shaped like a surf board that is used by lifeguards to paddle out and make a rescue.

Rescue tube – A 45- to 54-inch vinyl, foam-filled tube with an attached tow line and shoulder strap that lifeguards use to make rescues.

Respiratory arrest – A condition in which breathing has stopped.

Respiratory distress – A condition in which breathing is difficult.

Respiratory failure – When the respiratory system is beginning to shut down, which in turn can lead to respiratory arrest.

Resuscitation mask – A pliable, dome-shaped device that fits over a person's mouth and nose; used to assist with rescue breathing.

RID factor – Three elements—recognition, intrusion and distraction—related to drownings at guarded facilities.

Ring buoy – A buoyant ring, usually 20 to 30 inches in diameter; with an attached line, allows a rescuer to pull a victim to safety without entering the water.

Risk management – Identifying and eliminating or minimizing dangerous conditions that can cause injuries and financial loss.

Roving station – When a roving lifeguard is assigned a specific zone, which also is covered by another lifeguard in an elevated station.

Rules – Guidelines for conduct or action that help keep patrons safe at pools and other swimming areas.

Runout – The area at the end of a slide where water slows the speed of the riders.

Safety check – An inspection of the facility to find and eliminate or minimize hazards.

Scanning – A visual technique used by lifeguards to properly observe and monitor patrons participating in water activities.

Secondary responsibilities – Other duties a lifeguard must perform, such as testing the pool water chemistry, assisting patrons, performing maintenance, completing records and reports, or performing opening duties, closing duties or facility safety checks. Secondary responsibilities should never interfere with a lifeguard's primary responsibility.

Seiche – A French word meaning to sway back and forth. It is a standing wave that oscillates in a lake because of seismic or atmospheric disturbances creating huge fluctuations of water levels in just moments. Water sloshes between opposing shores within the lake basin, decreasing in height with each rocking back and forth until it reaches equilibrium.

Seizure – A disorder in the brain's electrical activity, marked by loss of consciousness and often by convulsions.

Shepherd's crook – A reaching pole with a large hook on the end. See also reaching pole.

Shock – A life-threatening condition in which the circulatory system fails to deliver blood to all parts of the body, causing body organs to fail.

Sighting – A technique for noting where a submerged victim was last seen, performed by imagining a line to the opposite shore and estimating the victim's position along that line. See also cross bearing.

Sink – To fall, drop or descend gradually to a lower level.

Soft tissue – Body structures that include the layers of skin, fat and muscles.

Spa – A small pool or tub in which people sit in rapidly circulating hot water.

Spasm – An involuntary and abnormal muscle contraction.

Speed slide – A steep water slide on which patrons may reach speeds in excess of 35 mph.

Spinal cord – A bundle of nerves extending from the base of the skull to the lower back and protected by the spinal column.

Splint – A device used to immobilize body parts; applying such a device.

Spokesperson – The person at the facility designated to speak on behalf of others.

Sprain – The stretching and tearing of ligaments and other tissue structures at a joint.

Standard of care – The minimal standard and quality of care expected of an emergency care provider.

Standard precautions – Safety measures, such as body substance isolation, taken to prevent occupational-risk exposure to blood or other potentially infectious materials, such as body fluids containing visible blood.

Starting blocks – Platforms from which competitive swimmers dive to start a race.

Sterile – Free from germs.

Stern – The back of a boat.

Stoma – An opening in the front of the neck through which a person whose larynx has been removed breathes.

Strain – The stretching and tearing of muscles or tendons.

Stress – A physiological or psychological response to real or imagined influences that alter an existing state of physical, mental or emotional balance.

Stroke – A disruption of blood flow to a part of the brain, causing permanent damage.

Submerged – Underwater, covered with water.

Suctioning – The process of removing foreign matter from the upper airway by means of manual device.

Sun protection factor (SPF) – The ability of a substance to prevent the sun's harmful rays from being absorbed into the skin; a concentration of sunscreen.

Sunscreen – A cream, lotion or spray used to protect the skin from harmful rays of the sun.

Superficial burn – A burn involving only the outer layer of skin, the epidermis, characterized by dry, red or tender skin. Also referred to as a first-degree burn.

Surveillance – A close watch kept over someone or something, such as patrons or a facility.

Thermocline – A layer of water between the warmer, surface zone and the colder, deep-water zone in a body of water in which the temperature decreases rapidly with depth.

Throwable device – Any object that can be thrown to a drowning victim to aid him or her in floating.

Throwing assist – A method of helping someone out of the water by throwing a floating object with a line attached.

Tornado warning – A warning issued by the National Weather Service notifying that a tornado has been sighted.

Tornado watch – A warning issued by the National Weather Service notifying that tornadoes are possible.

Total coverage – When only one lifeguard is conducting patron surveillance for an entire pool while on duty.

Universal precautions – Practices required by the federal Occupational Safety and Health Administration to control and protect employees from exposure to blood and other potentially infectious materials.

Universal sign of choking – When a conscious person is clutching the throat due to an airway blockage.

Vector-borne transmission – Transmission of a disease by an animal or insect bite through exposure to blood or other body fluids.

Ventricles – The two lower chambers of the heart.

Ventricular fibrillation (V-fib) – An abnormal heart rhythm characterized by disorganized electrical activity, which results in the quivering of the ventricles.

Ventricular tachycardia (V-tach) – An abnormal heart rhythm characterized by rapid contractions of the ventricles.

Waterfront – Open water areas, such as lakes, rivers, ponds and oceans.

Waterpark – An aquatic theme park with attractions such as wave pools, speed slides or winding rivers.

Wheezing – The hoarse whistling sound made when inhaling and/or exhaling.

Work practice controls – Employee and employer behaviors that reduce the likelihood of exposure to a hazard at the job site.

Wound – An injury to the soft tissues.

Xiphoid process – The lowest point of the breastbone.

Zone coverage – Coverage in which the swimming area is divided into separate zones, with one zone for each lifeguard station.

Zone of surveillance responsibility – Also referred to as zones, these are the specific areas of the water, deck, pier or shoreline that are a lifeguard's responsibility to scan from a lifeguard station.

REFERENCES

2010 International Consensus on Cardiopulmonary Resuscitation and Emergency Cardiovascular Care Science With Treatment Recommendations, *Circulation.* http://circ.ahajournals.org/content/122/16_suppl_2/S250.short. Accessed August 2011.

American Alliance for Health, Physical Education, Recreation and Dance. *Safety Aquatics.* Sports Safety Series, Monograph #5. American Alliance for Health, Physical Education, Recreation and Dance, 1977.

American Heart Association and the American National Red Cross, 2010 Guidelines for First Aid, *Circulation*, http://circ.ahajournals.org/content/122/18_suppl_3/S934.full.pdf. Accessed August 2011.

The American National Red Cross. *Adapted Aquatics: Swimming for Persons With Physical or Mental Impairments.* Washington, D.C.: The American National Red Cross, 1977.

——. *Basic Water Rescue.* Yardley, Pennsylvania: StayWell Health & Safety Solutions, 2009.

——. *CPR/AED for the Professional Rescuer and Health Care Providers.* Yardley, Pennsylvania: StayWell Health & Safety Solutions, 2011.

——. *Emergency Medical Response.* Yardley, Pennsylvania: StayWell Health & Safety Solutions, 2011.

——. *First Aid/CPR/AED.* Yardley, Pennsylvania: StayWell Health & Safety Solutions, 2011

——. *First Aid–Responding to Emergencies.* Yardley, Pennsylvania: StayWell Health & Safety Solutions, 2006.

——. *Lifeguarding Manual.* Yardley, Pennsylvania: StayWell Health & Safety Solutions, 2006.

——. *Lifeguarding Today.* Boston: StayWell, 1994.

——. *Safety Training for Swim Coaches.* Yardley, Pennsylvania: StayWell Health & Safety Solutions, 2009.

——. *Swimming and Water Safety.* Yardley, Pennsylvania: StayWell Health & Safety Solutions, 2009.

American Red Cross Scientific Advisory Council (SAC). *Advisory Statement on Aspirin Administration,* 2001.

——. *Advisory Statement on Asthma Assistance,* 2003.

——. *Advisory Statement on Epinephrine Administration,* 2001.

——. *Advisory Statement on Cervical Collar Application in Water Rescue,* 2000.

——. *Advisory Statement on Hand Hygiene for First Aid,* 2006

——. *Advisory Statement on Hyperthermia,* 2009.

——. *Advisory Statement on Lightning Safety for Pools,* 2009.

——. *Advisory Statement on Subdiaphragmatic Thrusts and Drowning Victims,* 2006.

——. *Advisory Statement on Voluntary Hyperventilation Preceding Underwater Swimming,* 2009.

Armbruster, D.A.; Allen, R.H.; and Billingsley, H.S. *Swimming and Diving.* 6th ed. St. Louis: The C.V. Mosby Company, 1973.

Association for the Advancement of Health Education. "Counting the Victims." HE-XTRA 18 (1993):8.

Baker, S.P.; O'Neill, B.; and Ginsburg, M.J. *The Injury Fact Book.* 2nd ed. Lexington, Massachusetts: Lexington Books, D.C. Heath and Co., 1991.

Beringer, G.B., et al. "Submersion Accidents and Epilepsy." *American Journal of Diseases of Children* 137 (1983):604–605.

Bierens, Joost J.L.M.; *Handbook on Drowning.* Berlin/Heidelberg: Springer-Verlag, 2006.

Brewster, C.B. *Open Water Lifesaving: The United States Lifesaving Association Manual.* 2nd ed. Boston: Pearson Custom Publishing, 2003.

Brown, V.R. "Spa Associated Hazards–An Update and Summary." Washington, D.C.: U.S. Consumer Product Safety Commission, 1981.

Bruess, C.E.; Richardson, G.E.; and Laing, S.J. *Decisions for Health.* 4th ed. Dubuque, Iowa: William C. Brown Publishers, 1995.

The Canadian Red Cross Society. *Lifeguarding Manual.* Yardley, Pennsylvania: StayWell Health & Safety Solutions, 2009.

Centers for Disease Control and Prevention. "Drownings at U.S. Army Corps of Engineers Recreation Facilities, 1986–1990." *Morbidity and Mortality Weekly Report* 41 (1992):331–333.

——. "Drownings in a Private Lake–North Carolina, 1981–1990." *Morbidity and Mortality Weekly Report* 41 (1992):329–331.

——. "Suction-Drain Injury in a Public Wading Pool–North Carolina, 1991." *Morbidity and Mortality Weekly Report* 41 (1992):333–335.

——. *Suggested Health and Safety Guidelines for Recreational Water Slide Flumes.* Atlanta, Georgia: U.S. Department of Health and Human Services, 1981.

——. *Swimming Pools–Safety and Disease Control Through Proper Design and Operation.* Atlanta, Georgia: United States Department of Health, Education, and Welfare, 1976.

Chow, J.M. "Make a Splash: Children's Pools Attract All Ages." *Aquatics International* (1993):27–32.

Clayton, R.D., and Thomas, D.G. *Professional Aquatic Management.* 2nd ed. Champaign, Illinois: Human Kinetics, 1989.

Committee on Trauma Research; Commission on Life Sciences; National Research Council; and the Institute of Medicine. *Injury in America.* Washington, D.C.: National Academy Press, 1985.

Consumer Guide with Chasnoff, I.J.; Ellis, J.W.; and Fainman, Z.S. *The New Illustrated Family Medical & Health Guide.* Lincolnwood, Illinois: Publications International, Ltd., 1994.

Council for National Cooperation in Aquatics. *Lifeguard Training: Principles and Administration.* New York: Association Press, 1973.

Craig, A.B., Jr. "Underwater Swimming and Loss of Consciousness." *The Journal of the American Medical Association* 176 (1961):255–258.

DeMers, G.E., and Johnson, R.L. *YMCA Pool Operations Manual.* 3rd ed. Champaign, Illinois: Human Kinetics, 2006.

Ellis, J., et al. *National Pool and Waterpark Lifeguard Training Manual.* Alexandria, Virginia: National Recreation and Park Association, 1993 and 1991.

Ellis & Associates. *International Lifeguard Training Program.* Burlington, Massachusetts: Jones & Bartlett Learning. 2006

Fife, D.; Scipio, S.; and Crane, G. "Fatal and Nonfatal Immersion Injuries Among New Jersey Residents." *American Journal of Preventive Medicine* 7 (1991):189–193.

Forrest, C., and Fraleigh, M.M. "Planning Aquatic Playgrounds With Children In Mind: Design A Spray Park Kids Love." *California Parks & Recreation* (Summer 2004):12.

Gabriel, J.L., editor. *U.S. Diving Safety Manual.* Indianapolis: U.S. Diving Publications, 1990.

Gabrielsen, M.A. "Diving Injuries: Research Findings and Recommendations for Reducing Catastrophic Sport Related Injuries." Presented to the Council for National Cooperation in Aquatics. Indianapolis, 2000.

——. *Swimming Pools: A Guide to Their Planning, Design, and Operation.* 4th ed. Champaign, Illinois: Human Kinetics, 1987.

Getchell, B.; Pippin, R.; and Varnes, J. *Health.* Boston: Houghton Mifflin Co., 1989.

Hedberg, K., et al. "Drownings in Minnesota, 1980–85: A Population-Based Study." *American Journal of Public Health* 80 (1990):1071–1074.

Huint, R. *Lifeguarding in the Waterparks.* Montreal: AquaLude, Inc., 1990.

Idris A.H.; Berg, R.; Bierens, J.; Bossaert, L, Branche, C.; Gabrielli, A.; Graves, S.A.; Handley, J.; Hoelle, R.; Morley, P.; Pappa, L.; Pepe, P.; Quan, L.; Szpilman, D.; Wigginton, J.; and Modell, J.H. Recommended Guidelines For Uniform Reporting of Data From Drowning: the "Utstein Style". *Circulation,* 108 (2003):2565–2574.

Kowalsky, L., editor. *Pool-Spa Operators Handbook.* San Antonio, Texas: National Swimming Pool Foundation, 1990.

Lierman, T.L., editor. *Building a Healthy America: Conquering Disease and Disability.* New York: Mary Ann Liebert, Inc., Publishers, 1987.

Lifesaving Society. *Alert: Lifeguarding in Action.* 2nd ed. Ottawa, Ontario: Lifesaving Society, 2004.

Litovitz, T.L.; Schmitz, B.S.; and Holm, K.C. "1988 Annual Report of the American Association of Poison Control Centers National Data Collection System." *American Journal of Emergency Medicine* 7 (1989):496.

Livingston, S.; Pauli, L.L.; and Pruce, I. "Epilepsy and Drowning in Childhood." *British Medical Journal* 2 (1977):515–516.

Marion Laboratories. *Osteoporosis: Is It in Your Future?* Kansas City: Marion Laboratories, 1984.

MayoClinic.com. Dehydration Overview. http://www.mayoclinic.com/health/dehydration/ds00561. Accessed August 2011.

Mitchell, J.T. "Stress: The History, Status and Future of Critical Incident Stress Debriefings." *JEMS: Journal of Emergency Medical Services* 13 (1988):47–52.

——. "Stress and the Emergency Responder." *JEMS: Journal of Emergency Medical Services* 15 (1987):55–57.

Modell, J.H. "Drowning." *New England Journal of Medicine* 328 (1993):253–256.

National Committee for Injury Prevention and Control. *Injury Prevention: Meeting the*

Challenge. New York: Oxford University Press as a supplement to the *American Journal of Preventive Medicine,* Volume 5, Number 3, 1989.

National Safety Council. *Injury Facts, 1999 Edition.* Itasca, Illinois: National Safety Council, 1999.

National Spa and Pool Institute. *American National Standard for Public Swimming Pools.* Alexandria, Virginia: National Spa and Pool Institute, 1991.

New York State Department of Public Health. *Drownings at Regulated Bathing Facilities in New York State, 1987–1990.* Albany, New York: New York State Department of Health, 1990.

O'Connor, J. "A U.S. Accidental Drowning Study, 1980–1984." Thesis, University of Oregon, 1986.

O'Donohoe, N.V. "What Should the Child With Epilepsy Be Allowed to Do?" *Archives of Disease in Childhood* 58 (1983):934–937.

Orlowski, J.P.; Rothner, A.D.; and Lueders, H. "Submersion Accidents in Children With Epilepsy." *American Journal of Diseases of Children* 136 (1982):777–780.

Payne, W.A., and Hahn, D.B. *Understanding Your Health.* 7th ed. St. Louis: McGraw Hill Companies, 2002.

Pearn, J. "Epilepsy and Drowning in Childhood." *British Medical Journal* 1 (1977):1510–1511.

Pearn, J.; Bart, R.; and Yamaoka, R. "Drowning Risks to Epileptic Children: A Study From Hawaii." *British Medical Journal* 2 (1978):1284–1285.

Pia, F. "Observations on the Drowning of Nonswimmers." *Journal of Physical Education* (July 1974):164–167.

———. *On Drowning,* Water Safety Films, Inc. (1970).

———. "Reducing Swimming Related Drowning Fatalities." *Pennsylvania Recreation and Parks* (Spring 1991):13–16.

———. "The RID Factor as a Cause of Drowning." *Parks and Recreation* (June 1984):52–67.

Quan, L., and Gomez, A. "Swimming Pool Safety—An Effective Submersion Prevention Program." *Journal of Environmental Health* 52 (1990):344–346.

Rice, D.P.; MacKenzie, E.J.; et al. *Cost of Injury in the United States: a Report to Congress 1989.* San Francisco, California: Institute for Health and Aging, University of California, and Injury Prevention Center, The Johns Hopkins University, 1989.

Robertson, L.S. *Injury Epidemiology.* 2nd ed. New York: Oxford University Press, 1998.

The Royal Life Saving Society Australia. *Lifeguarding.* 3rd ed. Marrickville, NSW: Elsevier Australia, 2001.

The Royal Life Saving Society UK. *The Lifeguard.* 2nd ed. RLSS Warwickshire, UK, 2003.

Spinal Cord Injury Information Network. Facts and Figures at a Glance—Feburary 2011. http://www.spinalcord.uab.edu. Accessed August 2011.

Spray Parks, Splash Pads, Kids-Cool! http://www.azcentral.com/families/articles/0514gr-mombeat14Z12.html. Accessed August 2011.

Strauss, R.H., editor. *Sports Medicine.* Philadelphia: W.B. Saunders Co., 1984.

Torney, J.A., and Clayton, R.D. *Aquatic Instruction, Coaching and Management.* Minneapolis, Minnesota: Burgess Publishing Co., 1970.

——. *Aquatic Organization and Management.* Minneapolis, Minnesota: Burgess Publishing Co., 1981.

United States Lifeguard Standards Coalition. *United States Lifeguard Standards.* January 2011. http://www.lifeguardstandards.org/pdf/USLSC_FINAL_APPROVAL_1-31-11.pdf. Accessed August 2011.

White, J.E. *Starguard: Best Practices for Lifeguards.* Champaign, Illinois: Human Kinetics, 2006.

Williams, K.G. *The Aquatic Facility Operator Manual.* 3rd ed. The National Recreation and Park Association, National Aquatic Section, 1999.

Wintemute, G.J., et al. "The Epidemiology of Drowning in Adulthood: Implications for Prevention." *American Journal of Preventive Medicine* 4 (1988):343–348.

World Waterpark Association. *Considerations for Operating Safety.* Lenexa, Kansas: World Waterpark Association, 1991.

YMCA of the USA. *On the Guard II.* 4th ed. Champaign, Illinois: Human Kinetics, 2001.

SPECIAL THANKS

Special thanks to Lead Technical Reviewers for video and photography: David Bell, Boy Scouts of America National Aquatic Committee and Shawn DeRosa, The Pennsylvania State University Manger of Aquatic Facilities and Safety Officer for Intercollegiate Athletics; Dan Jones and City of Norfolk lifeguards; Lauren Scott, Ginny Savage and the lifeguarding staff of Water Country U.S.A; Bill Kirkner, Mark Bonitabus, Sue Szembroth and the lifeguarding staff of the JCC of Greater Baltimore; Mike McGoun and the lifeguarding staff of the Coral Springs Aquatic Center; and Angela Lorenzo-Clavell and the City of Chandler lifeguarding staff for opening their facilities to us and providing their expertise with our photography and video shoots. We would also like to express our appreciation to Barbara Proud, Simon Bruty, Bernardo Nogueria, Primary Pictures crew, the Canadian Red Cross and the many volunteers who made the photos and videos a reality.

INDEX

1. Check scene for safts

2. Gloves

3. Child → ask parent

4. "Are u okas?"

5. Call 911

6. Breathing & pulse — 10 sec

{ 7. Adult - check for bleeding. Child - 2 breaths

{ 8. Adult - 2 breaths. Child - check for bleeding

{ 5 chest thrust
{ Check for object
{ 2 breaths

breathing & pulse → HAINES Recovers

no breathing & pulse → Rescue breathing
— adult: 1 breath/5 sec 12 breaths/2 minutes
— child/infant: 1 breath/3 sec 20 breaths/1 minute

no breathing & no pulse → CPR

1 adult: 30 com. 2 breaths → 3 → time
  child/infant: 30 comp. 2 breaths → 3 → time

2 adult: 30 com/2 breaths → 3 × 3
  child/infant: 15 comp./2 breaths/3